BORDERS OF BEING

BORDERS OF BEING

Citizenship, Fertility, and Sexuality in Asia and the Pacific

Edited by
MARGARET JOLLY
and
KALPANA RAM

Ann Arbor
THE UNIVERSITY OF MICHIGAN PRESS

Copyright © by the University of Michigan 2001
All rights reserved
Published in the United States of America by
The University of Michigan Press
Manufactured in the United States of America
⊚ Printed on acid-free paper

2004   2003   2002   2001   4   3   2   1

No part of this publication may be reproduced, stored in a retrieval system, or transmitted in any form or by any means, electronic, mechanical, or otherwise, without the written permission of the publisher.

A CIP catalog record for this book is available from the British Library.

Library of Congress Cataloging-in-Publication Data

Borders of being : citizenship, fertility, and sexuality in Asia and
   the Pacific / edited by Margaret Jolly and Kalpana Ram.
       p.   cm.
     Includes bibliographical references and index.
     ISBN 0-472-09755-5 (cloth : alk. paper) — ISBN 0-472-06755-9 (pbk. : alk. paper)
     1. Body, Human—Social aspects—Asia.   2. Body, Human—Social aspects—Oceania.   3. Sex role—Asia.   4. Sex role—Oceania.   5. Birth control—Government policy—Asia.   6. Birth control—Government policy—Oceania.   7. Women—Asia—Social conditions.   8. Women—Oceania—Social conditions.   9. Asia—Social life and customs.   10. Oceania—Social life and customs.   I. Jolly, Margaret.   II. Ram, Kalpana.
GN625 .B58   2000
306.4—dc21   00-10459

Contents

Illustrations   vii

Tables   ix

Acknowledgments   xi

INTRODUCTION
Embodied States—Familial and National
Genealogies in Asia and the Pacific   1
Margaret Jolly

CHAPTER 1
Government Agency, Women's Agency:
Feminisms, Fertility, and Population Control   36
Kathryn Robinson

CHAPTER 2
Her Body and Her Being:
Of Widows and Abducted Women in Post-Partition India   58
Ritu Menon and Kamla Bhasin

CHAPTER 3
Rationalizing Fecund Bodies:
Family Planning Policy and the Modern Indian Nation-State   82
Kalpana Ram

CHAPTER 4
Keep It in the Family:
Government, Marriage, and Sex in Contemporary China   118
Gary Sigley

CHAPTER 5
Doing God's Work:
Citizenship, Gender, and Sexuality in the Philippines   154
Anne-Marie Hilsdon

CHAPTER 6
Fecundity and the Fertility Decline in Bali   178
Lynette Parker

CHAPTER 7
Empowerment or Control?
Northeast Thai Women and Family Planning   203
Andrea Whittaker

CHAPTER 8
Mutual Goals?
Family Planning on Simbo, Western Solomon Islands   232
Christine M. Dureau

CHAPTER 9
Infertile States:
Person and Collectivity, Region and Nation in the Rhetoric   262
of Pacific Population
Margaret Jolly

Contributors   307

Index   311

Illustrations

Maps

Map 1	Location of countries and regions in Asia and the Pacific discussed in this volume	3
Map 2	The Solomon Islands, showing location of Simbo in the West	233
Map 3	The geographical distribution and classification of languages (and approximate Papuan Languages) across the Asia and Pacific regions, showing subregions of Melanesia, Polynesia, and Micronesia	265

Figures

Fig. 1	Family planning poster eulogizing the small family, Ujung Pandang, Sulawesi, Indonesia	40
Fig. 2	Family planning poster exhorting people to accept family planning, Ujung Pandang, Sulawesi, Indonesia	41
Fig. 3	Several stills from the documentary film *Something like a War,* showing Indian women being tagged before tubal ligation surgery, being escorted by doctors from the operating table, and recovering on the floor after surgery	51
Fig. 4	Many stages of the Balinese wedding ceremony, such as the Egg Rite, express the wish that the bridal couple be fertile.	181
Fig. 5	Statue at a crossroads in Klungkung, East Bali, advertising the Ten-Point Program at the PKK and the "Small Family Norm" of the Family Planning Program	192
Fig. 6	Monthly weighing of babies is now institutionalized, *banjar* "Anjingan," East Bali	192
Fig. 7	The introduction of toys to the "under-fives" (*anak balita*) at the monthly weighing meeting, *banjar* "Tirtawangi," East Bali	193

Fig. 8	Immunizations of babies are now routine in Bali	193
Fig. 9	Women and children waiting for MCH services at the local clinic	246
Fig. 10	Vai, suckling her third child while arranging upcoming UCWF activities with neighboring women	247
Fig. 11	Pacific Island populations, wall chart	269
Fig. 12	Pacific Island populations, wall chart, cont'd.	270
Fig. 13	Population pyramids for Melanesia, Micronesia, and Polynesia compared	271
Fig. 14	Population decline and recovery on Aneityum Island, Vanuatu, 1850–1990	276
Fig. 15	Indigenous patterns of housing on Bau, Fiji (original caption was "Roof Tops of Bau")	280
Fig. 16	High-ranking Fijians in European-style clothing after Christian conversion (original caption was "High Fijians")	281
Fig. 17	"Fijian Chiefs and Native Constabulary" (original caption)	283
Fig. 18	Sandstone sculpture in Janus form, with ancestral faces, used to ensure the fertility of crops in south Pentecost, Vanuatu	287

Tables

Table 1	Women's Relation to Nationalism	8
Table 2	Percentage of Couples Using Contraception, by Method, 1970–71 to 1986–87	87
Table 3	Common Side Effects Attributed to Contraceptives by Isaan Women	215
Table 4	Alleged Deleterious Influences and Causes of Depopulation and Racial Degeneracy	279

Acknowledgments

This volume derives from a conference on State, Sexuality, and Reproduction in Asia and the Pacific, which was organized by the Gender Relations Centre at the Australian National University. We thank the Research School of Pacific and Asian Studies for the support of this conference and the wider project. We thank the Australian Research Council for providing the research fellowship that has permitted Dr. Ram to present an early version of her chapter at Jawaharlal Nehru University in New Delhi, do fieldwork in Tamil Nadu, collect research material, and edit this volume. We also want to thank the authors of the several chapters in this volume for responding so positively to the suggestions for revision by ourselves as editors and the anonymous referees.

Material from a couple of the chapters has previously appeared, though in slightly different form. The chapter by Ritu Menon and Kamla Bhasin (chap. 2) draws on material from their book *Borders and Boundaries: Women in India's Partition* (1998), and we thank the publisher, Kali for Women, for permission to republish. Andrea Whittaker's contribution (chap. 7) draws on her essay "Women's Desires and Burden: Family Planning in Northeast Thailand" in *Asian Studies Review* 22 (2): 137–55. Again, grateful acknowledgment is made to Blackwell Publishers Limited for permission to republish.

We must also acknowledge the permissions for many of the photographic images that were not taken by our authors. We thank Deborah Hill for her photographs of family planning posters in Ujung Pandang, Sulawesi, Indonesia (figs. 1–2, chap. 1). We also thank the Mitchell Library, State Library of New South Wales, Sydney, for permission to reproduce three historical photographs from Fiji (figs. 15–17, chap. 9). We must also thank Bob Cooper of Coombs Photography for his superb photograph of the sculpture from Pentecost (fig. 18, chap. 9) and Kay Dancey of Coombs Cartography for her excellent maps. In addition, we gratefully acknowledge permission to reproduce stills from the documentary *Something like a War,* produced by D&N (India) in association with Equal Media (London) for Channel 4.

Permission was given by

Women Make Movies
462 Broadway, 5th Floor
New York, N.Y. 10013
tel: 212–925–0606 ext. 360
fax: 212–925–2052
email: info@wmm.com
http://www.wmm.com

We would both like to thank Annegret Schemberg for her meticulous attention to detail in copyediting and proofreading and Ria van de Zandt for her excellent word processing and formatting skills. They are always a formidable team. Finally, we thank each other for the creative work and commitment it has taken to edit another volume together. We trust readers will like it as much as we do.

INTRODUCTION

Embodied States—Familial and National Genealogies in Asia and the Pacific

Margaret Jolly

Borders of Being? The title of this volume is inspired by Ritu Menon and Kamla Bhasin's depiction of the poignant circumstances of the repatriation of women in the partitioning of India and Pakistan from 1947 (this volume, 1993, 1998; cf. Das 1995). The violence of these events poses in a stark and gruesome way the questions that prompted this book. First, how are the bodies of persons, the imagined edges of their corporeal being linked to the borders of countries, the partitioning of nation-states? And how are the flows from their bodies, their sexual desires and their children conceived as belonging within, or confined by, the borders of countries? Second, are such associations similar or different for women and men? There has been a long and productive debate about the gendering of nationalism and about the ways in which the subject positions of women and men differ, as citizens of states and as agents of nations. But closely connected to this are other questions, not of imagined charters nor of abstract political contracts but of the sex of bodies. Are women's bodies, especially in their sexual and maternal aspects, more often used to mark the boundaries or plug the dangerous porosities of nation-states?

Much has been written about the way in which a "family romance" connects embodied daily life with the imagined community of the nation and naturalizes the nation so that it appears not as a novel, fragile contingent creation, but as something ancient, robust, and real. In Asian and Pacific countries the family so romanticized may not be the nuclear family enshrined in the liberal political philosophies of some Western states but a rather more copious and extended family or lineage and its privileged head an older patriarch.[1] We offer an account of sexed subjectivities in the states of Asia and the Pacific by exploring the power of nation-states and the claims of citizenship in the realms of sexuality and reproduction, but we also consider the way state power is accommodated and resisted, complicit with, and contested by, other powers grounded in relations of kinship, ethnicity, religion, and class.

How far do nation-states thus reinscribe heterosexual reproductive relations as normative, extruding homoerotic, nonreproductive, even celibate sexualities as marginal, deviant, or threatening to the patriotic values of being a good citizen, man or woman? And how far do we as feminist scholars perhaps unwittingly reinforce both the heterosexist scripts of state power and the power of the state by concentrating on the familial (cf. Parker et al. 1992)?

Places and Positions, Regions and Disciplines

This volume addresses such questions through a consideration of the past and present experiences of two proximate regions—Asia and the Pacific (see map 1). Their proximity is not inconsequential: it relates to earlier ancestral affinities and more recent historical connections.[2] But the fashionable conjugation of the two regions as "Asia-Pacific" bears witness not so much to such connections *between* the two regions as to geopolitical imperatives emanating *beyond* them (see Dirlik 1992, 1993). Increasingly in the language of international fora dominated by economic and developmentalist paradigms, and even in some global women's conferences, they are yoked as Asia-Pacific. We prefer to distinguish them. This is not just because many people from the small states of the Pacific complain that through such rubrics they feel even smaller, less significant, and weaker through too proximate an association with the larger, more populous and stronger states of Asia. It is also because the differences in their histories are as important as their both being part of large, homogenizing categories like the "Third World" or "developing nations" (see Escobar 1995).

Although the peoples of both Asia and the Pacific were both subject to colonial rule and both have experienced the traumatic struggles of decolonization and of creating "new nations," Asia had an important prior history of indigenous states, whereas in the Pacific there were, arguably, no indigenous precursors.[3] And in these Asian states gender was inextricably connected not only with differences of lineage and rank, as in the Pacific, but with broader hierarchical relations between rulers and ruled, landowners and peasants, and different castes or classes. Moreover, decolonization in the Pacific has been both more recent and far more pacific and the independent states established there much smaller, poorer, and less powerful. Although most states in both regions presume to influence the sexual and reproductive lives of their citizens and to control fertility, there are important differences between the degrees of coercion and persuasion used and in the efficacy of the state power exerted. In general, in the Pacific there is little coercion, and even strenuous persuasion

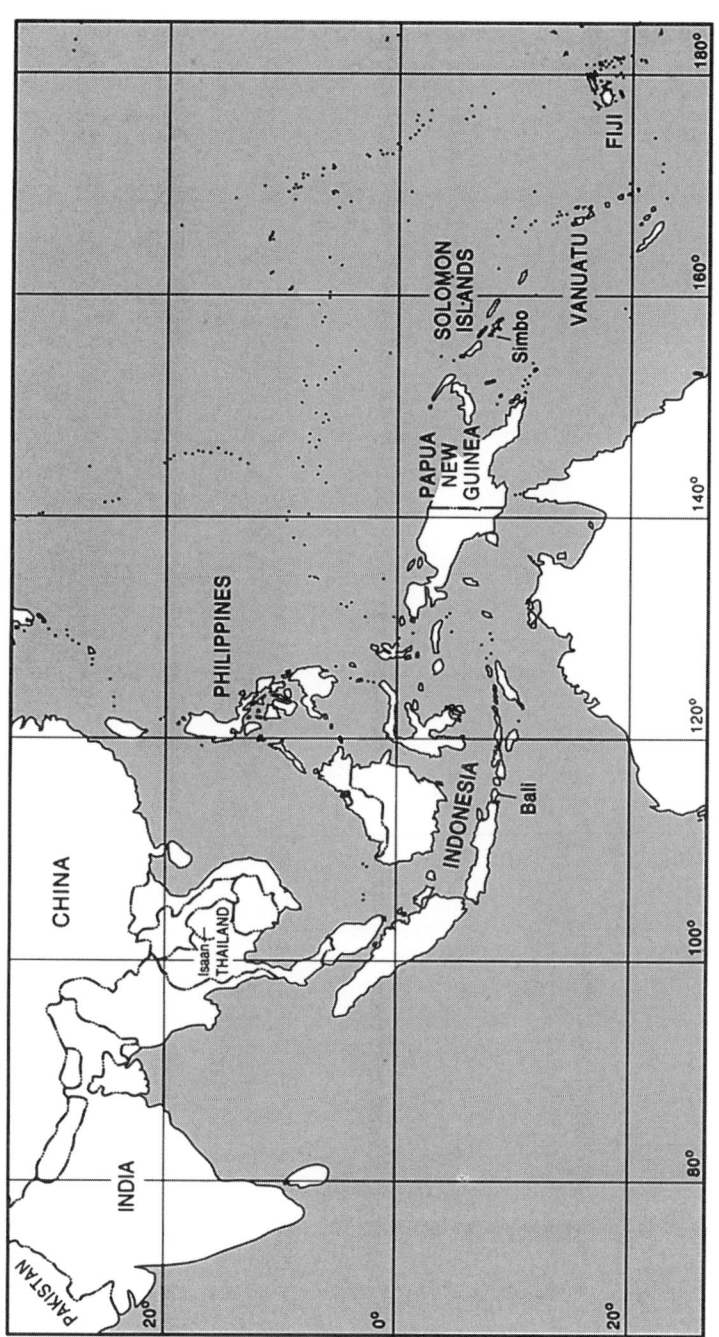

Map 1. Location of countries and regions in Asia and the Pacific discussed in this volume

often fails due to the lack of appropriate resources and powers as much as the resistance or indifference of women and men. Moreover, in very general terms nationalism in the Pacific is a far less compelling force for most of its citizens beyond a small urban elite and is not so strongly linked with projects of population control (see Dureau, this volume; and Jolly, this volume, chap. 9). Although local, regional, and religious communal bases of identity prevail in all states and often compete with national identities in deadly ways,[4] the power of nationalism is much stronger as both discursive force and military might in most Asian states. Such broad affinities and differences between the regions are important in how we frame the comparative project of this volume and our particular accounts of several countries.

Successive chapters address the relation of citizenship, fertility, and sexuality in Asia in general, India, China, Malaysia, the Philippines, Indonesia, Thailand, the Solomon Islands, and the Pacific region. Our authors write from a variety of positions and deploy a range of methodologies. Some are citizens of the states they write about. Ritu Menon is a well-known feminist author and publisher. She is cofounder of the feminist press Kali for Women in Delhi, India. Kamla Bhasin is a founder of Jagori, the Women's Resource and Training Centre in Delhi, where she lives. She works with the United Nations, publishes books, and writes political songs. Both have worked together on a project on women and Partition, initially with women from the other side of the border in Pakistan (see Menon and Bhasin 1998). Kalpana Ram migrated to Australia some twenty years ago but is as much connected to India by kinship and schooling as by her ongoing projects of research. Most of the other authors are based in Australia and relate to these countries and regions of study as foreign researchers, but researchers who have long experience, linguistic fluency, and textual knowledge of those places they write about.

Our authors use a rich mix of methodologies derived from anthropology, history, feminist theory, and cultural studies. Some chapters—most notably those by Andrea Whittaker on northeast Thailand, Lynette Parker on Bali, and Christine Dureau on Simbo in the Solomon Islands—are more grounded in the particularities of ethnography and deploy the methods of participant observation in an exemplary way. But even in these chapters the oral testimony of life histories, interviews, focus groups, and questionnaires is complemented by a critical reading of government documents and religious texts, indigenous narratives and the texts of earlier observers, be they travelers, missionaries, colonial officials, or ethnographers. Embodied, lived experience and intersubjectivity, however, underlies all of the chapters in different ways.

Hilsdon combines insights from her dangerous field experiences living with those who fought nationalist and separatist struggles in the Philippines and interviews with combatants and Catholic nuns with a broader appreciation of Philippine history and the recent texts of Catholic liberation and feminist theology. Ritu Menon and Kamla Bhasin combine their own perceptions of the continuing impact of Partition on communalism in South Asia with the voices of those who were involved in the repatriation of women and a careful appraisal of government archives. Kalpana Ram combines a reading of government plans and demographic policies with the insights of her own ethnographic and personal experiences and a theoretical framework derived from both feminism and postcolonial studies.

The chapter by Gary Sigley, though grounded in research in China, is primarily an exegesis and critique of official Chinese sources, academic analyses, and media debates. He moves between Chinese and English language sources, charting the fluid exchanges of theories of race, eugenics, and evolution between Europe and China. The more general chapter by Kathryn Robinson juxtaposes an interpretation of two television documentaries to talk about the differences between First World and Third World experiences of fertility control. Her comparative insights are situated in a critical review of the large global literature on family planning. Margaret Jolly combines insights derived from extended ethnographic and archival research in Vanuatu and Fiji with a critical review of representations of "population" in the discourses of foreign experts—missionaries, colonial officials, demographers, and anthropologists. The volume thus yields a cross-disciplinary as much as a cross-regional conversation.

Much has been written on the questions we address for South and East Asia but less for Southeast Asia and very little for the Pacific. Moreover, much of what has been published has been trapped *within* the discursive borders of regions or countries. There has been little comparative work that attempts to address such questions *between* countries and regions. But this volume tries not just to extend the debates beyond the usual disciplinary and geographic confines. We also explore some new thematic and theoretical connections. This collection is situated between the large literatures on gendering nationalism and citizenship and on population and fertility. Although both literatures have been burgeoning in recent time, they have too often been traveling on divergent paths. We try to make these paths intersect in Asia and the Pacific, where the creation of "new nations" and citizen-subjects has been often closely imbricated with concerns about population and where states have presumed, by force or persuasion, to influence the intimacies of the sexual and reproductive lives of their citizens. But, before reviewing the themes of the present volume, let me consider some questions emerging from both literatures, first on the gendering of nationalism and citizenship and second on state powers over population and fertility in the context of globalization.

Gendering Citizenship in the "New" Nation-States

The revitalized and bloody force of nationalism in Africa, Eastern Europe, and in Asia in recent times has been predictably accompanied by an intensification of academic analysis, witnessed in influential works such as Anderson (1991), Bhabha (1990), Chatterjee (1986, 1993), Gellner (1983), Hobsbawm (1990). And yet it is hard to reconcile the deeply felt emotions of nationalism, the primordial sentiments expressed on the basis of race and place with prevailing academic orthodoxies about nationalism—with the notion of nations as "imagined communities" or recent fictions. But so they are. Regardless of whether we trace the origin of nationalism in metropolitan Europe—in the emergence of Italy, France, and the United Kingdom out of a congeries of erstwhile principalities or small feudal states—or whether like Anderson (1991) we discern its origin in the colonies of North and South America, there seems little doubt that even "old" nations are rather new and that all are cultural creations. There are no natural nations, even though some may appear more natural than others.

And so we might ask: how are nations naturalized, how do their fictions persuade, what gives that compelling inflection to the narration of the nation?[5] Sometimes, compulsion is by the brute force of those who rule, the discipline imposed by arms and patriotic drilling. More often it is through more subtle processes of persuasion, of soliciting sentiments of attachment on the part of citizen-subjects. Very often such solicitations depend on the mobilization of emotions associated with blood and kinship and the melding of the model and values of the family to the nation. So we hear those oft-repeated clichés, the familial metaphors of nation—"motherlands" or "fatherlands" and leaders as "fathers" or "mothers of the nation" (see Jolly 1994; Heng and Devan 1992).[6] Through such language men and women are alike invited into the nation through the cozy values of heterosexual reproduction, through being part *of* the "family of the nation" and through making families *for* the nation. But are they interpellated in similar ways as citizen-subjects, and are all familial fictions deployed by nation-states identical?

Pateman has argued that notions of citizenship in European political philosophy and in the practices of nation-states are canonically masculine (1989).[7] For her this derives from the gendered separation and opposition between public and private spheres: the male public sphere transcends the female private sphere. The unequal social contract of the state is grounded in the unequal sexual contract in domesticity (Pateman 1988). Pateman's model has been much debated and criticized even for her theoretical heartland in Europe and North America.[8] The binary terms of her model—male public worker/citizen, female private wife/mother—may represent the ideals of certain conservative or liberal political philosophies but fail to do justice to the far more complex empirical relation and the permeability of these two spheres. Moreover, they fail to address the complex configurations of gender, ethnicity, and class in Europe and North America and still less so in regions like Asia and the Pacific, as we argue here. For in these places the dubious binary of female domestic and male public is linked in even more problematic ways with tradition and modernity.

Moreover, we might ask what purchase did nationalist ideals, liberal contracts, and Enlightenment visions have beyond Europe? Were they "derivative discourses, which simply transplanted the narratives of nationalism in Europe in new terrain?" Chatterjee (1986, 1993) and some others have persuasively argued not. He perceives Indian nationalism as neither identical with a European original nor merely a copy but a new and hybrid form or, rather, a tense conjunction that defies that organic imputation of conjoined essences imaged in "hybridity." Indian nationalism entails a contradictory combination of Western political philosophy with anticolonial resistance, a combination that generates a tension between liberal, emancipatory ideals and a collectivist vision that stresses Indian unity and progress against colonial decadence (Chatterjee 1993, 203–5; see Ram, this volume, for an important development of this argument). We might ponder, given this tension, how male and female subjects were differently located within its terms.

Drawing on examples from the Middle East and South Asia especially, Kandiyoti (1991) suggests that women are particularly caught in the tensions between the contradictory projects of nationalism in postcolonial states—expressions of cultural difference and affirmations of national identity often entail controls over women that compromise their rights as enfranchised citizens or promises of their "emancipation." She stresses the perduring Janus-faced character of nationalism that "presents itself both as a modern project that melts and transforms traditional attachments in favour of new identities and as a reaffirmation of authentic cultural values culled from the depths of a presumed communal past." Though this tension traps both male and female subjects, she argues that women are particularly caught in the cross-currents of anticolonial nationalism, being variously portrayed as "victims of social backwardness, icons of modernity and privileged bearers of cultural authenticity" (1991, 431). Such themes have been consummately developed in a recent collection focused on Egypt, Iran, and Turkey, in which Kandiyoti, Abu-Lughod, and others have combined to persuade us how central the idea of "remaking women" is to the projects of modernity and how obscuring have been those binaries that link tradition with oppressive domesticity and women's entry into the public sphere with emancipation and progress (Abu-Lughod 1998).

Kandiyoti's insights extend far beyond her regional focus, as I earlier suggested in a study of women in the independent state of Vanuatu in the southwest Pacific (see Jolly 1997). Indeed, for most of the countries discussed in this volume we might observe the gendered consequences of the contradictory demands of nationalisms that use the emancipatory language of the colonizers to oppose the colonizers and to gain independent statehood but then must try to reconcile national development with the promises of postcolonial freedoms. Such "freedoms" are not so transparent as the teleologies of certain prophets of progress might envisage. As Abu-Lughod has argued for the Middle East (1998), the *un*veiling of upper- and middle-class women a century ago was a sign of modernity and secular nationalism, but so, equally, the contemporary *re*veiling of women is an icon of modernity and of bourgeois nationalism as much as it is a sign of being a good Muslim woman in more global garb (see also Stivens 1998).

Moreover, as Yuval-Davis and Anthias stress in their influential early volume *Woman—Nation—State* (1989), women are not just signs in the language of nationalism but themselves subjects. They discern five major ways in which women are implicated in nationalism (see table 1). They not only signify the nation but embody it as subjects, as authors narrating the nation, as participants and leaders in nationalist struggles, and as those who bear and nurture children for nation-state projects. So, how do we connect these concerns about engendering the imagined communities of nations with the practical corporeal investments nations have in the reproductive lives of their citizens? This is effected in many of the essays in this volume, but let us now consider that second stream of literature on state power in the context of the global politics of reproduction.

TABLE 1. Women's Relation to Nationalism

1. As biological reproducers—in either pronatalist or antinatalist nations.
2. As reproducers of boundaries of national groups—restrictions on sexual and marital relation.
3. As signs and symbols of national difference.
4. As creators and narrators of national culture.
5. As active participants in nationalist struggles, organized nationalist parties.

Source: Yuval-Davis and Anthias 1989, 8.

State Power and the Global Politics of Reproduction

A number of important recent collections pursue the changing relations between the local, the national, and the global in the politics of reproduction, in sites in Europe, the Americas, Asia, and Oceania (Handwerker 1986; Jefferey, Jefferey, and Lyon 1989; Manderson and Rice 1996; Ram and Jolly 1998). Perhaps most notable and proximate to our own concerns are Ginsburg and Rapp's *Conceiving the New World Order* (1995) and Lock and Kaufert's *Pragmatic Women and Body Politics* (1998a). Both volumes have a truly global reach. The first endeavors to link the global processes of reproductive practices, policies, and practices with local cultural logics and social relations. For example, they note how understanding honor and shame in an Egyptian village may also require attending to how women are subjects in experiments with Norplant (Morsy 1995; cf. Whittaker, this volume). They also stress how the diversity of different local experiences is globally connected, how the illegality of abortion and the lack of contraception in Ceausescu's Romania, coupled with dire needs for foreign currency, led to Romanian babies becoming a commodity on the American adoption market (Ginsburg and Rapp 1995, 2).

They deploy the concept of stratified reproduction to describe the power relations whereby some people are empowered and others disempowered to nurture and reproduce. Such inequalities are nowhere clearer than in the new reproductive technologies, that both promote and control fertility. Insofar as these technologies always contend with what is defined locally as "natural," they are also implicated in political contests about who knows about and controls reproduction. They note that, although women's bodies are central to all reproductive regimes, such centrality is regularly effaced by churches, development agencies, states, scientists, and, indeed, the very language of biomedical "miracles."

This volume is less concerned with the new reproductive technologies that promote fertility (but see Arditti, Duelli Klein, and Minden 1984; McNeil, Varcoe, and Yearley 1990; Raymond 1994; Strathern 1992). This partly derives from our region, where, for the most part, the new reproductive technologies to restrict fertility predominate. But they are not entirely absent. So, in her study of China, Handwerker (1998) shows how the pressures of the one-child family policy has in fact increased pressure on infertile women to have children, and there has been some celebrated Chinese successes in conceiving "test tube babies." Indeed, the plight of childless couples and, especially, childless women is, if anything, even more poignant and denigrated in contemporary China. Women who are involuntarily infertile are subject to rejection, violence, and divorce, and those who are voluntarily childless are seen as deviant in both state and popular cultural representations. A policy dedicated to fewer children for the nation simultaneously imagines women as primarily procreators and harshly devalues those who, for whatever reason, are childless. New reproductive technologies to control or promote fertility combine with more ancient Chinese values to represent women as mothers by nature. So, Lock and Kaufert (1998b) argue in the introduction to their volume that, through a series of ironies, methods of "choice" deploy technological innovations to reveal women's deepest and primordial "nature."

The chapters that follow address many of the questions posed here, although our emphases vary. Let me now try to situate their insights in terms of these two major themes in the literature. First, I explore the engendering of anticolonial nationalisms and ask how far the "natural" hierarchy of the family is projected onto the nation-state, not just as familial metaphors but in bureaucratic practices and policies that impinge on sexed bodies. Related to this is the question of whether we can witness the transformations that Pateman (1988) discerned for European states, from traditional patriarchal to modern patriarchal/fraternal authority. Second, I consider how male and female, individual and familial, national and global interests relate in the present debates about population and family planning and how this bears on our prevailing models of choice and agency.

Engendering the Nation-State: Beyond the Citizen-Mother?

Are there important differences in the way in which women and men are citizen-subjects of those nation-states, forged from anticolonial struggles in Asia and the Pacific? Menon and Bhasin's analysis of the partition of India and Pakistan (this volume) suggests so. They note how the national narratives of independence, of valor and freedom, coexist with memories of massacres and of violent divisions between Hindus, Muslims, and Sikhs. In attempting to "fix" the mutually antagonistic identities of India and Pakistan at and beyond Partition, the bodies of women who were "abducted" and "unattached" were critical. This is most palpable in the forced repatriations of women who had formed marriages and had children across the border who were, regardless of their own volition, labeled as "abducted." For years after Partition, India "recovered" or "restored" such women to their places of origin, primarily in western Punjab.

As Menon and Bhasin (this volume; cf. 1998) and Das (1995) attest, the sexual honor of women was closely connected with notions of familial and national honor and purity. Both those who had been kidnaped and those who had voluntarily entered partnerships with men rendered foreign by Partition were seen as defiled and impure. This defilement was not something they could erase or nullify on their return. Such women and their children were often spurned by their extended families and their communities. But, for decades after, the Indian state still insisted on bringing them "home": dislocations and "forcible conversions" across the lines of states and of religions were not to be tolerated. These women were subject to a forcible "recovery" that denied both the humanity of their "abductors" and the agency of the women themselves.

Ultimately, their rights as citizens were sacrificed to the greater good of national and religious communal honor.

Those women who were "war widows" were in a rather different position vis-à-vis the nation-state. They were cast as the victims of the first national disaster, the first hapless subjects of state welfare. They were preferably housed in restricted ashrams or segregated agro-industrial settlements (akin to *purdah* in a nation-state preoccupied with moral hygiene). The state's aim was not just to save but to rehabilitate and train them for productive work and nation building. A nationalism that had been so influenced by notions of reform and enlightenment and which had, despite much opposition, outlawed the practices of child marriage and widow burning could not be seen to be deserting those "mothers of the nation," those widows who had been destituted by detachment from their own families.[9] The state thus assumed the status of paterfamilias, in the absence of their families and, more particularly, male kin. Thus, in relation to both abducted and unattached women, the newly independent state, though pursuing a secular and democratic program, also revealed how different male and female citizens were and how difficult it was to transcend patriarchal communal values. The nationalist project was saturated with communal anxieties, about conversions to Islam and Christianity and the loss of Hindu *dharma,* masculine potency, land, and sacred sites. This might be seen to be recuperated in the state's presumption to be the father of the large extended family of India, even as the patriarchs of different religious communities and castes threatened to tear the "motherland" apart.

What this history so poignantly reveals, then, is that women's sexual and reproductive bodies were privileged in the process of creating the borders of the Indian nation-state. Men's sexual and reproductive bodies were also defined by the boundaries of religious or national communities (see Ram, this volume), but, in marking national borders, women's bodies mattered more, just as they do in marking the borders of religion, ethnic, class, and caste distinctions.[10] Border crossing was more dangerous for women. Their very dislocation, their alleged vulnerability to the ravages of foreign men, and their ready pollution by sexual liaisons or marriages with strangers were not paralleled by similar concerns about Indian men moving across borders or relating to foreign women. Such liaisons or marriages do not seem to endanger national and communal integrity in a similar way. This echoes a pattern still prevailing in some nation-states, whereby the children of men who marry nonnationals automatically acquire citizenship, while those of women do not (Yuval-Davis and Anthias 1989, 22). It also accords with the view often emergent from the literature on the Middle East or South Asia that women's bodies are critical in the policing of communal boundaries. As Santi Rozario (1992) has shown so conclusively for the proximate case of Bangladesh, this preoccupation with women's purity is not just the preserve of Hindu communities, but of Muslims and Christians. The sexual purity of women signals the integrity of their community, their impurity the dangerous permeability or disintegration of its borders.

But, as is clear from Menon and Bhasin's discussion, more than sexuality is at issue here. Equally important is maternity. Much has been written about the images of Bengal and later India at large as a "mother," defiled and laid low by the British, and how nationalist men imagined themselves as warriors whose calling was to defend her and set her free. Probably even more has been written about the way in which women were imaged as mothers of the emerging nation (Bagchi 1990; Chatterjee 1989; Katrak 1992; Kishwar 1985; Sen 1993; Thapar 1993). Not only did Gandhi deploy the canonically feminine and maternal values of domestic self-sufficiency and stoic suffering in the practices of *satyagraha* (truth force), but women active in such struggles were often allowed passage into public places out of *purdah,* so long as they conformed to this image of devout mothers. Apart from being both signs and subjects of nation, mothers were also critical in the more quotidian corporeal terms of bearing babies, and especially sons for the nationalist struggle and beyond that the independent state, although the indigenous and exogenous forces of pronatalism were later to be opposed by antinatalist programs whereby fecundity had to be restrained and rationalized, as Ram (this volume; and see later discussion) lucidly shows.

Images of fecund, modest mothers might be counterposed with the way in which childless, celibate[11] women, such as nuns, subvert the usual ways in which we think of gender and citizenship (see Hilsdon, this volume). Catholic nuns have been crucial agents of nationalist and separatist struggles in the Philippines, not just as proponents of liberation theology and fighters for justice and poverty but also as allies, envoys, and even soldiers in armed insurrection. Both Catholic liberation theology and Filipino nationalism have been seen as the local precipitates of global processes. Liberation theology, as elsewhere in the Third World, was in part a radical response to several statements emanating from the Vatican and the Catholic hierarchy in the 1960s and 1970s. But, as Hilsdon attests, Catholic theologians in the Philippines were not always liberationist, and those who were often tried to remodel what they perceived as a disembodied universalist theology with an Asian or a feminist form. Resurgent nationalism in the Philippines was in part a response to the complicity between conservative elites and the military and economic interests of the United States. From the 1960s armed resistance to the state was diverse— embracing communists (the New People's Army) and Muslims (Moro National Liberation Front), private militias, and army factions who had seceded from the state. The Catholic Church was a protagonist not just in peaceful resistance but in violent struggles. After Vatican II, Filipino nuns shed their habits and their seclusion to become central figures in movements for human rights and national liberation, such as the National Democratic Movement and the National Democratic Front.

As Hilsdon points out, this history poses problems for those who subscribe to the conventional gendered narratives of nation, who imagine women's citizenship as relentlessly compromised by their sexuality and maternity. There is no doubt that sexual chastity and maternal modesty are as critical in the Philippines as they are in Indian and Malay communal and national imaginaries and that the lives of most women are still subject to such strictures. But the image of the Madonna has been remodeled and embraced by radical nuns as chaste militant and as martyr, suffering with and helping the poor and oppressed, as protagonists and as victims in armed struggle. Both the convent and the habit of nuns became signs of resistance, and nuns were often subject to suspicions of concealing weapons. Paradoxically, for a period, nuns were safer if they assumed the civilian attire of ordinary women. Their celibate status did not exempt them from abuse. Ordinary women were subject to sexualized forms of torture, and nuns likewise suffered sexual torture and rape.

Such figures of celibate, childless women clerics thus deserve to be juxtaposed alongside the dominant images of women as sexual and maternal beings in religious national imaginaries. But is the active agency of nuns as fighters in nationalist struggles to be contrasted with the experience of other Filipino women who are domestically confined and whose relation to the state is mediated by men, the fighters and the workers? Such a view would occlude the huge, diverse public movements of women in the Philippines, strenuously concerned as citizens in the affairs of their state, and actively involved as fighters, not just as envoys and allies in violent armed struggles in nationalist and dissident causes (see also Gaitskell and Unterhalter 1989; and McClintock 1991, on South Africa; Sparks 1997, on dissident activism and women's citzenship).

The example of the Philippines, like the earlier cases of India and Malaysia, challenges some of the orthodoxies in that wider literature about gendering nationalism, through a critical interrogation both of the predominant image of the female subject as citizen-mother and the male subject as citizen-warrior or worker. Are we in danger of reinscribing the very binary oppositions between male and female, public and private, state and family, that we aspire to deconstruct? There has been a burgeoning discussion of the issue of maternal citizenship in Europe, in North America, in Australia, and now to a lesser extent in Asia. Following Pateman (1988), it is suggested by many commentators that, whereas men are the exemplary models of citizens, acting in canonically public contexts as workers or warriors, women are imagined by many nation-states as being lesser or unequal citizens who rarely transcend domesticity and whose relation to the state is vicarious and mediated by men—as the wives or mothers of workers or fighters.

So, Marilyn Lake (1993) talks of the contradictions of maternal citizenship in Australia. Some early-twentieth-century feminists claimed that women's service to the state as mothers be acknowledged, since childbirth was as dangerous as war. Following federal legislation in 1912, maternity allowances were paid to white women, but not to Aboriginal, Asian, or Pacific Islander residents, who were not seen as appropriate citizen-mothers for a white Australia. Such victories, however, were not just racially but sexually discriminatory, since arguments for women's difference justified work inequalities and an industrial system predicated on a notion of a family wage in which men were the breadwinners and women dependents, wives of men rather than mothers of the nation. Lake concludes, following Pateman, that within patriarchal states neither sameness nor difference can produce a "genuine democracy" for women but that what is needed is the "effective reformulation of the meanings of citizen, worker and mother" (1993, 393). Such rhetorical proclamations contend with obdurate masculinist structures still embedded in the practices and policies of many states in Asia and the Pacific, even where there are intentions to emancipate women.

Kathryn Robinson (1994) has observed a similar contention between the ideals of sameness and difference in the Indonesian context. She observes that in independent Indonesia there are two national holidays that commemorate women: Hari Kartini, which commemorates the life of a Javanese noblewoman who sought emancipation through education and literacy, and Hari Ibu, the National Mother's Day, which celebrates the first National Women's Congress. The juxtaposition of these two days for her signals the difference between women who claim their place in the imagined community of the Indonesian nation as equals with men, as against those who claim it on the basis of their difference as mothers and wives. She asserts that the notion of a family foundation (*azas keluargaan*) imputes a natural hierarchy that connects the authority of the father and the New Order government of Suharto, which prevailed between 1967 and 1998.

Such Indonesian state familism, founded in New Order ideology, is analyzed by Lynette Parker (this volume) for the island of Bali. Here, as elsewhere in Indonesia, the charter of the PKK (Family Welfare Organization) envisages women's relation to the state foremost as producer and educator of children, as wife and faithful companion to her husband, and as manager of the household.

Her status as citizen is listed last. Women in Bali lack local public power in the community organizations of *banjar,* which are composed only of married men. The *banjar* head, perforce a married male, though technically not a civil servant, is increasingly seen as a state functionary. His wife has a role and responsibility derived from him, as unpaid leader of the appropriate stratum within the PKK.[12]

And yet it would be important not to perceive this conservative state ideology of female citizenship focused on being a wife and mother as the *only* model of women's relation to the state, especially since the collapse of the New Order government. As Robinson (1994) suggests, there is a long tradition of Indonesian feminism, from the nationalist movement onward, which offers an alternative view of women as active public citizens, who are advancing through the liberating forces of education and public employment (cf. Jayawardena 1986). Balinese girls are staying longer at school, and women have moved dramatically over the last twenty years out of unpaid family labor in *sawah,* or rice fields, into paid work as laborers in construction and, more particularly, textile and garment industries. Some better-educated, high-caste women have jobs as teachers, doctors and nurses, businesswomen, and civil servants. Although the Balinese women who are Parker's interlocutors hardly embrace a self-conscious feminism, there is the clear sense that younger women in particular experience travel to schools or to jobs as "freedom." And, perhaps even more remarkable, they perceive the Balinese pattern of land tenure, whereby men own *sawah* and women do not, as unjust.

Parker's analysis graphically poses the question of how far there has been a transformation of male control from the patriarchal forms of kinship collectivities and families to the more "fraternal" civil forms of male control that Pateman (1989) suggests are characteristic of contemporary nation-states in Europe and North America. Parker—like Menon and Bhasin, and Dureau (all in this volume)—suggests, rather than a transformation from one to the other, that they coexist in the contemporary states of Asia and the Pacific. This coexistence can shift between complicity, tense accommodation, and contest between these two different loci and configurations of male control.[13]

Parker claims that the indigenous forms of collectivity in Bali—patrilineages, caste groups, and *banjar*—were all male dominated. Patriarchal control over sexuality and fertility was pronounced. Women's sexuality and fecundity were, as in India, used to mark the purity and vitality of groups. Notions of purity and pollution defined the boundaries of endogamous caste groups and were particularly expressed through protocols about women's bodies. Sexual double standards prevailed—women were enjoined to be chaste or faithful, men were expected to be promiscuous. Divorce was rare but especially traumatic for women, since they would lose not only rights of access to family wealth but their children—to the husband's patrilineage. Men thus had a heavy investment in their wives' fertility, and women were blamed for infertility and feared to have the potential to take revenge against the husband by aborting or contracepting.[14]

Parker depicts a past pattern whereby fecundity was highly valued and where men were critically engaged in promoting the fertility of their wives but also, more broadly, of their kinship and caste groups. How, then, might we explain the very dramatic recent decline in fertility in Bali, from 5.96 in the period 1967–70 to 2.28 in the period 1986–89? Bali is exemplary, the model province within the Indonesian family planning program, in terms of the theory and the goal of "demographic transition." Parker finds the answer not just in the distinctive form of the program, the *sistem banjar* (the *banjar* system), or the rapid socioeconomic transformations of Bali. Clearly, both were important. The *sistem banjar* offered a Balinese inflection to the national program, while it perpetuated male control of fertility by making *banjar* heads responsible for drawing up reproductive censuses and maps of all eligible couples and for fulfilling contraceptive targets in their areas. They, like clinic staff, were rewarded credits and prizes for good rates of "acceptance" (compliance), while recalcitrant couples were subject to ostracism, communal vilification, and inspections by government officials.[15]

The broader transformation from a familial agricultural system to one dominated by compulsory schooling, wage labor, and commodity relations has no doubt transformed the value of children from economic benefits to burdens. Women, like men, have a powerful economic incentive to have fewer children; they say that with only two or three children they are "free" to pursue money. Parker sees women's pursuit of money and engagement in family finances not as a sign of their economic autonomy (as others have done) but, rather, as a sign of their dependency on men, who alone still own the main property, the *sawah* (rice fields). This particular example, then, suggests that women do perceive contraception as a route to freedom, although women's desires have not been a prominent feature of family planning in Bali and the choice of available methods has been negligible. (The major method of contraception promoted has been the IUD, a method less likely to be discontinued and more amenable to biomedical and state control.) This, then, poses in graphic form the very notions of freedom and of choice in global debates about fertility. I now focus on this question in considering the configuration of individual, national, and global interests in the family planning debate, in relation to several other chapters on family planning.

State Power and the Global Politics of Reproduction

Most of these countries discussed in this volume are committed to controlling fertility; they are antinatalist rather than pronatalist states. Malaysia, an important exception to this pattern, is, alas, not discussed here (but see Omar 1996; Ong 1990; Stivens 1998). In this they conform to what Robinson (this volume) has depicted as the Third World, or developing country, configuration as opposed to that of the First World, or developed country, pattern. In her latter category there are many states with pronatalist policies or preferences: witness the protracted struggles over abortion law reform in both North America (Ginsburg 1989), Europe (Kligman 1992; Petchesky 1990), and Australia. Moreover, as Robinson stresses, Third World states in general exert far more agency in antinatalist programs than any government would presume in North America, Europe, or Australia. The rights of the individual person and especially the agency of women assume far greater prominence in such countries. There is a stress on individual choice, on self-fulfillment in sexual and reproductive life, and the rights of individuals to be biological parents, even if their bodies are infertile. Hence, the terms of the cultural and political debates over the new reproductive technologies, which, as Strathern and others have stressed, carry the biologistic obsessions of Euro-American theories of kinship and the individual compulsion to "choose" to ever greater heights (Franklin 1995; Strathern 1992, 1995; see also Jolly, this volume, chap. 9; and later discussion).

And yet the horrors of eugenic control over people whose ethnicity, intelligence, or physical integrity were thought deficient are quite recent memories in several such states—including Sweden and the United States of America. The contemporary reality of coercive state control over reproduction in Romania (see Kligman 1995) is not so easily marginalized as totalitarian or Eastern European barbarism. It may be that the exterminations and the forced sterilizations that were part of fascist state practices in Europe yield haunting memories of the Holocaust and constrain any similar violence by European and American states to the bodies of their citizens. But a focus on fascism occludes how routine and normal were eugenic interventions in the policies and practices of many Western European and American states until recent decades.

Moreover, as the several chapters in this volume make clear, there are other ways in which this clear dichotomy between Third World antinatalist coercion and First World pronatalistic choice is problematic. There is not only the important exception of pronatalist Malaysia but also a great variety in the power of states to exert their agency. At one extreme we have the example of China with its draconian one-child family policy and on the other those Pacific states where state incapacity, economic insufficiencies, and inappropriate means often combine to ensure that family planning programs falter and fail. In the Solomon Islands total fertility rates remain some of the highest in the world, and, while national programs are now committed to restriction, many contraceptive forms that are locally desired are unavailable (see Dureau, this volume; and Jolly, this volume, chap. 9). Such diversities pose difficult questions about the very language of choice and the way in which we tend to pose such stark oppositions between the agency of states and of individuals, or of men versus women (see later discussion; and Jolly, this volume, chap. 9).

The relation between female and national interests in family planning is directly addressed both by Andrea Whittaker for Thailand and Christine Dureau for the Solomon Islands (this volume). Both focus their attention on women's bodies and women's motivations for, and responses to, contraception. Both pose dilemmas of analysis and of practical implementation, which ultimately converge on the question of why family planning is almost exclusively "women's business."

For Whittaker the dilemma is whether modern, state-sponsored forms of fertility control are empowering women or disempowering them through entrenched state control. Thailand, like Bali in Indonesia, has had a "successful reproductive revolution" with pronatalist policies giving way to antinatalist policies by 1970 and the free availability of the contraceptive pill, IUD, and (female) sterilization at government health stations from 1976. State efforts were complemented by vigorous NGO activity. But in the subsequent national plans for human resource development and population control, the ethnically distinct peoples of the northeast were seen as marginal and obdurate obstacles to the reproductive revolution. Whittaker stresses how their ethnic and linguistic distinction from central Thai speakers, coupled with the region's representation as both backward and politically insurgent, makes this a particularly fraught site for the struggle between female and state agency. This is a region that is a prime target because of its high birth rates, its endemic poverty, and patterns of out-migration to the affluent cities further south. Unsurprisingly then, this is a site where women's autonomous desires might be opposed to state interests and where there is a particular tension over the persistence of abortion, which, though "traditionally" legitimate, is now illegal.

But such a picture of women's autonomy poses the question of autonomy from whom? From their husbands, male-dominated groups, or from the state? Unlike Bali, descent groups are here matrilineal, but women still move to live with their husbands and bride-price is paid. Indigenous forms of fertility control—barks, clay, and herbal distillations—were primarily in the hands of women, especially midwives. In contrast to Hindu Bali, women were perceived in popular Buddhism to have more investment in children than men, who were rather enjoined to reject their sexuality and fertility for a time to become monks in pursuit of merit. Such female control of fertility has been diminished with the introduction of modern contraception, the main forms being tubal ligations, contraceptive pills, Depo Provera, and increasingly Norplant. In this, women are not just the "targets" of increasing state and patriarchal control; they are, Whittaker insists, "enthusiastic volunteers." Women desire fewer children than was typical of the recent past; younger women especially echo the clinic credo: "two children is enough." Parents face financial burdens in providing for children and sending them to school, rather than deriving income from their work in the rice fields as before. As in Bali, women stress that fewer children "frees" them for paid work, albeit menial jobs in the towns of the northeast and in Bangkok.

Yet women also experience such freedom with ambivalence. They perceive a loss of their indigenous status as valued mothers of many children and report morbid symptoms as a result of contraception—in particular disruption of the humoral balance of the body. Contraceptives that disturb the menstrual cycle are thought to reduce vitality and the ability to work hard. This sense of enervation is compounded by the lack of information and support and frequent humiliation experienced at clinics and hospitals, typically staffed by Central Thai or Chinese Thai people, who assume both class and ethnic superiority. So, Whittaker concludes that, although women's and state desires coincide, in the medicalization of their bodies women *lose* power and are rendered weaker in both social and corporeal terms. Medicalization combines with ethnic and class marginalization. Doctors and nurses typically perceive those Isaan women who are their clients as dirty, ignorant villagers and are abrupt and perfunctory in consultations with them. Such unequal relations are most pronounced when Isaan women seek abortions, which are regularly denied (even when rape or an illicit sexual relation resulted in pregnancy) as being contrary to both Buddhist principles and state laws. In choosing illegal abortions, Isaan women resist such controls but also risk their lives. Finally, Whittaker notes, it is women who are the targets of fertility control. Family planning programs are integrated with maternal and child health services, condoms and vasectomies are rarely mooted as alternatives, and men are hardly involved.

In many respects Dureau (this volume) detects rather similar patterns in Simbo, a small remote island, in the Western Province of the archipelago of the Solomon Islands. Here, too, family planning is women's business, and women's and state interests coincide in desires for fewer children, but mutual expectations are continually frustrated. This is typical of much of the

Solomons, where total fertility rates continue to be very high by global standards and neither demographic transition nor reproductive revolution appears imminent (see Dureau, this volume; and Jolly, this volume, chap. 9). This may be as much due to the slower pace of capitalist development as to the shortcomings of family planning. The Solomon Islands continue to have a predominant pattern of customary land tenure, with predominantly subsistence but some cash cropping. Despite increasing urbanization, foreign revenues are derived primarily through extractive industries, like logging, rather than the development of capitalist agriculture or industry.

Moreover, the ethnic situation of Simbo within the Solomon Islands is rather different. The extreme cultural and linguistic diversity of this nation does not afford such clear hegemony to one ethnic group, although in some respects the people of the western Solomons are perceived as the first modernizers, since they were very early and rapidly affected by the influences of foreign traders, Methodist missionaries, and the British colonial state. In contrast to both Bali and Thailand, Dureau stresses how in the past uncontrolled fecundity was not valued. Although both men and women attained adult status by becoming parents, fertility was tightly controlled, through practices of abstinence and sexual sequestration of couples as well as the use of indigenous contraceptives and abortifacients, by those daring sex outside conjugal confines. Such techniques were women's business, and, although they afforded some autonomy for women from their husbands, ultimately their sexuality and fecundity was under the violent control of their *luluna,* or "brothers."

The rates of fertility soared with Christian reformation of conjugality and a Pauline model of family hierarchy that conferred on the husband corporeal control of his wife, with a legitimated violence akin to that of brothers in the past.[16] "Custom medicine" is now seen to have lost its potency as contraceptive or abortifacient, and abortion, as in Thailand, is illegal. Women have a strong desire for family planning, and in this their interests coincide with recent antinatalist state policies. But, despite these common goals, there is constant disappointment. Women lack the available means to fulfil their desires and, in Dureau's view, are regularly opposed by their husbands. Although men, like the agencies of the state, construct fertility as a female problem, they still attempt to control fertility both through the legitimacy conferred on them by conservative interpretations of the Bible and by state edicts that require a husband's permission for family planning.

And yet this very idea that husbands must give their "permission" for their wives' contraception is predicated on two premises that, Jolly suggests (this volume, chap. 9), pervade family planning programs in the Pacific. The first is that in the recent programs addressing overpopulation, as in the earlier programs addressing depopulation, women are the privileged targets of state control. Contraception is typically offered, as in Thailand, in the context of maternal and child health programs. Although MCH clinics and hospitals have been central in the dramatic reduction of infant and maternal mortality, and the delivery of primary health care, the very conjugation of family planning and maternal and child health, patent in the coupling of acronyms MCH/FP, suggests that this is not men's domain. Indeed, as Jolly argues, it might be suggested that men have been extruded from family planning programs until recent times, when the female and family centric bias of sexual and reproductive health has been challenged but, still, rarely redressed.

Such extrusion of men from contemporary family planning must be juxtaposed with their central involvement in ancestral, indigenous regimes of fertility. Ancestral regimes throughout the southwest Pacific, as in Simbo, valued fewer, healthy children. The indigenous ideal of two children that Dureau reports for Simbo is very close to the ideal promoted in family planning campaigns today. Postpartum abstinence coupled with protracted breastfeeding often meant that children were spaced two to three years apart. And, although men were vitally interested in children in affirming their own adult status and ensuring the vitality and growth of descent groups, it is hazardous to impute to men an unquenchable desire for many children and a natural hostility to birth control. As Jolly asserts (this volume, chap. 9), this is not to deny that many men oppose their wives seeking contraception, fearing both the loss of their power as husbands and the risk of undetected infidelity by contracepting wives. But male opposition to fertility control is often too readily presumed in demographic analyses and family planning practice. So, in the Pacific there is often not so much a clear opposition between women's agency and government agency but, rather, as in Thailand, a sense of ambiguity and ambivalence. Women and states may have convergent desires for fewer children, but either through technical and economic insufficiencies or through the excesses of state power their desires ultimately diverge. Moreover, in the Pacific, as in many parts of Asia, there is often rather a triangulation of interests; male and female interests are seen to diverge precisely at the point where state or global interests promise an alliance with women.

This raises further questions about the very notions of choice and rationality that pervade debates about family planning—questions that are directly addressed by Ram and Sigley (this volume). Ram notes the particular way in which the Indian state has aspired to a lofty and idealist modernity in relation to its citizen-subjects. Family planning has become central to the legitimacy of the state and has entailed a concordance between the rationality of state planning and the rationality of the conjugal couple, the combined reason of governing and governed bodies. Unlike China, liberal precepts of the democratic state and the sanctity of individual rights were early applied to family planning with a stress both on the participatory democracy of collectives and the value of informed consent on the part of the "acceptors." But such principles are both "continually reiterated and equally constantly eroded" by targets, by financial incentives, and of course the promotion of sterilization, in some instances forcibly, most notably the mass sterilizations of poor men during the Emergency. But, Ram insists, the extremity of Emergency coercions should not hide the quotidian limits on choice. Despite the illusion of a "cafeteria" of contraceptive choice, in fact the state tended to favor one method at a time and typically promoted methods that diminished the power to choose and especially to discontinue: sterilization and, later, hormonal implants. There was very little information disseminated about the contraceptive pill, which was seen as a technology appropriate only to the rich or the well educated. Ram imagines that the typical Indian family planner believes that the consumer cannot be trusted. Increasingly, external "motivators" are needed—health care workers who themselves need motivating with incentives and targets—to drive the engine of development while reducing population.

Ram suggests, elaborating on Chatterjee (1986, 1993) in novel and important ways, that there is a tension between two progressivist projects of the Indian state: its liberal charter and its drive toward development, which can readily sacrifice individual agency to state agency. Although its adherence to liberal goals distinguishes India from many other Asian states (most notably China but also Indonesia and Malaysia), it shares the imperative of economic progress. As in Thailand, those who reject family planning are seen as "backward" and lacking a sense of national responsibility. This applies not only to the rural poor but also to those who champion individual or communal rights of difference or resistance. Some planners see India's very diversity, liberalism, and electoral politics as obstacles to development: diversity and particularity must be transcended through a rationality that conjoins state and conjugal planning.

Interestingly, men are not so marginal to the projects of family planning in India. Gandhi, in his vision of moral rather than technological control, enjoined men to abstain from sex and to relinquish selfish desires to possess women (see Caplan 1987). But, even when moral instruments gave way to technological and chemical means, men were not extruded from the process so much as in the Pacific. Intriguingly, there was an early preponderance of male sterilizations until later in the 1980s, when, with new surgical techniques, female sterilizations became more frequent. Men were enjoined to plan, to defend the weaker members of the family (women and children), just as the state presumed to defend the welfare of backward castes, the rural poor, and widows (see Menon and Bhasin, this volume).

But, ultimately, Ram sees this as a fanciful wish, a kind of "dream formation" by the state that reconciles the contradictory imperatives of liberalism and development in the hope that individuals will freely choose to limit their children, in harmonious synchrony with the state's desires. This fancy pushes back, into the premodern and the irrational, not just women but the poor and those still marked as "backward" by caste, class, ethnicity, or language. Muslim minorities in particular are the contemporary exemplars of a refusal to be "suitably modern" in a high-caste, Hindu way, continuing to insist on their personal laws and still "overbreeding."

China, of course, offers an example of a state whose developmentalist and progressivist goals seem little compromised by liberal ideals of the sanctity of the private sphere or of the freedom of individuals to choose. As distinct from "coercion in a soft state" such as India (Vicziany 1982a, 1982b), this is coercion in a hard, muscular state. As is well-known, China's one-child family policy is a blunt instrument of population control. But, although we must acknowledge both the corporeal and "euphemized violence" that the Chinese state deploys, there is, even in this extreme situation, a question of how the subjectivity of male and female citizens is formed and how their desires for an elusive modernity are shaped (cf. Anagnost 1995).

Anagnost poses the question of why in post-Mao China there is "popular acceptance of such a painfully austere policy which appears to restore the statist ambitions of party leadership" (1995, 23). She argues that since the one-child family policy was proclaimed in China in 1987 there has been a shift from an emphasis on the quantity to the quality of bodies. Like Sigley (this volume), she sees this new stress on quality as having ancient roots in notions of being Chinese, being Confucian, and in eugenic theories from earlier this century. But, increasingly, the idea of "quality" is concentrated in the wealth and intellectual elites of the coastal provinces, which as they become increasingly integrated with the global market, strand the inland regions in backwardness and poverty. The crisis imagined if the mass of poor peasants do not limit their children is not famine but cultural and political chaos. There is a strong connection drawn between a modernizing state and a body that is strong, supple, aware, and moving forward. This, Anagnost suggests, is linked to an idea of transforming consuming passive bodies into producing and active ones, especially in those disciplined sites of new factories in the coastal provinces, where labor itself becomes consuming. And such self-sacrifice for collective good is mirrored in the hard work of coercions inherent in the work of birth control officials (Anagnost 1995, 32–35).

Sigley detects ancient Confucian roots, imported eugenics theories, and modern Communist ideals of a harmony connecting the bodies of family and state. Eugenics theory, though disavowed by Mao as imperialist, is now communist common sense. Moreover, Sigley suggests that, although reproductive coercion is palpable, the contemporary conversations about conjugality in marriage manuals, magazines, and on hot lines also stress the pleasures of sex and of domesticity. This is not to suggest a preoccupation with sex or that sex is the secret of an interior Chinese subject. The celebration of sex is confined to conjugal heterosexual relations. Infantile, adolescent, extramarital, and homoerotic sexuality are all pathologized. The harmony of Chinese domesticity is seen to be threatened both by such pathologies but also by pernicious foreign or Western influences. Anagnost suggests that, alongside the othering of China's non-Han minorities, there is also an increasing sense of the dangers of the floating population and even the traffic in bodies associated with growth. Itinerant people, like Gypsies, can escape the inspections of state bureaucracy and household registration (1995, 38).

Moreover, Sigley suggests there is a sense not just of a loosening of spatial but of temporal anchors. There is the threatened loss of Chinese values of filial respect and piety combined with the state's ambivalence about elders and particularly the control of the patriarchs. Although the state desires the legitimacy of the power of elders, feudal forms, such as arranged marriages, must be opposed. Thus, the Chinese state at the same time as it rigidly controls the number of children born to couples can also promise women "emancipation," in the new forms of marriage for love and consequent domestic bliss. Evoking women's energetic pleasure in sensuality and their newfound freedoms in choosing partners constructs women both as willing subjects as well as ciphers and conduits of state family policy.

The Globalizing Rhetoric of Choice

This final example of women's subjectivity and agency in China poses yet again the fundamental question of the relation between collective and individual rights, male and female bodies, and the importance of reconceptualizing agency in terms that transcend the notions of choice inherent in ideas of the market and of individual consumers. It has been often claimed that such ideas of choice are indissociable from Western notions of individuals, embedded in capitalist notions of property, production, and consumption.

Insofar as demographers imagine agency, there is often in the family planning literature an imputation of an individual imbued with an entrepreneurial rationality that assimilates having children to the logic of capitalism, whereby children are human "resources" and parents invest in them. This productionist presumption has its consumerist counterpart in a tendency to present an array of models of birthing and contraception as a supermarket or a cafeteria of choices (cf. Ram 1994, 20; see Ram, this volume; and Jolly, this volume, chap. 9). But, of course, this abstract ideal of choice and a free and abundant market is radically at variance with the realities of options that are limited and hierarchized by the family planning programs of states and international agencies, most palpably in those states where fertility is tightly controlled and sterilization is forced. But, even where ostensibly more choice can be exercised, the range of contraceptions locally available or promoted may be those more in the interests of the state or international agencies, because they are cheaper, less reversible, and confer greater control on biomedical personnel. Thus, Whittaker (this volume) ponders whether Isaan women in northeast Thailand are being empowered or controlled through state-promoted family planning.

In discerning the limits of choice, the deeply gendered character of choice in reproductive politics is also exposed. There is no doubt that the development of "modern" contraceptive and reproductive technologies has been very asymmetrical, with chemical and instrumental devices designed for women's bodies—the pill, the diaphragm, IUDs, tubal ligations, Depo Provera, and now Norplant. With the exception of condoms and vasectomies, and the long promised male pill, most modern contraceptive technologies intervene in women's reproductive biologies. Some radical feminist opponents of both modern contraceptives and the new reproductive technologies see all this as an expression of the patriarchal, masculinist character of biomedicine and science and urge a return to indigenous, ancestral, or natural methods (see Robinson, this volume). Some liberal feminists see it as appropriate that women should be the privileged agents of reproductive choice. If women bear children, they should be the ones who decide whether to conceive or not, whether to bear or abort. Other feminists warn that this risks exempting men not only from the burdens of chosen fatherhood but from the responsibilities of controlling fertility.

It is perhaps those new technologies that "assist" rather than restrict fertility (artificial insemination, in vitro fertilization, surrogacy) that most poignantly reveal some of the underlying notions about gender, nature, and choice that inform biomedical models and pervade Euro-American notions of kinship.[17] What infertile person would adopt if they could choose to be "assisted" in their reproduction? Natural kinship rather than preexisting, being taken-for-granted, is increasingly chosen or selected (Strathern 1992, 20). Such "enabling" technologies thus help "persons fulfil themselves" (32). Tissue techniques reproduce the choices, the desires of the parents; the child is thus not so much the product of social relations but the embodiment of the desire to have a child. This language of choice, she stresses, does not just affect those who use such technologies. Thus, in her subversive comments on "enterprise culture," Strathern notes how the market analogy is being extended to more areas of life and how that analogy is "less than benign." There is, then, a hidden prescription that we *ought* to act by choice (36).

> The sense that one has no choice not to consume is a version of the feeling that one has no choice not to make choice. Choice is imagined as the only source of difference: this is the collapsing effect of the market analogy. (37)

We are witnessing a new globalization of such notions of choice, especially in the domain of reproductive politics. This process is nowhere clearer than in the complex pattern whereby fertility is perceived as increasingly a global problem to be addressed in international fora, such as the International Conference on Population and Development in Cairo in 1994 (Johnson 1995), and by mobilizing armies of international organizations and multilateral agencies that are poised to cross between states as necessary to shape, to challenge, or to implement population plans. Simultaneously, we witness, especially in the developing countries of Asia and the Pacific, more strenuous national interventions in the sexual and reproductive lives of their citizens, often at the behest of international agencies. Whether state policy be antinatalist or pronatalist, whether the programs be coercive or cajoling, the contemporary nation-state is usually seen to have a legitimate stake in surveying and shaping the reproductive lives of its citizens, because this is what all responsible nation-states should do. In more conservative garb, family planning programs enlist the imputed rationality of the conjugal couple (and especially the wife) with the alleged reason of state in a conjunction of "plans" between governed and governing bodies and the governmentality of an imagined globe. In more recent rhetoric, the stress is on the sexual and reproductive "rights" of individuals and of choices, but still a connection is assumed between the person's capacity to "choose" and the way in which nations or international agencies affirm or control such choices.

The spread of this global language is nowhere clearer than in the documents of the International Conference of Population and Development

(ICPD), held in Cairo in 1994. The resolutions of the conference and the program of action are laudable, especially in plans to reduce infant, child, and maternal mortality, to enhance education, especially for girls, and to prevent and control the HIV/AIDS pandemic (see Johnson 1995, 211–47). As is clear in Johnson's (1995) summation of the preparations, the meeting, and its outcomes, that conference was unprecedented in its declaration of reproductive rights and especially in its commitment to gender equality and the empowerment of women (cf. Corrêa 1994). The bold visionary document drafted by the ICPD's preparatory committee under the leadership of Dr. Nafis Sadik supplanted talk of numerical goals and women as targets or "objects" of family planning programs by insisting on women as subjects who can make choices. As was widely reported, the forces of religious conservatism combined to try to thwart such a global exercise of choice: Islamic states and the Vatican forged an alliance, especially to oppose abortion. But, despite this alliance, strong resolutions and a program of action were passed. The essence of the new strategy was on meeting the "needs of individual women and men rather than on achieving demographic targets." The key was "empowering" women and offering them "more choices," in the process of making family planning universally available by 2015 or sooner.

It is hard to resist the ringing emancipatory claims of such language, but how then to deal with the critical cautions and the deconstructive insights of feminists like Strathern who are alert to the shuffling between "subjects" and "objects" in Western constructs of the person and how both are predicated on commodity logic? Increasingly in developed capitalist societies, the body, like property, can be owned. And we impute to the severed mind not just that dubious entrepreneurial rationality of choice but, even more severely, the compulsion that, like a good consumer, it *must* choose.

So let me in conclusion ponder Petchesky's (1995) feminist revisioning of the notion of the body as property and the way in which she and Corrêa (Corrêa and Petchesky 1994) approach notions of reproductive and sexual rights. Petchesky suggests that the notion of women owning their bodies has been too summarily equated with the notion of the body as property in a narrow Lockean paradigm. Through a recuperation of the histories of radical groups like the Levellers in England, early European feminist writings, and Strathern's own depiction of the Highlanders of Papua New Guinea (1988), she attempts to suggest that notions of property are like those of persons and bodies, much more labile than the capitalist and masculinist conceptions of private property that attach things to autonomous male persons. She suggests that ideas of women "owning" their own bodies do not necessarily partake of the processes of control and traffic that make women's bodies into commodities or things. Rather, as with her essay on sexual and reproductive rights, coauthored with Corrêa, Petchesky (1994) perceives the contemporary challenge as one of recapturing the notion of rights from the strictures of a liberal, individualist, masculinist paradigm. She hopes that notions of self-propriety might, like those of rights, become inclusive rather than exclusive, might be broadened to include the moral space of community as well as the interiority of possessive selves.

One can witness the global proliferation of a language of women owning their bodies being used in movements for reproductive freedom across Asia and the Pacific, a process that Petchesky sees as their *dis*covery rather than *re*covery of the idea of self-ownership (which is what she discerns in Europe and North America) (1995, 401). In so distinguishing *dis*covery from *re*covery of emancipation, her history still starts the story in the West and still privileges notions of freedom originating there. There is perhaps a future story to be told of how in struggles about reproductive rights, as in related struggles and debates about human rights, Asian and Pacific women are using the language of rights in a way that far exceeds the Eurocentric, individualist, and masculinist limits that many criticize (see Hilsdon et al. 2000; Jolly 1996). Whether associating women's agency in their sexual and reproductive lives with the notions of choice, of owning their bodies, and claiming their rights achieves the global effects that Petchesky envisions is a question that haunts both this volume and the futures of women in Asia and the Pacific.

NOTES

1. On this point I owe a debt to a recent discussion with Dipesh Chakrabarty. Some of his thoughts about this are elaborated in his book *Provincializing Europe* (Chakrabarty 2000).

2. Prehistorians trace the original homelands of many Pacific peoples to southern China or Taiwan. There are important ancient links that are witnessed still in the cognacies of those Austronesian languages stretched across the insular Pacific and much of insular Southeast Asia. There have been more recent Asian influences in the Pacific— Chinese traders in most ports and towns; Indian, Vietnamese, Filipino indentured laborers working on plantations; and Japanese laborers, settlers, and rulers. Cultural and political connections between the Pacific and Asia have reached their highest velocity and most exquisite tension in the contemporary ethnic politics of the state of Hawai'i.

3. I say arguably, since some would suggest that the kingdom of Hawai'i prior to European colonization was a proto-state, and similar arguments have been elaborated for Tonga. But the formation of centralized polities and kingdoms was often entangled with early processes of European colonization, and so I concur with the view that states were not indigenous to the region. Although the larger size, greater centralization, and

intensified hereditary hierarchy of polities characterized Polynesia and Micronesia in contrast to those in Melanesia, which were usually smaller, less centralized, and less hierarchical, recent scholarship has been critical of strong distinctions between the regions (see Jolly and Mosko 1994).

4. I here allude to the violence of religious communal and separatist movements, especially in India, but also in more recent time—since the collapse of the Suharto regime—in Indonesia, and in the Pacific to both secessionist struggles in Vanuatu in the 1970s as well as the long and bloody war about Bougainville's independence from Papua New Guinea and the 1990s struggles between Malaitans and locals on Guadalcanal in the Solomons.

5. The phrase, of course, derives from a book by Bhabha (1990), although the idea of narrating the nation has become quite popular in the literature since then. See, for instance, Radhakrishan 1992; and Otto and Thomas 1997.

6. Although the gender of the parents evoked seems to vary between states, both may be evoked and may signify epochal shifts or portend transformations in state borders. Thus, Suharto's repressive New Order regime was distilled in his image as strict father of the nation, while Megawati Sukarno recently authored herself as "Indonesia, the mother" in an extraordinary speech given in Dili before the elections were held that decided the choice of East Timorese for independence rather than their autonomy as part of Indonesia. She suggested that to "let East Timor go" would be like a mother abandoning her children. In October 1999, when she accepted the vice president's position in relation to the new president and her old ally in reform, she deployed the more egalitarian language of siblinghood, by affirming him as her brother in struggle. A more humorous personal anecdote might illustrate the popular power of the metaphors linking families and nations. While traveling in India in 1980, there was a moment of uncertainty about whether the railway carriage in which I was departing the cantonments of Delhi would be designated a women-only carriage. An older woman, a captain in the Indian army, got on. She agreed that it was fine for my partner to join me in the carriage and urged me to summon him from the hallway with the words: "Tell your husband to come in. He is standing outside like Bangladesh."

7. Pateman (1989, 33ff.) suggests that most discussions of the classic social contract theories of the seventeenth and eighteenth centuries fail to acknowledge that the contract is inherently patriarchal. The Enlightenment credo of liberty, equality, and fraternity needs to be understood as just that—instituting liberty and equality through a fraternal pact. Pateman (1988, 1989) offers a more complex reading of the contest between patriarchalists like Filmer and contract theorists like Locke and suggests that the triumph of Locke's political philosophy should not be read as the defeat of patriarchy but the supplanting of one form of patriarchy by another. The historical rupture in the claim to liberty and equality by the sons against the authority of the fathers, of a public polity separate from the naturalized hierarchy of the family, elides the continuity of the naturalized subordination of women. The liberal political right of individual sons/brothers is as much dependent on male domination as the natural familial right of fathers. The inequality of the sexual contract is the predicate of the alleged equality of the social contract. Although Pateman interrogates the domain distinctions of public and private and the variable relation of state, civil society and domesticity conjured by these terms, her theory often seems to reinscribe those very domain distinctions she is

criticizing. There is a problematic relation between her discussion of political philosophies and the practices of those Western capitalist democracies that are her purview, a problem further compounded if we consider not just the "woman" of a certain kind of Western theory but "women" in more plural cultural and historical accounts. In an excellent critique of Pateman's fixation on origins rather than on critical genealogical history, Gatens (1996) suggests that Pateman ultimately relies on an essentialist notion of sexual difference in her undue focus on heterosexuality and her unwarranted equation of heterosexuality with male domination. In a persuasive rebuttal of some strategic essentialisms that have proved catastrophic for feminism both theoretically and politically, she highlights how women's bodies have often been seen as "unfit" for citizenship and how "women's bodies are often likened to territories whose borders cannot be defended" (1996, 33). This echoes, if rather distantly and perhaps dissonantly, the concerns of the present volume.

8. These are too many to list, but a significant critique appears in Gatens (1996), considered in the previous note. Unfortunately, a collection devoted to a critical review of Pateman's work, edited by Gatens and Tapper and based on an Academy of Social Sciences of Australia conference, was never published.

9. The authors note that, although both were classified as "war widows," there was a difference between those whose male kin had been killed, who were seen as a lifelong state responsibility, and those who were simply unable to maintain them, who might at some point become self-sufficient or be able to be maintained by kin.

10. I am grateful to Kalpana Ram for her insistence on the inextricable connections between how women's bodies are critical in drawing the borders of these several imagined communities.

11. Because of a reader's query, I perhaps should say notionally celibate but, like Hilsdon, have no basis on which to posit that nuns she interviewed were not in fact adhering to their vows, and so leave this unmarked.

12. This pattern, whereby wives of government officials assume a vicarious role in national development, prevailed nationally in the PKK at all levels and across the nation.

13. And it is a moot point whether the familial language of the state always deploys an image of a new modern nuclear family founded on love and companionship as against the image of an extended family in which arranged marriage and male domination prevails. Chakrabarty's recent book (2000) suggests that for Bengal and then India the extended family was as much a part of the nationalist imaginary as the modern nuclear family.

14. As in many parts of Indonesia and throughout the Pacific (see Jolly, this volume, chap. 9), the fertility of humans and of crops was associated and linked to broader preoccupations with cosmic fecundity and regeneration. In this ancestral schema sexuality and fertility were fused: desire for sex and children were inseparable, but women's and men's desires for both were differentially legitimized.

15. This echoes how Fijian chiefs were held responsible for promoting the fertility of couples in their area and awarded bonuses for more babies and penalties to those who failed to procreate quickly (see Jolly, this volume, chap. 9; Lukere 1997).

16. We might note in passing that, contrary to the teleology Pateman plots for Western history, we have here a shift from a patriarchy dominated by brothers to one

dominated by the father/husband. An associated question is posed by Foucault's corpus. Has there been a shift toward a novel biopower distinguished by the interpellation of new kinds of persons, summoned up by state interest in sexuality and fertility under the novel concept of "population" (Foucault 1980)? Does this entail, as Foucault's paradoxical formulation suggests, a heightened sense of an abstract mass coupled with an enhanced sense of the autonomy and particularity of individuals, so that a person relates to the collectivity more as one of a series of individuals rather than as part of a hierarchical form like a family or lineage?

17. Older models tended to privilege mothers rather than fathers as the natural and rightful possessors of their children, but the advent of the new reproductive technologies has—in detaching ova, wombs, and nurture—yielded some interesting new paradoxes in Euro-American notions of kinship (Strathern 1992). Who is the real mother and who the surrogate? Is she the one who gave the egg or the womb? As specular and microscopic technologies discern smaller elements and particles of matter as constitutive of human persons, the biological basis of kinship seems ever more compelling.

REFERENCES

Abu-Lughod, L., ed. 1998. *Remaking women: Feminism and modernity in the Middle East.* Princeton, N.J.: Princeton University Press.

Anagnost, A. 1995. A surfeit of bodies: Population and the rationality of the state in post-Mao China. In *Conceiving the new world order: The global politics of reproduction,* ed. F. D. Ginsburg and R. Rapp, 22–41. Berkeley: University of California Press.

Anderson, B. 1991. *Imagined communities: Reflections on the origin and spread of nationalism,* rev. ed. London: Verso.

Arditti, R., R. Duelli Klein, and S. Minden, eds. 1984. *Test-tube: What future for motherhood?* London: Routledge and Kegan Paul.

Bagchi, J. 1990. Representing nationalism: Ideology of motherhood in colonial Bengal. *Economic and Political Weekly.* Review of Women's Studies 35 (42–43): WS65–71.

Bhabha, H., ed. 1990. *Nation and narration.* London: Routledge.

Caplan, P. 1987. Celibacy as a solution? Mahatma Gandhi and *brahmacharya.* In *The cultural construction of sexuality,* ed. P. Caplan, 271–95. London: Tavistock.

Chakrabarty, D. 2000 *Provincializing Europe: Postcolonial thought and historical difference.* Princeton, N.J.: Princeton University Press.

Chatterjee, P. 1986. *Nationalist thought and the colonial world: A derivative discourse?* Delhi: Oxford University Press.

———. 1989. The nationalist resolution of the women's question. In *Recasting women: Essays in Indian colonial history,* ed. K. Sangari and S. Vaid, 233–53. New Delhi: Kali for Women.

———. 1993. *The nation and its fragments: Colonial and postcolonial histories.* Princeton, N.J.: Princeton University Press.

Corrêa, S., with R. Reichmann. 1994. *Population and reproductive rights: Feminist perspectives from the South.* London and New Jersey: Zed Books in association with DAWN.

Corrêa, S., and R. Petchesky. 1994. Reproductive and sexual rights: A feminist perspec-

tive. In *Population policies reconsidered: Health, empowerment, and rights,* ed. G. Sen, A. Germain, and L. C. Chen, 107–23. Boston: Harvard School of Public Health.
Das, V. 1995. National honor and practical kinship: Unwanted women and children. In *Conceiving the new world order: The global politics of reproduction,* ed. F. D. Ginsburg and R. Rapp, 212–33. Berkeley: University of California Press.
Dirlik, A. 1992. The Asia-Pacific idea: Reality and representation in the invention of a regional structure. *Journal of World History* 3 (Spring): 55–97.
——., ed. 1993. *What is in a rim? Critical perspectives on the Pacific region idea.* Boulder: Westview Press.
Escobar, A. 1995. *Encountering development: The making and unmaking of the Third World.* Princeton, N.J.: Princeton University Press.
Foucault, M. 1980. *The history of sexuality: An introduction,* vol. 1. Trans. R. Hurley. New York: Vintage Books.
Franklin, S. 1995. Postmodern procreation: A cultural account of assisted reproduction. In *Conceiving the new world order: The global politics of reproduction,* ed. F. D. Ginsburg and R. Rapp, 323–45. Berkeley: University of California Press.
Gaitskell, D., and E. Unterhalter. 1989. Mothers of the nation: A comparative analysis of nation, race and motherhood in Afrikaner nationalism and the African National Congress. In *Woman—nation—state,* ed. N. Yuval-Davis and F. Anthias, 58–78. Basingstoke: Macmillan.
Gatens, M. 1996. Sex, contract and genealogy. *Journal of Political Philosophy* 4 (1): 29–44.
Gellner, E. 1983. *Nations and nationalism.* Oxford: Basil Blackwell.
Ginsburg, F. D. 1989. *Contested lives: The abortion debate in an American community.* Berkeley: University of California Press.
Ginsburg, F. D., and R. Rapp, eds. 1995. *Conceiving the new world order: The global politics of reproduction.* Berkeley: University of California Press.
Handwerker, L. 1998. The consequences of modernity for childless women in China. In *Pragmatic women and body politics,* ed. M. Lock and P. A. Kaufert, 178–205. Cambridge: Cambridge University Press.
Handwerker, W. P., ed. 1986. *Culture and reproduction: An anthropological critique of demographic transition theory.* Boulder, Colo.: Westview Press.
Heng, G., and J. Devan. 1992. State fatherhood: The politics of nationalism, sexuality, and race in Singapore. In *Nationalisms and sexualities,* ed. A. Parker et al., 343–64. New York and London: Routledge.
Hilsdon, A., M. Macintyre, V. Mackie, and M. Stivens, eds. 2000. *Human rights and gender politics in the Asia-Pacific.* London and New York: Routledge.
Hobsbawm, E. J. 1990. *Nations and nationalism since 1780: Programme, myth, reality.* Cambridge: Cambridge University Press.
Jayawardena, K. 1986. *Feminism and nationalism in the Third World.* London: Zed Books.
Jefferey, P., R. Jefferey, and A. Lyon. 1989. *Labour pains and labour power: Women and childbearing in India.* London: Zed Books.
Johnson, S. 1995. *The politics of population: The International Conference on Population and Development, Cairo, 1994.* London: Earthscan Publications.
Jolly, M. 1994. Motherlands? Some notes on women and nationalism in India and Africa. In *Women's difference: Sexuality and maternity in colonial and postcolonial*

discourses, ed. M. Jolly. *The Australian Journal of Anthropology*, special issue 5 (1–2): 41–59.

———. 1996. Women ikat raet long human raet o no? Women's rights, human rights and domestic violence in Vanuatu. In *The world upside down: Feminisms in the antipodes*, ed. A. Curthoys, H. Irving, and J. Martin. *Feminist Review* 52 (Spring): 169–90.

———. 1997. Woman-nation-state in Vanuatu: Women as signs and subjects in the discourses of *kastom*, modernity and Christianity. In *Narratives of nation in the South Pacific*, ed. T. Otto and N. Thomas, 133–62. Amsterdam: Harwood Academic Publishers.

Jolly, M., and M. Mosko, eds. 1994. *Transformations of hierarchy: Structure, history and horizon in the Austronesian world. History and Anthropology*, special issue 7.

Kandiyoti, D. 1991. Identity and its discontents: Women and the nation. *Millennium: Journal of International Studies* 20 (3): 429–43.

Katrak, K. H. 1992. Indian nationalism, Gandhian "satyagraha," and representations of female sexuality. In *Nationalisms and sexualities*, ed. A. Parker et al., 395–406. New York and London: Routledge.

Kishwar, M. 1985. Gandhi on women. *Economic and Political Weekly* 20 (40) (5 October): 1694–99.

Kligman, G. 1992. *When abortion is banned: The politics of reproduction in Ceausescu's Romania*. Washington: National Council for Soviet and East European Studies.

———. 1995. Political demography: The banning of abortion in Ceausescu's Romania. In *Conceiving the new world order: The global politics of reproduction*, ed. F. D. Ginsburg and R. Rapp, 234–55. Berkeley: University of California Press.

Lake, M. 1993. A revolution in the family: The challenge and contradictions of maternal citizenship in Australia. In *Mothers of a new world: Maternalist politics and the origins of welfare states*, ed. S. Koven and S. Michel, 378–95. New York and London: Routledge.

Lock, M., and P. A. Kaufert, eds. 1998a. *Pragmatic women and body politics*. Cambridge: Cambridge University Press.

———. 1998b. Introduction. *Pragmatic women and body politics*, ed. M. Lock and P. A. Kaufert, 1–27. Cambridge: Cambridge University Press.

Lukere, V. 1997. Mothers of the Taukei: Fijian women and "the decrease of the race." Ph.D. diss., Australian National University, Canberra.

Manderson, L., and P. L. Rice, eds. 1996. *Maternity and reproductive health in Asian societies*. Amsterdam: Harwood Academic Publishers.

McClintock, A. 1991. "No longer in a future heaven": Women and nationalism in South Africa. *Transition* 51:104–23.

McNeil, M., I. Varcoe, and S. Yearley, eds. 1990. *The new reproductive technologies*. London: Macmillan.

Menon, R., and K. Bhasin. 1993. Abducted women, the state and questions of honour: Three perspectives on the recovery operation in post-Partition India. Working paper no. 1. Canberra: Gender Relations Project, Research School of Pacific Studies, Australian National University.

———. 1998. *Borders and boundaries: Women in India's partition*. New Delhi and New Brunswick, N.J.: Kali for Women and Rutgers University Press.

Morsy, S. A. 1995. Not only women: Science as resistance in open door Egypt. In *Pragmatic women and body politics*, ed. M. Lock and P. A. Kaufert, 77–97. Cambridge: Cambridge University Press.
Omar, R. 1996. State, Islam and Malay reproduction. Working paper no. 2. Canberra: Gender Relations Project, Research School of Pacific Studies, Australian National University.
Ong, A. 1990. State versus Islam: Malay families, women's bodies, and the body politic in Malaysia. *American Ethnologist* 17 (2): 258–76.
Otto, T., and N. Thomas, eds. 1997. *Narratives of nation in the South Pacific*. Amsterdam: Harwood Academic Publishers.
Parker, A., et al., eds. 1992. *Nationalisms and sexualities*. New York and London: Routledge.
Pateman, C. 1988. *The sexual contract*. Cambridge: Polity Press.
———. 1989. The fraternal social contract. In *The disorder of women: Democracy, feminism and political theory*, by C. Pateman, 33–57. Stanford, Calif.: Stanford University Press.
Petchesky, R. P. 1990. *Abortion and woman's choice: The state, sexuality and reproductive freedom*. Rev. ed. Boston: Northeastern University.
———. 1995. The body as property: A feminist re-vision. In *Conceiving the new world order: The global politics of reproduction*, ed. F. D. Ginsburg and R. Rapp, 387–406. Berkeley: University of California Press.
Radhakrishnan, R. 1992. Nationalism, gender, and the narrative of identity. In *Nationalisms and sexualities*, ed. A. Parker et al., 77–95. New York and London: Routledge.
Ram, K. 1994. Medical management and giving birth: Responses of coastal women in Tamil Nadu. *Motherhood, fatherhood and fertility. Reproductive Health Matters*, special issue 4:20–26.
Ram, K., and M. Jolly, eds. 1998. *Maternities and modernities: Colonial and postcolonial experiences in Asia and the Pacific*. Cambridge: Cambridge University Press.
Raymond, J. 1994. *Women as wombs: Reproductive technologies and the battle over women's freedom*. North Melbourne: Spinifex Press.
Robinson, K. 1994. Indonesian national identity and the citizen mother. In *Communal/Plural 3: Pluralising the Asia-Pacific*, ed. G. Hage, J. Lloyd, and L. Johnson, 65–81. Nepean, N.S.W.: Research Centre in Intercommunal Studies, Faculty of Humanities and Social Sciences, University of Western Sydney.
Rozario, S. 1992. *Purity and communal boundaries: Women and social change in a Bangladeshi village*. Sydney: Allen and Unwin.
Sen, S. 1993. Motherhood and mothercraft: Gender and nationalism in Bengal. *Gender and History* 5 (2): 231–43.
Sparks, H. 1997. Dissident citizenship: Democratic theory, political courage and activist women. *Citizenship in feminism: Identity, action and locale. Hypatia*, special issue 12 (4): 74–110.
Stivens, M. 1998. Modernizing the Malay mother. In *Maternities and modernities: Colonial and postcolonial experiences in Asia and the Pacific*, ed. K. Ram and M. Jolly, 50–80. Cambridge: Cambridge University Press.
Strathern, M. 1988. *The gender of the gift: Problems with women and problems with society in Melanesia*. Berkeley: University of California Press.

———. 1992. *Reproducing the future: Essays on anthropology, kinship, and the new reproductive technologies.* New York: Routledge.

———. 1995. Displacing knowledge: Technology and the consequences for kinship. In *Conceiving the new world order: The global politics of reproduction,* ed. F. D. Ginsburg and R. Rapp, 346–63. Berkeley: University of California Press.

Thapar, S. 1993. Women: A study of the Indian Nationalist Movement. *Feminist Review* 44:81–96.

Vicziany, M. 1982a. Coercion in a soft state: The family planning program of India. Pt. 1: The myth of voluntarism. *Pacific Affairs* 55 (3): 373–402.

———. 1982b. Coercion in a soft state: The family planning program of India. Pt. 2: The sources of coercion. *Pacific Affairs* 55 (4): 557–92.

Yuval-Davis, N., and F. Anthias, eds. 1989. *Woman—nation—state.* Basingstoke: Macmillan.

CHAPTER 1

Government Agency, Women's Agency: Feminisms, Fertility, and Population Control

Kathryn Robinson

The advent of second-wave feminism in the late 1960s coincided with an explosion in the numbers of women in the world using modern technical contraception to control their fertility. The year 1960 marks the beginning of "the era of modern contraception," with the introduction of oral contraceptives and the reintroduction of (modern) intrauterine devices (IUDs) (Rosenfield 1989). In the view of some feminists, it is the invention of the pill, a relatively safe, reliable contraceptive, that provided the enabling conditions for a new wave of feminism, initially announced as "women's liberation."[1] Rosi Boycott, founder of the feminist magazine *Spare Rib*, eulogized the pill as "the most significant change of this century. . . . The pill has given [women] different lives. We sit here doing different things [in her case editing *Esquire* magazine] and this was made possible by that one invention" (ABC 1992). The inventors of the pill, however, intended it not as a liberatory vehicle for Western women but, rather, as a device to facilitate the control of "overpopulation" in the developing world (ABC 1992).

Today, the majority of women using modern contraceptives are not in the wealthy, industrial societies, where control of fertility through improved access to safe reliable contraception and abortion was tied by early second-wave feminists to women's quest for autonomy, expressed in terms of personal liberation. Most of the world's women using contraception or permanent forms of fertility control live in Third World countries, where contraception is most likely to be available through state-sponsored programs (see Population Reports 1992; Rosenfield 1989, 386, table 1). That is, they begin using modern technical contraception, such as the pill, the IUD, or hormonal implants, in the context of a government program whose goal is population control and which offers restricted choice of methods and possibly coercion.

In a few developed countries, like Australia, government policy is pronatalist, manifested, for example, in the expressed concern to maintain replacement levels of population. In contrast, most developing countries have antinatalist policies. Where a fully formulated population control policy exists (as, e.g., in Indonesia, China, and India), the national government sets goals for fertility decline and establishes some formal mechanisms, usually a family planning program that distributes contraceptive devices and/or provides sterilization to achieve this. Such programs inevitably integrate incentives and disincentives against more than the permitted number of births for each woman (the most controversial being China's one-child policy), and the programs are administered in terms of achieving "targets."

Gender, Population, and Development

Much of the support for population programs in developing countries is from international aid donors; some of the poorest countries are dependent on aid funds for contraceptives, which in most cases have to be brought from scarce foreign exchange, as they lack the industrial capacity to produce their own supplies.[2] Government policies are necessarily responsive to the policies of international donors. Ostensibly, development assistance serves humanitarian ends of alleviating poverty, but it is now broadly acknowledged that development assistance benefits the rich countries in the global economy, for example by expanding trade opportunities.[3] The Rockefeller Foundation, which pioneered public health programs in developing countries, saw the goals of its philanthropic work thus: "to raise the productivity of the workers in underdeveloped countries" and to "reduce the cultural resistance of 'backward' and 'uncivilized' peoples to the domination ... [of] industrial capitalism" (Brown 1982, 3). Family planning became a component of development interventions in the 1960s. The failure of "trickle-down" effects to radically alter the economies of the poor countries led to a specific focus on curbing population growth to achieve that end. In the 1970s family planning was incorporated as a key element of primary health care initiatives (Golley 1982), that is, as fundamental to ensuring the health of Third World populations. Delicate diplomacy was needed to sell the idea to governments of poor countries that they should, with foreign assistance, limit their populations. In Southeast Asia

> direct visits to the Thai and Philippine rulers by John D. Rockefeller III himself and less than subtle suggestions by the World Bank to Indonesia and Malaysia constituted adequate incentive to those governments to find creative ways to promote the concept of population control for the first time in history. (1982, 12)

Rockefeller's view was that "the relation of population to material and cultural resources of the world represents one of the most crucial and urgent problems of the day" (SBS 1993). The Rockefeller Foundation sponsored the establishment of the Population Council in 1952 as an international research organization to facilitate the development of methods and strategies for fertility control.

Most donors channel their funds through multilateral organizations, in particular the United Nations Fund for Population Activities (UNFPA) and the International Planned Parenthood Federation (IPPF), due to the controversial nature of issues of contraception and abortion in their domestic electorates. Ten major donors[4] provide 90 percent of global assistance in this sector, the United States being the largest (Conly and Speidel 1993, 44). Hence, the approaches to population issues adopted by donors and multilateral agencies are critical to the manner in which poor women gain access to contraceptive information and supplies.

The strategies adopted by governments and donors in addressing issues of fertility regulation reflect underlying assumptions and philosophies about the relation between population and development (see Harvey 1974). Neo-Malthusianism has had a resurgence in recent years, as a consequence of growing concern about depletion of the world's resources. This argument holds that unchecked population growth is a fundamental cause of poverty in the Third World: even if gains can be made in achieving economic growth, these could be wiped out by population growth. The Malthusian notion of "overpopulation" has a high profile in developed country discourse about the Third World. There have been attempts to link rates of population growth and rates of economic growth,[5] to provide a scientific basis for the argument that direct interventions to reduce fertility are critical to reducing poverty. Population programs are technical programs, the aim being to achieve the highest possible prevalence of contraceptive use in order to bring down fertility and hence population growth.

The demographer Jack Caldwell has commented, "There is no theory of population outside of demography" (1982, 298). While economists, anthropologists, and historians might wish to challenge this assertion (see, e.g., Greenhalgh 1990), demography has been dominant in the formulation of population programs and policies. Demography as a science engages with a body understood in purely biological terms. Societies not using modern technical contraception are described as having "natural fertility regimes," that is, without modern artificial contraception fertility is perceived as uncontrolled, a biological property of human populations (see also Jolly, chapter 9 in this volume). Fertility is thus represented as a natural property of a biological body, which can be controlled with modern technology. Demographic understanding of fertility does not engage with a body that is socially inscribed. Policy arising from this view focuses on the manipulation of "proximate and intermediate variables" that influence fertility. Inevitably, this technical approach valorizes fertility rates and their manipulation as the measure of success. Women who are the bearers of children become part of the problem, to be targeted, educated, persuaded to use the kinds of modern contraception that population programs provide (usually a limited range). The goals of the interventions and the means to achieve those ends are always technically defined—for example, in terms of a limit to family size rather than in terms that engage with the human experience of fertility, such as removing fear of unwanted pregnancy, and of death and disablement, which can color the joyful experience of childbirth and parenthood. In the "worst-case" population programs, coercive strategies have been used to persuade women (and sometimes men) to be sterilized or utilize forms of contraception they feel uncertain about—most commonly due to fear of side effects. There is often a thin line between incentives, such as the material rewards given to long-term "acceptors" in Indonesia, and coercion. For example, the offer of credit to contraceptive users who join "integrated family planning" projects conflates women's decision making about contraceptive use or choice of method, with economic incentives, in a subtle exercise of state power.[6]

The dominant discourse in population assistance talks of "overpopulation" and population control sees fertility as a failure of rational control and fecundity as an enemy of humankind to be controlled and constitutes women as the objects of policies. Almost all the available methods, or at least the ones being heavily promoted, are female methods and are invasive of women's bodies (see Greenhalgh 1990).

Women's Status and Family Planning

Just as the Women in Development (WID) or, more recently, gender analysis literature has provided a specifically feminist voice in development debates, so research on population has its own liberal feminist discourse. The "status of women in family planning" literature points to associations between fertility rates and social indicators of women's "status." That is, improvements in the position of women, measured in terms of variables such as economic participation, education, and literacy, are linked to declines in fertility. Hence, the rationale for improving women's access to resources becomes one of facilitating the achievement of "development," measured in terms of statistical indicators such as changes in the gross national product (GNP) rate, through reducing fertility. These arguments are developed in terms of models of independent and dependent variables. In some cases, however, it is argued women's status

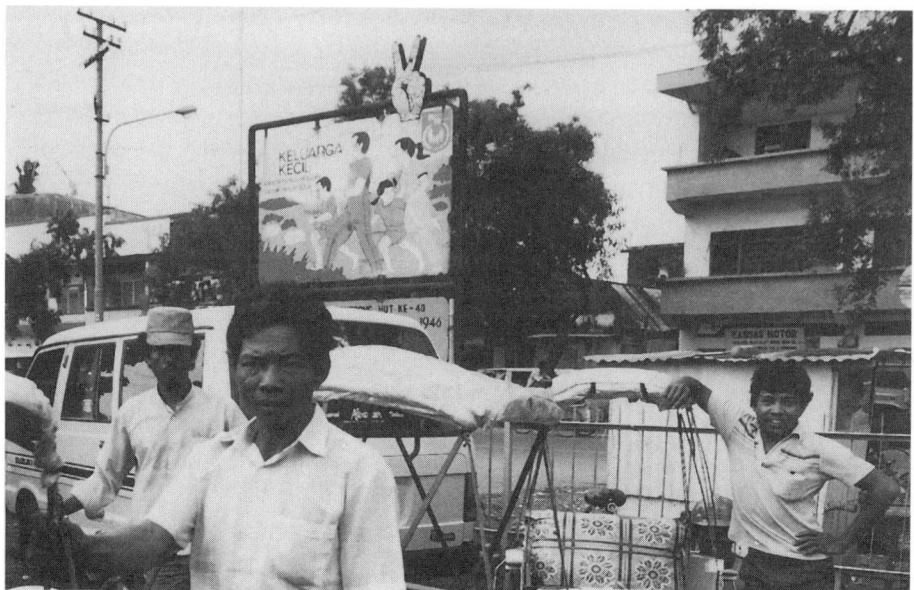

Fig. 1. Family planning poster eulogizing the small family, Ujung Pandang, Sulawesi, Indonesia

must improve in order for fertility to decline and, hence, for development to take place. In other cases, this is turned on its head and it is assumed that fertility must decline in order for there to be improvements in their status.

These arguments assume that the relation between variables identified in such studies are universal, indicative of underlying structurally determined relations between the variables indicative of "women's status" and those indicative of the state of development. They ostensibly provide a link between a feminist celebration of women's rights and state-sponsored family planning programs.

The concept of women's status is a tricky one; even more difficult to operationalize is the idea that it is possible the rank the position(s) of women (in one or several locations!) in a unilinear scale in terms of a single (necessarily synthetic) variable (Quinn 1977). More problematic is a single variable chosen as a surrogate for the synthetic dimension, to assume a primacy of one variable in determining women's status or social position. In an example of this genre, Kathryn Ward (1985) analyzes economic, fertility, and status of women data from twenty-nine developed and seventy-six developing countries, and women's level of education is the surrogate variable for women's status. She

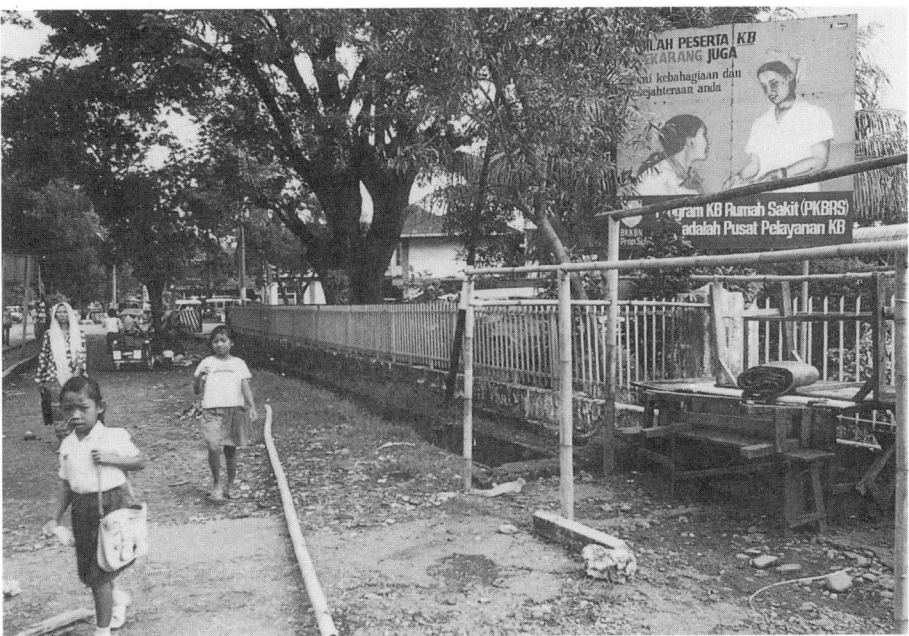

Fig. 2. Family planning poster exhorting people to accept family planning, Ujung Pandang, Sulawesi, Indonesia

argues that the higher the level of foreign investment, the lower women's share of the labor force, which is an impediment to them taking up initiatives offered by family planning programs. Therefore, family planning programs "can be more effective if instituted with changes in the patterns of investment/dependency and the economic status of women" (Ward 1985, 588). Her conclusion has the instrumentalist cast common to this debate: equity goals for women should be pursued, because they can provide a means to delivering the all-important declines in fertility, seen as a fundament of development. Safilios-Rothschild uses a more comprehensive set of variables for her statistical analysis of the relation between fertility and women's status in an article written for the Population Council but concludes with a policy recommendation that "only when the improvements in the status of women reach the majority of women . . . can a significant decline in fertility take place" (Safilios-Rothschild 1985, 20). The taken-for-granted desirable social outcome is declining fertility, and improving women's status is addressed as a means to achieving this. There is an unquestioned assumption that women benefit from access to modern contraception.

In the foundations of Safilios-Rothschild's argument, however, there is evidence that fertility limitation can be antithetical to women's interests. The question arises: What if high fertility is important to women's status (in the sense of social valuation) or to their economic security or to their sense of well-being and the positive meanings people create in their daily lives? Safilios-Rothschild writes that in societies where "women's access to valued resources" is blocked due to the "sex stratification system . . . children become women's most valued resource that can be controlled by them and constitute an important power and prestige base" (1985, 2). Still, she proceeds to a conclusion which valorizes changes in women's status not as a good in itself, but as a way of achieving another (more noble) goal: fertility decline.

The Rockefeller Foundation ran a dedicated research program on the status of women and family planning in the 1980s. In this context Mason prepared an essay on women's status in relation to fertility to provide background to applicants for funding under the program. In it she problematizes simple, unidimensional models of women's status, arguing status is both "multidimensional" and "multilocational," and discusses the problems of measuring poorly defined concepts (variables), which is the case with much of the literature she reviews (Mason 1985, 25–26). She particularly criticizes the demographic literature for confusing the effects of class and gender. While acknowledging that "in the abstract, it is difficult to specify what the most appropriate comparisons are for studying some particular aspect of female status in relation to fertility and mortality" (31), nonetheless she presses on with the task of identifying appropriate areas for study. Her list includes: "Links between different aspects of gender inequality" (73), "The meaning of female education and labor force participation" (74), and "The contexts in which female status influences fertility or mortality" (75). Although her critique of the literature is exhaustive and comprehensive, the validity of the central proposition is not challenged: that it is possible and desirable to explore the ways in which female status influences fertility.

These studies may appear to represent feminist practice, resting on a body of feminist literature and appearing to put women on center stage. But they take for granted that development is a good thing, manifesting an assumption common in much liberal feminist writing that it is not development per se that is the problem for poor women, but rather that benefits are unevenly distributed between men and women. It is also commonly argued, however, in literature that draws on the framework developed by Boserup (1970), that development can lead to a worsening of women's position; further, development can have the effect of increasing fertility, as poor families struggle to meet the new economic and cultural logics of a capitalist order.

The "status of women in family planning" literature accepts the premise that women's fertility is a problem, to both themselves and the world at large, and that it is legitimate to pursue equity goals for women with the intention of achieving a more generalized goal (a goal that principally serves the interests of the wealthy countries). This position does not question that women benefit from access to modern contraception. But there is a contending radical feminist critique that opposes technical contraception as an encroachment of patriarchal power, via masculinist science, on women's bodies.

Radical Feminist Critiques: The Natural Body and Its Technological Adversary

The growth in possibilities promised by reproductive technologies has elicited opposition from an increasingly voluble radical feminist voice that sees all reproductive technologies, from those that limit fertility through technical contraception to those that promote fertility (through new reproductive technologies, such as in-vitro fertilization [IVF]), as necessarily harmful to women. In this view, technology is inherently masculinist, a manifestation of patriarchal power, whereby men gain control over what is distinctively feminine: women's reproductive capacities. Hence, reproductive technology can never be an instrument of women's agency by providing ways for women themselves to exercise choice. These feminist antitechnology arguments have drawn on the arguments found in other emancipatory discourses, which see technology as synonymous with control and in the service of controllers, represented, for example, in the view of the era of Taylorism[7] as "the control revolution."

The most consistent and sustained radical feminist position in regard to reproductive technology is in the substantial body of writings from feminists identified with Feminist International Network of Resistance to Reproductive and Genetic Engineering (FINRRAGE).[8] All take the view that medically and pharmaceutically based technologies of reproduction are inherently antithetical to women's interests. Their critique has linked hormonal contraceptives (e.g., the pill and Norplant implants) with technologies of assisted reproduction (like IVF and related practices, such as surrogacy and genetic screening) and, most recently, the use of the hormonal abortifacient RU486.[9]

It is true that the methods being promoted in developing countries, especially under the auspices of international organizations, such as the Population Council, IPPF and UNFPA, are those most invasive of the body. Preferred are those that give maximum control to the provider: sterilization, IUD, injectables, implants (see also Dureau and Whittaker, this volume). In Indonesia, the most popular method is the pill, but the government is promoting the IUD as the method of first choice for initial users. According to an Indonesian family planning official this is to "upgrade the quality of consumers." Farida Akhtar, one of the most vociferous and energetic promoters of the FINRRAGE position with regard to contraceptive technology, has, according to Mies and Shiva, "shown convincingly that population control programmes were devised to serve the commercial interests of the multinational pharmaceutical companies; [used as a precondition of aid and credit] . . . and that, increasingly, coercion is applied in [their] implementation" (1993, 292). The political context of population control programs in the Third World means that women are seen as a means to an end and are not given the same degree of information nor provided with the same degree of health scrutiny and maintenance as is regarded as the norm for users of technical contraceptives in Australia.[10] For the FINRRAGE critics, modern technical methods are inexorably associated with patriarchal control and cannot be utilized in a way that facilitates women's freedom of choice, because of this political context.

Maria Mies and Vandana Shiva have developed a variant of this antitechnology position in their exposition of *Ecofeminism* (1993, chap. 19). They are critical of the population control perspective that identifies the poor and their fertility as the problem for global survival and, more particularly, that it is poor women and their fertile bodies who are held responsible for the action necessary to achieve a slowing down in rates of population growth. This leads to a situation where "women of the South . . . are increasingly reduced to numbers, targets, wombs, tubes and other reproductive parts by the population controllers" (282–83). Within this debate, they do not deny that there may be valid issues about controlling fertility, but argue that current methods are inappropriate. Apart from creating problems of scarcity in the South by imperialist exploitation, removing people from access to productive resources, another effect of imperialism is "the history of colonial intervention into people's reproductive behaviour." Sometimes these are represented as diverse pronatalist policies: urged breeding in order to increase the supply of labor, hence leading to colonialist and missionary campaigns against the "methods and sexual practices which, women in particular, had used for centuries to regulate their procreative potential to maintain a balance with the ecological limits of their region that provided their livelihood" (285). This romanticized rationality is reproduced, but with a mystical edge in a speech that Shiva gave in Rio in 1992. On the one hand she uses the rationality of the "value of children" argument to reinforce her point that the conditions of British colonial exploitation had the consequence of high fertility: "It makes sense for people displaced from their life support system and livelihood system, and turned into mere labour to be sold in the market, to multiply themselves" (Shiva 1993, 4). On the other hand, however, she argues that this consciously increased fertility is coupled with a breakdown of women's knowledge, capacity and skills "to decide whether they will [get] pregnant or not, whether they will have children or not." Evidence of this

> erasure of collective memory for decisions about reproduction is probably most conspicuous in the hearts of industrial society. It is not anywhere more conspicuous than in the downtown areas of the US cities, where there is an epidemic of teenage pregnancies.... [This is] an indication of a society that has forgotten how to culturally and socially reproduce itself. (1993, 5)

Her argument, which invokes a kind of "race memory," comes close to asserting the notion of an essentially biologized humanity, as the very predicate of the concept of "natural fertility" that she and Mies so powerfully critique (Mies and Shiva 1993, 286).

It is not necessary, however, to assert a loss of ability by women to exercise control of their bodies in order to understand the reason for the secular connection between capitalist domination in the form of imperial power and increasing fertility in the Third World. Capitalism leads to changes in the material circumstances of peoples' lives (as Shiva has so powerfully demonstrated) that, for example, lead to a reorganization of labor within the household. We do not have to see missionaries as knowing agents of pronatalist policies: the moral sensibilities of Christian doctrine motivated them to exercise their civilizing mission through "detoxifying" communities of barbaric customs that may (intentionally or incidentally) have had consequences for fertility (see Dureau, this volume). This included practices such as postpartum sex taboos, facilitated by customary practices—for instance, men's houses, which in some parts of Papua New Guinea were felt necessary because of the antagonistic relation of semen and mother's milk, to protect the child. In my own research in Indonesia, late age at marriage (for men and women) was explained to me as "ensuring the seeds were mature," in order to produce healthy children (see Jolly, this volume, chap. 9).

Moreover, economic changes associated with the encroachment of capitalism can displace the social and cultural practices that have had consequential effects on fertility. For example, increased labor demands that fall on adult women can necessitate the reorganization of household labor, which mean children can no longer suckle as frequently or for as long. Breastfeeding regimes have been the most significant factor limiting fertility in many societies, but their effectiveness depends not just on biological factors, but on the social and cultural factors influencing frequency and duration (see Alexander 1986). In summary, capitalist forms of social organization and the moral regimes of missionaries can interfere with practices that supported sexual abstinence and other behavioral norms that had the effect of limiting fertility.

Indeed, modern technical contraception is only one such factor that transforms our seemingly given world of reproduction. In many instances, the use of technical contraception merely substitutes for prior practices, such as postpartum abstinence, which served as a check on fertility. So capitalism works not just by erasing traditional knowledge but also by interpellating us within new forms of production relations, which shape the social arrangements and power relations within which people act. It also throws up new imagined possibilities that ensnare our consumer selves, for example, the promise of bottle feeding allowing more modern "intimate" marriage relations or a modern sexualized femininity leading to a desire to do away with sexual abstinence, prenuptially and postpartum. Many "traditional" methods, unlike "modern" technical methods, were not entirely the responsibility of women; they also placed an obligation on men, for example, to exercise sexual restraint.

The wholesale opposition to technical methods of controlling or promoting fertility is based on an assumption that they have been developed by masculinist science and, hence, serves the ends of male power. But technological change does not work in such a simple unilinear fashion. In the case of new reproductive technologies, such as IVF, Sawicki (1991) argues for their potential to provide a basis for opposition to normative definitions of family life and sexuality that they are so often used to reinforce, for example, allowing the possibility for women to conceive outside of heterosexual relationships. In a similar way, some Third World women point to the possibility that a contraceptive method like Depo Provera can be used by women without their husbands' knowledge and consent and, hence, increase their power in controlling their own sexuality. Lynette Parker (this volume) describes the ways in which twenty years of the pill in Bali is transforming the way women experience their own sexuality.

The demonizing of technology rests on the creation of phantasmic opposition: a romanticized past in which women controlled their own fertility and reproduction. This romanticism ignores the fact that women died in childbirth and as a consequence of abortion in times past. In a telling example of this, the women of Soroako in Indonesia (who speedily availed themselves of both hospital-based birth services and modern contraception provided in the context of the development of a mine) responded to my request to think about how their lives as women had been changed by industrial development by saying "Our babies don't die anymore."[11] Population planners make much of the phenomenon of "unmet need" for contraception; demographic surveys (including the World Fertility Survey) inevitably show that women want no more children than they have or hold to ideal family sizes that are the same or less than the number of children they have. Modern contraception holds out the promise of realizing such ambitions. Its failure to do so relates to problems with methods (inevitable side effects) that make it difficult for women to wholeheartedly embrace them. For increasing numbers of women, modern contraception is part of their taken-for-granted world, but one that creates problems as well as solutions. For the radical opponents of technical contraception, there is no possibility for a feminist intervention in the international population arena, on the basis of an argument about increasing possibilities for women to make choices about their fertility. The choice for modern methods is seen as inevitably entailing a relinquishing by the woman of control of her body to patriarchal power.

Third World Women and Their Fertility

In all societies, reproduction is imbued with social significance and cultural meaning. Adult social identity (for both men and women) is inevitably tied up with issues of marriage and parenting and these interact with phases of a woman's life cycle in terms of her social experience, including her social power. There are negative outcomes for women in terms of their reproduction (e.g., poor health from repeated childbearing, increased risk of death for high-parity mothers). But mothering always has cultural and social value and can be a principal means of social identity/social status in some communities. Women may have many unmet needs in regard to reproduction, but they are as likely to be concerned with reproductive health and the health of the children they bear as they are to be with simply limiting family size. In some societies, changes associated with the modern world have eroded traditional practices that allowed birth spacing. For example, a trend to single family dwellings puts pressure on methods of child spacing that relied on abstinence, and the desire for the intimacy of the separate marriage bed erodes practices that allowed around-the-clock breastfeeding. The introduction of modern contraception must take account of this changed context.

Family planning programs have tended to operate very much in terms of a Western model of a conjugal pair whose decision making is a rational expression of self-interest. The way this model couple perceives its interests in relation to fertility, however, may not be the same as the state's. Decision making occurs in specific economic circumstances and in particular social and cultural contexts.

Women do not live as social isolates; they belong to families, kin groups, status groups, classes, villages, nations, all of which encompass power relations that may impact on fertility (directly or indirectly). Women in societies with patrilineal kinship, who live in their husbands' households, will be very differently empowered in their domestic relations than women in matrilineal and uxorilocal societies, where they reside with their own families. Women may experience pressure from other women or from men other than their husbands to have more children.

Second-Wave Feminism, Fertility, and Female Autonomy

There have been other feminist voices that have emphasized and celebrated the possibilities of women gaining control of the means of reproduction through technology and have seen nature itself as the oppressor. Firestone (1971), as the most radical of these voices, provided a vision of a world in which artificial wombs could free women from the constraints imposed by their biological nature. In a less apocalyptic vision, O'Brien saw the "rational control of reproduction" as a cornerstone of the feminist emancipatory project, but was more sanguine than Firestone about the limitations of the current state of technical knowledge (1981, 205). These debates reflect a particular view of the relationship between fertility, femininity, and freedom that is presumed to be universal. This approach was exemplified in the BBC documentary discussed at the start (ABC 1992). This celebrated the contraceptive pill and eulogized this technological advance as the cornerstone of the liberation of women in the late twentieth century—a telling reversal of technophobic forms of liberationist discourse.

It documents the development of the pill by two American doctors, its early trial on women in Puerto Rico (because they were not permitted to have large-scale trials on American women) and the jubilation that a solution to the "population problem" had been found. It asserts that an unanticipated consequence of the new technology was the manner in which it was embraced by women in the industrial countries, as a way of controlling their fertility to allow liberation of their sexuality. In the documentary, a number of British women who used the pill in those early days describe its effects on their lives. In an excerpt from a 1965 BBC *Panorama* program, a woman responds to the question of the difference it has made to her marriage: "To me it's complete freedom. You've never got to worry to plan." Another comments: "I don't think I really enjoyed sex in the modern sense until well after my children were born" (linking her ability to explore her sensuality to the pill). A third woman reflects on her life as a single girl in the 1960s: "I did enjoy sex. I thought sex was quite wonderful. And it [the pill] allowed me to indulge myself. . . . The pill really enabled me to live my life as I wanted." She talks of her constant fear of getting pregnant, a motif that comes up in many of the interviews: fertility as an enemy of well-being, as life threatening (as in the case of the woman who feared she could be like her grandmother, who had eight children and died at forty), or fertility as a barrier to living the way you wanted to, which included freedom of sexual expression.

One of the women eulogized the technology of the pill and its transformatory effect on their lives:

> It fitted in so well with the era: we had miniskirts, we had moon landings, everything was an atmosphere of freedom, so the pill really did fit in absolutely marvellously with that. Because the technology of it, the pristine cleanliness of it—you just popped it out of the packet and popped it in your mouth and then you went out boogying all night. It really did give the impression of being totally an instrument of its age. (ABC 1992)

In this epoch, before the threat of HIV/AIDS, the assumption was that one could only achieve personal liberation through unrestricted sexual expression. Fertility and freedom were seen as being at odds: for these women fertility is an enemy, an aspect of their natural female body that needs to be held in check in order to achieve the realization of true selfhood. This view foreshadows the feminist position (e.g., Raymond 1994) in which it is argued that motherhood has been constituted as a "patriarchal institution":

> The mind-body split makes the mother into an inhuman monster by dividing the human realm of culture, politics and history from the realm of love and the body where mother carries, bears and tends her children. (Gallop 1988, 2)

This eulogizing of the revolutionary effects of the pill not only occludes some of the more negative effects, but shares the medical view of the body as irreducibly material or a machine whose systemic properties can be regulated by the pill.

Modern hormone-based "noncoital" contraceptive technology is seen by policy makers as the most desirable, because it is the most efficacious (see Rosenfield 1989). The pill is "probably the most widely used systemic medication in modern history" (388). These drugs are often felt by users to be intrusive, because of side effects that are often dismissed by service providers, and even medical researchers. Side effects that may not be defined medically as harmful are still negatively experienced by women (see Whittaker, this volume). This may be due to their perceived physical experience, shaped by inscribed notions of femininity. For example, the problems of the "menstrual chaos" associated with the injectable contraceptive Depo Provera is especially troubling in cultures where there are intimate, even sacral, associations of femininity and menstruation. Women's bodies are already sites for the inscription of femininity in terms of expectations about dress, posture, demeanor. The use of modern contraception inscribes bodies in a different way, locating them within different sets of power relations, which may intersect with the old. For example, men may be reluctant for women to use IUDs because of concerns about female modesty, as women are exposed to and touched by medical personnel during insertion. In my own research in Sulawesi, Indonesia, however, I found that women may be more pragmatic about such "compromises" of their modesty.

The War on Women? Indian Women—Fertility, Sexuality, and Population Control

The expressed attitudes of the British women in *The Pill* (ABC 1992) are in contrast to those of a group of Indian women who speak in a documentary about the Indian family planning program. The documentary, entitled *Something like a War* (SBS 1993), was made by Indian feminist critics of the national program. In this instance, the war is not between the women and their own bodies, but between women and the state. The title is taken from a comment, in 1976, by an Indian family planning official: "If some excesses appear, don't blame me. You must consider it something like a war. There has been pressure to show results. Whether you like it or not there will be a few dead people." The pressure he feels, the national climate within which he is acting, can be understood perhaps through a comment from Indira Gandhi in 1970: "We must act decisively to bring down the birthrate speedily. We should not hesitate to take steps which might be described as drastic. Some personal rights have to be kept in abeyance for the human rights of the nation" (SBS 1993).

This film documents a population control program in abundant excess: it moves between scenes of a small group of women discussing themselves, their lives and their bodies, and horrendous scenes of mass sterilization camps held in school halls. The obstetrician who sees himself as performing a service to the state bemoans the fact that he is limited by government regulation to a hundred procedures a day. "I question that . . . any industrialist—is he told how much business he can do? So when an experienced person is ready to do some more work for his country, his hands are tied" (SBS 1993). In the film, the images are of women being herded in like animals to an abattoir, sterilized and laid down to recover on the hallway outside the operating room, where several

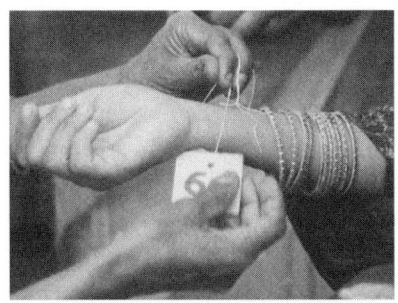
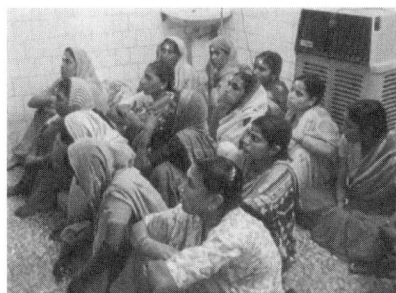
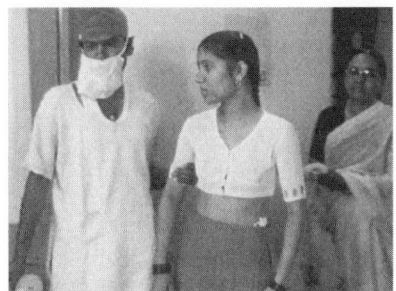
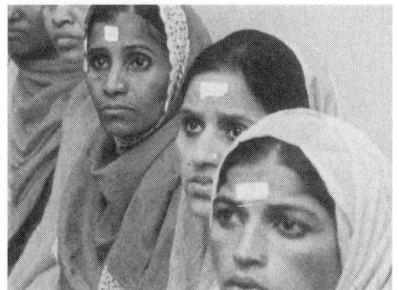
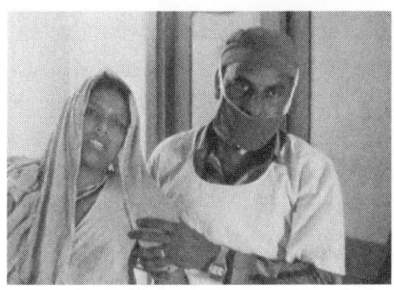

Fig 3. Several stills from the documentary film *Something like a War*, showing Indian women being tagged before tubal ligation surgery, being escorted by doctors from the operating table, and recovering on the floor after surgery

procedures are being conducted simultaneously. The women appear passive, frightened, and the motivation is often not merely a concern to regulate their fertility but a response to money and other material incentives offered by the state officials or indeed to coercion. A bewildering array of government departments compete for "targets," the very term indicating the denial of agency to the women who are sterilized. The film also documents the frustration of regional officials whose salaries are dependent on their achieving targets and the villagers complaining about the consequent bribery and deception by which they are induced to become sterilized.

While medical researchers and family planning officials talk of improving women's choices by increasing available methods (with hormonal implants, vaccinations, IUDs), the filmmakers interview women who complain of a failure of procedures of informed consent for clinical trials of new methods, and of family planning workers who are deaf to their complaints of side effects. The women who speak express an awareness of the political basis of the government programs. One of them comments:

> I keep asking myself what the government is up to when it tells us . . . get operated . . . get injected . . . insert this! What is behind the government's interest in this? We have no land and they are not going to even things up to allow us any. In these conditions our poverty is not about to disappear. They're killing the poor, not poverty. (SBS 1993)

In contrast to the construction of women's fertility in the official discourse, as the enemy of the nation, the women in the discussion group present their fertility in more complex social and cultural terms. For them, fertility is understood within kin-based power relations, such as pressure to have male children from in-laws and husbands; the value of child labor; the reality of infant death for the poor; but also as a fundamental aspect of their feminized being. For these women, their fertility is not the enemy of their selves, of their sexuality (as it is for the English women in *The Pill*), but rather an integrated part of it. Sexuality and fertility are expressed as part of their everyday being. One of the women comments:

> When I start to ovulate I feel sort of . . . I feel happy. I feel a change in my whole body and in my mind. . . . Yes, I like it a lot, I mean during that period the pleasure of experiencing my sexuality is more intense. I like my womb, it pleases me. It is thanks to this womb that I have born children.

A childless woman comments:

I enjoy having sex. I feel happy when I get my periods. I suppose my hopes are reactivated when I get my period. That's the shape of my womb (drawing it on a chart). That's where I feel pleasure. Still, I must admit that being childless I have a complaint against my womb. (SBS 1993)

For these women, their fertility is experienced integrally related to their sexuality and as intimately connected to the social and economic circumstances of their everyday lives. The rationalizing message of the government family planning propaganda "We are two, we have two" cuts across their more complex engagement with motherhood and femininity. As one of them comments: "The government does not see us. We do not exist for them."

International Conference on Population and Development—Cairo

The 1994 International Conference on Population and Development in Cairo was marked by the success of women activists and policy makers in getting the issue of women's reproductive rights and reproductive health on the international population agenda. The document approved by the conference stresses the importance of improving women's social participation, in particular through improved access to education as part of a strategy for reducing fertility. The efforts of women's groups who saw the conference as an opportunity to press feminist agendas were challenged, however, by the antitechnology radical feminists, who deny that the context of international population assistance can ever promote women's interests.[12] Feminists in both these camps were engaged in meetings and lobbying to put their case in the period leading up to the conference. The United States' delegation (which included Jane Fonda) brought liberal feminist concerns, of women's reproductive rights, to the international forum, and also was critical in getting the issue of rights to abortion (on which there was unsurprisingly no consensus) on the agenda.

The Cairo conference reflected the growing concern with ethical issues in population programs (see, e.g., Bankowski, Barzelatto, and Capron 1989) and in particular the often fine line between incentives and coercion. The final document, however, endorses the linking of population to issues of sustainable development, a resurgence of neo-Malthusianism in a new guise. While this paradigm underlies population policy, there is always the danger of women being subsumed as targets for initiatives justified as "in the common good." There are also echoes of the "status of women in family planning" approach: the necessity of attending to equity issues for women in order to achieve population goals. The resolutions, many of which were hotly contended, still need to be ratified by member governments in order for them to be put into practice. It will be interesting to see if the conference does usher in a new era of "family planning" for women, in which there *is* a greater choice of methods, a greater focus on women's reproductive health, and population targets are relegated to the background. Also of significance, the Cairo resolution is the acknowledgment of the importance of rights to contraception for the unmarried and for youth, freeing the issue of rights to contraception from marital status (see also Whittaker, this volume; and Jolly, this volume, chap. 9).

Conclusion

The idea of "overpopulation" is a manifestation of what Said (1978) has called the "imaginative geography" through which we know the world. There are too many of "them," which threatens the well-being of "us." This fiction allows an obfuscation of the lived experience of the poor of the world, where "we" are, to a great extent, the source of "their problems" (see also Escobar 1995, 210–11). This discourse imposes itself on international population policy, which provides the political order within which poor women gain access to modern contraception. Women experience powerlessness, which all too often prevents them from acting on their own desires in relation to their fertility. Those desires are not a timeless aspect of tradition, however, but are transformed through their insertion into the regimes of power of the contemporary world. Modern contraception involves overwhelmingly female methods—it implies a definition, and often a redefinition, of female sexuality as ever-ready to suit male needs. Modern methods displace older methods that, in many cases, placed responsibility on the man, for example by requiring him to be abstinent or practice noncoital sex. In the village of Soroako in Indonesia men whose wives had too many children or children too close together were scorned as lacking control and lacking in love for their wives (see Robinson 1989). Contraceptives accessed through state-controlled programs allow the operation of state power through women's bodies, a vehicle for inscription in terms of new forms of power that relate to international/global relations rather than the kin- and community-based power relations that were previously so significant in ordering women's lives.

There have been many feminist voices that claim to speak for all women and their reproductive rights, some of which reinforce the prevailing wisdom of these women and their bodies as the problem and others that deny that the population establishment has anything to offer them. We cannot assume that the position of First World women, with their different situation of power and their different "framework," can be automatically mapped onto the lives of Third World women. While the goals of population policies and programs are defined in terms of targets for reducing fertility rather than as vehicles for the goal of improving women's reproductive health, and facilitating expanded choice in the area of reproductive decision making, women will always be part of the problem to be solved. In order to achieve societal goals without compromising women's agency, they need to be subjects at the center of the process.

NOTES

1. For an account of "women's liberation," or early second-wave feminism, see Mitchell 1971.
2. China and Indonesia are notable exceptions to this.
3. There is a long tradition of Marxist and crypto-Marxist critiques of the manner in which "development" ultimately serves the economic and political interests of the industrial nations (see, for example, Larain 1989). Escobar (1995) extends this critique through a Foucauldian analysis of the "colonization of reality" through development discourse, allowing the exercise of power over the Third World.
4. The ten major donors are the United States, Germany, Japan, Norway, the United Kingdom, Sweden, the Netherlands, Canada, Finland, and Denmark (Conly and Speidel 1993, 10).
5. This was the issue canvassed by an Australian government inquiry in 1993, precipitated by the intervention of independent Senator Brian Harradine. The findings of the "expert enquiry" were equivocal, arguing for population control as an important part of the "package" of development assistance, although not sufficient in itself.
6. See Warwick 1986, for an overview of the Indonesian family planning program.
7. *Taylorism* is the term given to a form of scientific management named for F. W. Taylor, whose goal was to transform the administration of the workplace so as to increase profitability.
8. For example, Arditti, Duelli Klein, and Minden 1984; Raymond 1994.
9. Women identified with FINRRAGE were at the forefront of opposition to trials of RU486 in Australia.
10. It is interesting that as women in Australia refuse to use IUD (because of negative publicity) Third World women are denied adequate information on side effects. If one were very cynical, one could imagine that the insertion of am IUD under less than ideal conditions is likely to produce secondary infertility as a consequence of infection, because it has been found in Australia that there is a direct relation between the skill and experience of the inserter and the likelihood of side effects.
11. For an account of my research on the Soroako Nickel Project, see Robinson 1986.
12. See the journal *People's Perspectives,* published by UBINIG in Bangladesh. Issues in 1993 and 1994 carried ongoing critiques of the ICPD as well as of the feminist organizations engaged with the preparation process in the hope of influencing the agenda.

REFERENCES

ABC Television. 1992. *The pill: Prescription for a revolution.* BBC production; screened ABC [Australian Broadcasting Corporation] TV series *True stories.*

Alexander, P. 1986. Labor expropriation and fertility: Population growth in nineteenth century Java. In *Culture and reproduction: An anthropological critique of demographic transition theory,* ed. W. P. Handwerker, 249–62. Boulder and London: Westview Press.

Arditti, R., R. Duelli Klein, and S. Minden, eds. 1984. *Test-tube women: What future for motherhood?* London: Pandora Press.

Bankowski, Z., J. Barzelatto, and A. M. Capron, eds. 1989. *Ethics and human values in family planning.* Papers from the 22nd CIOMS Conference, Bangkok, Thailand, 19–24 June 1988. Geneva: Council for International Organizations of Medical Sciences.

Boserup, E. 1970. *Woman's role in economic development.* New York: St. Martin's Press.

Brown, R. E. 1982. Public health in imperialism: Early Rockefeller programs at home and abroad (adapted from the article in *American Journal of Public Health* 66(9), 1976). *Southeast Asia Chronicle* 84:2–4.

Caldwell, J. C. 1982. The failure of theories of social and economic change to explain demographic change: Puzzles of modernization or Westernization. *Research in Population Economics* 4:297–332.

Conly, S. R., and J. J. Speidel. 1993. *Global population assistance: A report card on the major donor countries.* Washington: Population Action International.

Escobar, A. 1995. *Encountering development: The making and unmaking of the Third World.* Princeton, N.J.: Princeton University Press.

Firestone, S. 1971. *The dialectic of sex: The case for feminist revolution.* London: Paladin.

Gallop, J. 1988. *Thinking through the body.* New York: Columbia University Press.

Golley, L. 1982. Health policy in ASEAN: Addressing human needs or protecting the status-quo? *Southeast Asia Chronicle* 84:7–19.

Greenhalgh, S. 1990. Towards a political economy of fertility: Anthropological contributions. *Population and Development Review* 16(1):85–106.

Harvey, D. 1974. Ideology and population theory. *International Journal of Health Services* 4(3):515–37.

Larain, J. 1989. *Theories of development: Capitalism, colonialism and dependency.* Cambridge: Polity Press.

Mason, K. O. 1985. The status of women: A review of its relationships to fertility and mortality. Paper prepared for the Population Sciences Division, The Rockefeller Foundation.

Mies, M., and V. Shiva. 1993. *Ecofeminism.* Melbourne: Spinifex.

Mitchell, J. 1971. *Woman's estate.* Harmondsworth: Penguin Books.

O'Brien, M. 1981. *The politics of reproduction.* Boston: Routledge and Kegan Paul.

Population Reports. 1992. *The reproductive revolution: New survey findings.* Series M, no. 11, December. Baltimore: Population Information Program, Johns Hopkins University.

Quinn, N. 1977. Anthropological studies of women's status. *Annual Review of Anthropology* 6:181–225.

Raymond, J. 1994. *Women as wombs: Reproductive technologies and the battle over women's freedom.* Melbourne: Spinifex.

Robinson, K. 1986. *Stepchildren of progress: The political economy of development in an Indonesian mining town.* Albany, N.Y.: SUNY Press.

———. 1989. Choosing contraception: Cultural change and the Indonesian family planning programme. In *Creating Indonesian cultures,* ed. P. Alexander, 21–38. Sydney: Oceania Publications.

Rosenfield, A. 1989. Modern contraception: A 1989 update. *Annual Review of Public Health* 10:385–401.

Safilios-Rothschild, C. 1985. The status of women and fertility in the 1970–1980 decade. Working Papers, no. 118. New York: Center for Policy Studies, The Population Council.

Said, E. W. 1978. *Orientalism.* London: Routledge and Kegan Paul.

Sawicki, J. 1991. *Disciplining Foucault: Feminism, power and the body.* New York: Routledge.

SBS Television. 1993. *Something like a war.* D&N Productions (India) in association with Equal Media (London) for Channel 4; screened Australian SBS [Special Broadcasting Service] TV series *The cutting edge,* 15 June.

Shiva, V. 1993. Population and the question of carrying capacity. *People's Perspectives* 4–5:2–6.

Ward, K. B. 1985. The social consequences of the world economic system: The economic status of women and fertility. *Review* 8(4):561–93.

Warwick, D. P. 1986. The Indonesian family planning program: Government influence and client choice. *Population and Development Review* 12(3):453–90.

CHAPTER 2

Her Body and Her Being: Of Widows and Abducted Women in Post-Partition India

Ritu Menon and Kamla Bhasin

This chapter is set against the background of the partition of India in 1947, the creation of Pakistan, and the ensuing turmoil as both countries struggled to cope with the aftermath of division. As an event of shattering consequence, Partition retains its preeminence even today, despite three wars on India's borders and wave after wave of communal violence. It marks a watershed as much in people's consciousness as in the lives of those who were uprooted and had to find themselves again, elsewhere. Chronologies are still qualified with "before Partition" or "after Partition," personal histories are punctuated with references to it, so much so that it sometimes seems as if two quite distinct, rather than concurrent, events took place at independence, and that Partition and its effects are what have lingered in collective memory. Each new eruption of hostility or expression of difference swiftly recalls that bitter and divisive erosion of social relations between Hindus, Muslims, and Sikhs, and each episode of brutality is measured against what was experienced then. The rending of the social, political, and emotional fabric that took place in 1947 is still far from mended.

There is no dearth of written material on the partition of India: official records, documents, private papers, agreements and treaties, political histories, analyses, a few reminiscences. A vast amount of newspaper reportage and reams of government information exist on the resettlement and rehabilitation of refugees from Punjab and Bengal; on negotiations between India and Pakistan on the transfer of power and division of assets; and there are hundreds of pages of parliamentary debates on the myriad issues confronting both countries and both governments. Nationalist historiography has generally seen Partition as the unfortunate outcome of sectarian and separatist politics, and as a tragic accompaniment to the exhilaration and promise of a freedom fought for with courage and valor. Historical analyses over the last three or four decades, however, have uncovered the processes and strategies that led to the successful manipulation of Muslim perception in favor of a separate homeland, based on ineluctable differences between Hindus and Muslims.

We began our project as an oral history of how women experienced Partition.[1] To the best of our knowledge there has been no feminist historiography of the partition of India, not even of the compensatory variety. Women historians have written on this cataclysmic event but from within the parameters of the discipline and still well within the political frame. Consequently, the importance of such a historic moment has been evaluated not with specific reference to them, but with reference to the movement in question. Yet the story of 1947, while being one of the successful attainment of independence, is also a gendered narrative of displacement and dispossession, of large-scale and widespread communal violence, and of the realignment of family, community and national identities as people were forced to accommodate the dramatically altered reality that now prevailed.

Partition fiction has been a far richer source both because it provides popular and astringent commentary on the politics of Partition and because, here and there, we find women's voices speaking for themselves. But the most useful material for our purpose has been the very few first-hand accounts and memoirs by women social workers who were involved in the rehabilitation of women, and the oral testimonies we set out to obtain from them and other women in ashrams and refuges in Punjab and Haryana, the field of this research.

Forty years after Partition, there were no "communities" of women we could identify whom we might find, waiting to be found. Families had dispersed, resettled, moved many times over and, initially at least, we were not looking for women in families. We were looking for those who had been left quite alone. People we spoke to said, "Partition? What do you want to talk about that for? Anyway, it's too late—they're all dead." This was true; many were undoubtedly dead, but we persisted. "Speak to so-and-so," people said, "she'll know." Sometimes she did, sometimes she did not and sometimes she would say, "I'm not the person you want, but ask—." Eventually we found that there did exist communities of sorts, of women in ashrams or homes, set up where the first of the refugee camps had been established in erstwhile East Punjab.

But this was not enough. We needed to know what the women could not tell us, the how and why of the ashrams and of rehabilitation, of what happened to the widowed women, to those whose husbands were missing, whose families could not be traced. "Speak to—" the women told us, "she was the warden there for twenty years." We traveled to different cities to meet them; we lived with them; we went back to them, sometimes once or twice, sometimes more often. We spoke mainly to women, but also to men, to Hindus, Muslims, and

Sikhs. We talked to senior government and police officers, politicians, doctors, and social workers.

We went back to the records to find what we could of the women's stories there, as disaggregated data, memoranda, reports, official statements, government documents. We did this not because we wanted to corroborate what they said, but because it was important to locate their stories in a political and social context, to juxtapose the official version with the unofficial ones.

In this chapter we propose to examine the response of the Indian state and government[2] to this altered reality: we examine the contrastive policies toward two groups of women for whom it assumed responsibility in the wake of Partition. The first are the women who were dislocated, destituted, widowed—these were collectively described in policy terms as "unattached." The second group were those who had been separated from their families, picked up while fleeing to safety, taken hostage or kidnaped—these women were called "abducted." Both groups of women were obvious subjects for government intervention and beneficiaries of rehabilitation programs, but their significance transcends this simple humanitarian concern: in a crucial way their very condition, which became their identity—abducted or unattached, in turn became the touchstone by which the government formulated and implemented policies with regard to their "recovery" and "resettlement." For both groups, the common factor now was the rupture of normal familial arrangements and the absence of male kin, necessitating the state's stepping in as the surrogate paterfamilias and inheriting the mantle of protector. As protector, one of the state's principal concerns was with the sexuality of the women. This concern was quite explicitly manifested in the case of abducted women, whose sexuality was perceived as available for exploitation by any transgressor, and had to be zealously guarded. The concern was implicit in the case of widows (the majority of "unattached" women) who were now assumed to be sexually inactive, but in need of rehabilitation—social and economic, for they were now without families or menfolk who would vouch for them. As abducted women, they were sexual property but also upholders of honor, symbols of sacred motherhood, definers of community and national identity. As widows, they had to be liberated from the traditional stigma of widowhood and its consequent social death and activated as economic beings, part of the mainstream of national life.

Through its policies and programs for both categories of women the government not only undertook its first major welfare and legislative responsibility as an independent state; it revealed the complexity of its relationship to gender and community, and secularism and democracy. In those early post-Partition years when the Indian state was defining its own political character and priorities, drawing up an egalitarian constitution and safeguarding pluralism through a modified secularism, the intersection of gender, community, and state acquired particular importance for women. It highlighted the critical role played by the state in mediating gender and community rights in moments of political crisis as well as the differential approximations to citizenship of its male and female members. It exposed the tremendous internal dissonances in terms of how women were categorized and dealt with. Finally, it demonstrated the state's ambivalence regarding its own identity as secular and democratic. Even if it had been zealous in pursuit of such goals, it was very nearly impossible for it to be free of patriarchal, communal, and cultural biases.

The Widows

> With tears in her eyes, a few days ago, a refugee woman went to see Pandit Nehru at his residence. Before India's partition, she belonged to a prosperous family in Pakistan, but now she was homeless, with no money to buy food and no relations to comfort her in her distress: her only hope was her country's Prime Minister.
>
> "I want a job," she pleaded with Panditji. The Prime Minister recommended to the Women's Section of the Ministry of Relief and Rehabilitation that she should be given a sewing machine. In addition, he paid her a sum of Rs. 20.
>
> Almost every day Pandit Nehru receives such appeals and there are hundreds of women in free India with the same tearful demand.
>
> The Women's Section has opened destitute homes and relief centres for such women, but then there are other problems worse than "unemployment." To find solutions for some of them would be a difficult task.
>
> "What shall I do about utensils?" asked a destitute refugee woman who came to the Women's Section the other day. Her son had been shot, her husband murdered and daughter abducted. She did not know where to turn for support. The Officer-in-Charge of the Homes for Destitute Women and Children offered to help her.
>
> "You will have a place to live where you will be provided with utensils and you can cook your meals," said the officer.
>
> "But how shall I cook my meals with these hands," the woman replied, weeping, showing her right hand which had been chopped into half during disturbances. The woman is now at one of the Homes for Disabled Persons started by the Women's Section. (*Hitavada* 1948)[3]

In 1988, forty years after the partition of India, we found eleven widows still living in the Mahila Ashram in Karnal. They had a room each to live and cook in, received subsidized rations and a stipend of a hundred rupees a month. If they wished, they could continue to do the occasional bit of embroidery or tailoring for the ashram and get paid for their labor; if not, they were not obliged to work in order to avail of the ashram's facilities—as Partition widows, they had a right to stay there for the rest of their lives.

The dislocation of roughly twelve million people that took place in 1947–48, as a result of the massive exchange of populations in the border states of India and Pakistan, also made for a phenomenon without precedent: mass widowhood. As families got separated in the upheaval, and the foot caravans, trains, and road convoys were ambushed and men slaughtered, by all communities, thousands of women were destituted and widowed. Many did get reunited with their families eventually and were claimed by their next-of-kin from camps and homes, but several thousands lived and worked for years in ashrams and rehabilitation centers, where they brought up their children and strove to attain some kind of social and economic equilibrium.

The scale and incidence of this widowhood was so immense—as was the related task of resettling and rehabilitating refugees—that it resulted in the Indian government setting up what was to be almost its first major welfare activity as an independent state: the rehabilitation of what it called "unattached" women. Never before in the country's experience had a *sarkar* (ruler, "government"), either feudal or colonial, been called upon to take social and economic responsibility for a circumstance as problematic as widowhood: a condition ritually inauspicious, socially stigmatized, traditionally shunned. It is true that throughout the nineteenth century the colonial state had been compelled, by social reformers, to address the issue of widow remarriage and child widows, and so intervene in social and cultural practice, but that exercise was qualitatively different from what the Indian state was now called upon to do. Rather than reform them to the community or family to deal with as they thought appropriate, the government now assumed direct responsibility for what it conceded were victims of a national disaster. They were deserving of government intervention much as flood or war or famine victims would be.

In a note dated December 1949, Rameshwari Nehru stated that the number of "unattached" women looked after by the government in October 1948 was 45,374 (Nehru n.d.). Although not all of these women were widows, a very large percentage were; indeed, it was the very size of this category that persuaded the government to set up a special section within the Ministry of Relief and Rehabilitation to administer to their needs. Rameshwari Nehru, who had been looking after the evacuation of women and children from West Punjab during the worst disturbances, took over as honorary director of the Women's Section in November 1947, responsible for the "care, maintenance, and rehabilitation of uprooted women and children from Pakistan."

In a sense, the Women's Section of 1947 can be seen as a forerunner of the many government agencies that now exist for the welfare of women and children, for the disabled, for disaster victims, and for the destitute. But it had an added, and important, dimension as part of the government's program of resettlement. Apart from being an immediate and urgent necessity in the aftermath of Partition, this rehabilitation was a crucial aspect of the state's *perception* of itself as benign and paternalistic, and in its *definition* of itself as socialist, democratic, welfarist—and secular. Stephen Keller, who did extensive fieldwork among Punjab's refugees in the seventies, has observed that "in Punjab and other areas of north India government has always been characterized as *ma-baap* (mother-father). As [such] it is duty bound to provide a rich, warm, nurturant relationship (the *ma* part) as well as paternal protection from the dangers of life (the *baap* part)" (1975, 47). In times of national disaster, particularly, the more maternal aspect is emphasized.[4] It was obviously such an event that galvanized it into responding. But having said that, it is worth examining both the conceptual dimension of the project of rehabilitating widows and its implementation, to arrive at some understanding of how, through government intervention, their status underwent some change.

The critical shift that took place was that the widows of 1947 became the responsibility of the state. In acknowledging this, and by stepping in to mediate their reabsorption into the social and economic life of the country, it had, simultaneously, to perform two functions: that of custodian and guardian—*parens patriae*—in the absence of actual kinsmen; and of an apparently benign, neutral, and secular agency that could not be seen to be subscribing to or reinforcing traditional biases against widowhood. The tensions between the two functions of the state resulted in a historically unusual, if not unprecedented, situation where widows were in a direct relationship with state authority. However distant that authority may have seemed in relation to the women, it was nevertheless a decisive one.

Since the widows of 1947 were, ironically, widowed by history—or, as the government put it, "victims of a struggle that might well be regarded as a war"—it was proposed by the government that they be classed as war widows and treated as such. This particular definition of widows, and of the circumstances of Partition, enabled the government to deal with the crisis as a national emergency and, more important, to look upon the widows not as *individual women* inviting social ostracism, but as a *community* of hapless survivors to be accorded the same status as other refugees.

Important distinctions were made, however, within this newly formed community of survivors. In addition to being classified as "war widows" they were further classified as (1) those whose husbands and sons and other breadwinners were killed during the riots, and (2) those who—though "unattached"—had relatives alive who, having lost their jobs and possessions, were unable to maintain them. These two categories were to be treated differently: the responsibility for the first had to be shouldered by the government *for the rest of their lives,* while that for the second could extend either until the time they became self-supporting or till their relatives were able to maintain them. Further, those in the first category who were not willing to lead the regulated (read: restricted) life of the homes should be given allowances *sufficient to maintain themselves* because, it was thought, there would be very few of them. In a report on the work done by the Women's Section from 1947 to 1949, Rameshwari Nehru noted:

> At the very outset the Section realized that rehabilitation is an intricate process and can be achieved only if adequate attention is paid to the psychological, educational and emotional needs of the women. It is of utmost importance to make them self-reliant and self-supporting and restore their sense of dignity and worth. (Nehru n.d.)

The best way to do this, in the view of the Women's Section, was to treat them to a course of occupational therapy, to pay attention not only to their physical needs but to "their intellectual and vocational development."

Without wishing to belabor the point or to put too fine a construction on stated intent, we would like to put forward the view that it was such an approach that in fact enabled a large number of widows to be drawn into some form of economically productive activity. Despite the many shortcomings in the actual workings of the rehabilitation program, which became especially evident after the mid-1950s, the formal recognition of the fact that "the care and maintenance of destitute women *is a task in social reconstruction*" indicates another critical shift in perception, namely, that the rehabilitation of widows was as much an economic as it was a social or "welfare" activity.

The first endeavor of the Women's Section was to free the widows from economic dependence. It was hoped that, in the long term, specially planned women's settlements would develop, embracing not only the refugees of Partition but other categories of destituted women as well. State and central governments were therefore requested to make available suitable land, open and extensive, near the large cities, for this "new experiment": it was a matter of some conviction that, with proper facilities, the women could be prepared for dairy farming and agriculture and for those "advanced industries which require meticulous training and skill in execution." Underlying this conviction, or experiment, was the hope that they would be absorbed into the economic reconstruction of the country. Renuka Ray, member from West Bengal, made the point in the Legislative Assembly thus:

> I want to note some specific points with regard to the rehabilitation of women. I do not think that the establishment of homes where some little occupation is given . . . is enough. In this country there is a very great dearth of women who come forward to be trained in different fields of nation-building. . . . This great tragedy has left thousands of women homeless and alone. . . . The opportunity should be taken to train [them] to become useful and purposeful citizens. Tinkering with the problem by doing a little here and there will not be sufficient. What is required is a properly planned scheme of vocational training on a long-term basis. (Constituent Assembly of India 1948)

Women with some educational qualifications were offered training in "useful professions," like nursing, midwifery, teaching, stenography, accounts, and office management. Those with very little or no literacy could take up the usual embroidery, tailoring, or minor handicrafts, although it was well understood that the scope for economic independence through such skills was quite limited: the market was already glutted with fancy leather work and luxury articles. This excess of produce opened the way to exploitation of women's labor, and they were paid ridiculously low wages for their work. But the women's own inclination had also to be considered and, as the report notes, "despite our best efforts, it was not possible to enlist women's interest in any other work" (Nehru n.d.).

Women who were able-bodied and able to do some physical labor were to be settled in what were called "agro-industrial" settlements. It was proposed that they be built up on a few acres of land outside towns and cities and women be trained in such activities as vegetable and dairy farming and oil pressing. A beginning was made by giving sixty acres of land near Kilokheri to the Kasturba Seva Mandir. In all the work of training and vocationalizing, the Women's Section worked with a range of training centers, academic institutions, voluntary and social work organizations including the Tata Institute of Social Sciences, the vocational training centers of the Ministry of Labour in Bombay and Delhi, the Kasturba Gandhi Memorial Trust, and Lady Hardinge Medical College in Delhi. An employment bureau was set up, in cooperation with the Employment Exchange of the Labour Ministry, for placing women once they were trained. In March 1949 the report noted that five hundred women had secured employment through the employment bureau.

From an age-based classification of four hundred widows in the Gandhi Vanitha Ashram in Jallandhar we learn that the oldest was seventy and the youngest fifteen years old. By far the greatest number were in their twenties, thirties, and forties, many with very young children. Since there is no disaggregated data on the widows available (and most of the records of the homes and ashrams in East Punjab are now untraceable), we have had to rely on verbal accounts and some official documents to get a general impression of their background. Important class differences were apparent. Most of the women in homes and ashrams came from urban areas, from petty trade or very small landholding families. By and large, those from rural backgrounds resettled with some male members of their family in India when their land compensation claims came through. Of those who initially came to homes and ashrams from the camps, many were reclaimed by their relatives within a couple of years—between October 1947 and December 1948 the number dropped from approximately seventy-three thousand to forty-five thousand. Again, not all may have been widows, but a great many were. Here is a story of a young widow, with three daughters, we call by the pseudonym Maya Devi:

> I was twenty or twenty-one years old when my husband died. I came to Delhi by train—my own family and my in-laws were still in the camps. My father brought me here. I lived in Western Court for a year. We were two to a room, which was free, and the government gave us a stipend of Rs. 45 a month. There were about 250 of us learning typing, pickle-making, basketry, tailoring—all kinds of skills were taught. We were all refugees; they didn't accept anyone else.

Maya Devi worked in the Karnal ashram till she retired from service in the early 1980s. She may not have been the typical rehabilitated Partition widow—or again, she may have. It is not easy to know. In the course of her working life, she married off her two sisters-in-law, and got her share of 12.5 acres of land when their claims were finally settled about six years after Partition. But, according to her, the land never fetched her much of an income: Rs. 300 a month sometimes, at other times less. She educated her daughters, built her own house where she now lives and, according to her, never thought of remarrying. We asked her what course her life would have taken had she not been widowed, remained with her husband, perhaps had more children; after a long while she replied, "I think that life would have been more difficult." Her greatest satisfaction, she says, lies in the fact that "*maine kisi ke age haath nahin phailay*" (I asked no one for charity)—not even her own family.

It would be incorrect to hold (perhaps even to expect) that the rehabilitation program of the government of India in fact accomplished all it set out to, either in spirit or in letter. In our interviews with women still resident in ashrams in Karnal and Jallandhar there was enough disquiet to suggest that, over the years, bureaucracy and budget cuts—and an absence of urgency on the part of new social workers—vitiated much of the spirit that characterized the period immediately following Partition.[5] But there was also enough remembrance of things past for them to underline the difference between women like Premwati Thapar, Kamla Mehra, Krishna Thapar, and others and those who followed.

Financial allocations apart, the entire responsibility for implementing the rehabilitation of destituted women was in the hands of women who were not cast in the mold of government employees;[6] rather, they were themselves either personally (many had been similarly widowed themselves), politically or vocationally impelled into a kind of social work that they recognized as being difficult and demanding, and complicated by extraordinary factors. This called for grit and dedication, of course, but it also required an ability to innovate, to be flexible, to use every opportunity to advantage, and to overturn precedent if necessary. It is entirely likely that in the bargain they simultaneously reinforced certain social biases regarding widowhood, remarriage, even women's subordinate status. We have argued that this has to be seen as a two-way process: of attempting to free women from their disability and destitution through economic sufficiency and imbuing them with a sense of worth; and restoring them to social "acceptability" through a reiteration of restrictions on sexuality (permissible only through remarriage if the woman was still in the ashram's charge), interaction with other males, socialization of children, and mobility (see Menon and Bhasin 1998a, 169ff.). Yet, even here, as we were told by many social workers, flexibility was preferred. "Of course we realized that they had their 'needs' and there were those who struck up friendships with men they met outside the ashram. To them we used to say: 'Stay outside the ashram if you insist on continuing your relationship. We'll still give you work, but we can't allow this kind of freedom if you're living with us.'"[7]

Underlying some of this regulation was a concern that the women would be drawn into prostitution and a strong desire to provide them with the "security" of a simulated "family"—the female community of the ashram and its overseers. This extended to providing child care while the women worked or trained, special nurturing of those who were feeling more traumatized than others. We were told how, often, such women would move into the ashram superintendent's living quarters till they felt able enough to cope on their own. At least four social workers told us that, to this day, they receive letters or visits from women they helped rehabilitate immediately after Partition; and, indeed, we met several women who spoke warmly of the support and special strength they derived from them.

The disruption of life and livelihood, post-Partition, made for another more traumatic disruption as far as the women who were widowed were concerned: loss of family, of residence, of community, of social and economic status. But this very disruption meant that ritual and customary sanctions against widows were temporarily suspended in the absence of family and social constraints, and even though the state stepped in as guardian and paterfamilias, so to speak, the nature and scale of rehabilitation compelled it to facilitate the reassimilation of widows into the economic and social mainstream as expeditiously as possible.

The Abducted Women

> We know that the crimes committed were crimes against humanity. Providence will never forgive those who have been guilty of them and we must do everything that lies in our power to restore the abducted women and children to their relations. . . . What unspeakable and inexpressible joy must it be of those persons who have been virtually under confinement . . . when they are restored to their own families.
> —Jaspat Roy Kapoor (Constituent Assembly of India 1949)

In the aftermath of Partition and during the huge exodus of people from one country to another, very large numbers of women were kidnapped or abducted by men or families of the "other" community. This "kidnapping" could have taken place by force or deceit; while families were fleeing and women or young girls got separated; in the confusion of the refugee camps; or simply by promising safe transit to distressed families in exchange for their women.

The incidence of such abductions was so great that the governments of India and Pakistan were swamped with complaints of "missing" women by relatives seeking to recover them through government, military or voluntary effort. The official estimate of the number of abducted women was placed at fifty thousand Muslim women in India and thirty-three thousand non-Muslim women in Pakistan. Although Gopalaswami Ayyangar (minister of transport, in charge of recovery) called these figures "rather wild," Mridula Sarabhai believed that the number of abducted women in Pakistan was ten times the 1948 official figure of one hundred and twenty-five thousand (Basu 1995).

The material, symbolic, and political significance of the abduction of women was not lost either on the women themselves and their families, on their communities, or on leaders and governments. As a retaliatory measure, it was simultaneously an assertion of identity and a humiliation of the rival community through the appropriation of its women. When accompanied by forcible conversion and marriage it could be counted upon to outrage both family and community honor and religious sentiments. The fear of abduction, or of falling into the hands of the enemy, compelled hundreds of women to take their own lives or be killed by their own families and literally thousands of others to carry packets of poison on their persons in the eventuality that they might be captured. Our own interviews confirmed that very many committed suicide after they were released by their captors for having been thus "used" and polluted.

Political leaders expressed their concern and anger at the "moral depravity" that has characterized this "shameful chapter" in the history of both countries; the fact that "our innocent sisters" had been dishonored was an issue that could not be looked upon with equanimity. "If there is any sore point or distressful fact to which we cannot be reconciled under any circumstances, it is the question of abduction and nonrestoration of Hindu women. We all know our history," said one member of parliament, "of what happened in the time of Shri Ram when Sita was abducted. Here where thousands of girls are concerned, we cannot forget this. We can forget all the properties, we can forget every other thing, but this cannot be forgotten." And again, "as descendants of Ram we have to bring back every Sita that is alive" (Constituent Assembly of India 1949).

On 6 December 1947 an Inter-Dominion Conference was held at Lahore at which the two countries agreed upon steps to be taken for the implementation of recovery and restoration, with the appointment of Mridula Sarabhai as chief social worker. The primary responsibility of recovery was that of the local police, assisted by a staff of one additional inspector-general (AIG), two deputy superintendents of police (DSP), fifteen inspectors, ten subinspectors, and six assistant subinspectors (ASI) (Rai 1965). Between December 1947 and July 1948 the number of women recovered in both countries was 9,362 in India and 5,510 in Pakistan (about a fifth and a sixth of the number abducted respectively in each country). Recoveries dropped rather drastically after this date and it was felt that a more binding arrangement was necessary for satisfactory progress. Accordingly an agreement was reached between India and Pakistan on 11 November 1948 that set out the terms for recovery in each dominion.

Until December 1949 the number of recoveries in both countries was twelve thousand for India and six thousand for Pakistan. At the Constituent Assembly (Legislative) session held in December 1949, considerable dissatisfaction was expressed at the low rate and slow pace of recovery in Pakistan, especially from Sind, Baluchistan, Azad Kashmir and the "closed" districts of Gujarat, Jhelum, Rawalpindi and Campbellpur. To facilitate recovery and because the ordinance in India expired on 31 December 1949, Gopalaswami Ayyangar moved a bill in parliament on 15 December, called the Abducted Persons (Recovery and Restoration) Bill, for consideration by the House. It extended to the United Provinces of East Punjab and Delhi, the Patiala and East Punjab States Union (PEPSU), and the United State of Rajasthan and consisted of ten operative clauses, which the minister termed "short, simple, straightforward—and innocent."

A brief summary of its main clauses is in order, for three reasons: First, the act was one of the first pieces of legislation attempted by the independent Indian government, preceding even the constitution and raising important questions on the rights and responsibilities of the state and its citizens. Second, it was remarkable for the sweeping powers and immunity from legal action that it conferred on its police officers and inspectors. Third, the terms and context in which it defined "abducted persons" saw them solely as missing members of naturalized communities of families or religious groups, never as citizens.

The act defined *abducted person* as "a male child under the age of sixteen years or a female of whatever age who is, . . . or was . . . a Muslim . . . and who had become separated from his or her family and is found to be living with or under the control of any other individual or family, and in the latter case, includes a child born to any such female" (cl. 2[a]). It empowered any police officer, not below the rank of an ASI, "on mere suspicion of the presence of an abducted person 'in' any place" to enter without warrant, search and take into custody any person who "in his opinion" is an abducted person. Should a dispute arise on whether such a person was in fact abducted, the case would be referred to a (police) tribunal, constituted by the central government for this purpose. The decision of the tribunal would be final. The detention of abducted persons in a camp till such time as they were handed over to their relatives could not be "called in question in any Court" and "no suit, prosecution or other legal proceeding whatsoever shall lie against the Central Government, the Provincial government or any officer or authority for, or in respect to, any act which is in good faith done or intended to be done in pursuance of this Act" (cl. 8). All the above provisions were made "notwithstanding anything contained in any other law for the time being in force."

As is evident, the bill—although it may indeed have been short—was not as simple, straightforward or innocent as the minister would have the House believe. More than seventy amendments were moved by twenty members in an extended debate on the bill that took a full three days to pass. Every clause, subclause, and section was discussed threadbare, and serious objections were raised on everything, from the preamble to the operative clauses. The main objections related to the definition of abductors and the time-frame that the bill referred to (1 March 1947 and 1 January 1949); the virtually unlimited powers given to the police with complete immunity from inquiry or action and no accountability at all; the denial of any rights or legal recourse to the recovered women; the question of children; the constitution of the tribunal; camp conditions and confinement; forcible return of unwilling women; unlimited duration for the bill to remain in force; and the unequal and disadvantageous terms of the agreement for India vis-à-vis Pakistan.

Jaspat Roy Kapoor, quoted at the beginning of this section, put it succinctly:

> Let not our enthusiasm to do the right thing get the better of our judgment. . . . Legislation must be fair, just and equitable. Judged from this standard, I find that this legislation is very defective. . . . What do we find in this Bill? We find that after release [the women] will have absolutely no say about . . . where they are to live, in the matter of their companions with whom they are to live, in the matter of the Dominion where they would like to live, and in the matter of the custody of their children . . . these women have been given no voice. (Constituent Assembly of India 1949)

The amendments moved by members sought to mitigate many of the gross irregularities they pointed out, and to qualify or modify certain other procedural aspects that were set out. But, despite their strenuous efforts and the strong dissenting voices like that of Roy Kapoor, the honorable minister declined to incorporate a single amendment or modification proposed (bar one, limiting the duration of the bill to December 1951), and it was passed, unchanged, on 19 December 1949 and notified in the official *Gazette* on 28 December 1949.

Elsewhere we have elaborated on implications of the bill in terms of the actual recovery work and its harrowing consequences for women (Menon and Bhasin 1996; 1998a). Here, we would like to focus on the use and definition of the term *abducted* and its ramifications both for policy making and in constructing the figure of woman-as-victim, in need of recovery and restoration by the state-as-parent/protector.

In the context of worsening Hindu-Muslim relations, the term *abducted* was first used in November 1946, after the Noakhali riots, in the Indian National Congress session at Meerut. A resolution was passed that stated:

> The Congress views with pain, horror and anxiety the tragedies of Calcutta, East Bengal, Bihar and some parts of Meerut district . . . These new developments in communal strife are different from any previous disturbances and have involved . . . mass conversions . . . abduction and violation of

women, and forcible marriage. (Cited in Constituent Assembly of India 1949, 634)

Communal tension and the ensuing violence escalated at such a rapid pace, especially after March 1947, that leaders and representatives of the Indian and Pakistani governments met in Lahore in September 1947 and resolved that steps be taken to "recover and restore abducted persons." On 17 November 1947 the All-India Congress committee passed a resolution that said:

> During these disorders large numbers of women have been abducted on either side and there have been forcible conversions on a large scale. No civilized people can recognize such conversions and there is nothing more heinous than the abduction of women. (Constituent Assembly of India 1949)

It is important to note here that, from the very beginning, the concern with abducted women or persons went hand in hand with alarm at "forcible conversions." This preoccupation continued throughout the debates and, in fact, underlined another important factor in India's relationship with Pakistan: the loss of Hindus to Islam, through such conversions, in addition to the loss of territory. Abduction and conversion were the double blow dealt to the Hindu "community," so that the recovery of "their" women, if not of land, became a powerful assertion of Hindu manhood, at the same time as it demonstrated the moral high ground occupied by the Indian state. Nothing like this concern was evident with regard to the abduction of Hindu women by Hindu men, or Muslim women by Muslim men, leading one to conclude that this was so because here no offence against community or religion had been committed, nor anyone's "honor" compromised.

Although there seemed to be a general consensus, on both sides, that large numbers of women had indeed been abducted, a working definition of who was an abducted person was attempted by the Indian government only in 1949 in the bill under discussion. The looseness of the definition ("had become separated from his or her family and is found to be living with or under the control of any other individual or family") as well as the arbitrariness of its scope ("If any police officer . . . has reason to believe that an abducted person resides or is to be found in any place") provoked intense debate in the Assembly and many members were justifiably disturbed by its implications. Pandit Thakur Das Bhargava made his disquiet clear:

> In my humble opinion, this word "abducted person" . . . is a misnomer. . . . I know of thousands of good Hindus who gave protection to such Mus-

lim girls. I know in Pakistan also there are good Mohammadans who gave protection to innocent Hindus. They can by no manner be called abductors if they give protection. The proper word should have been "separated persons." (Constituent Assembly of India 1949)

Members demurred at the absence of any judicial recourse available either to abducted persons or to their families; others drew attention to the significant departures made in this definition from the legal definition of *abduction* (to kidnap; to carry away illegally or by force or deception) and the consequent culpability of the government in a court of law.

Their misgivings were often fully borne out not only by the actual process of recovery (see Menon and Bhasin 1998a) but by the very impossibility of establishing, beyond reasonable doubt, that the person/woman recovered had in fact been abducted in the first place. As we learned in the course of our interviews, the circumstances of their abduction varied widely. Some were left behind as hostages for the safe passage of their families; others were separated from their group or family while escaping, or strayed and were picked up; still others were initially given protection and then incorporated into the host family; yet again, as in the case of Bahawalpur State, all the women of a single block were kept back. Some changed hands several times or were sold to the highest or lowest bidder, as the case might be (the going rate, we were told, was two rupees for non-Muslim girls, four annas for Muslims, in Pakistan); some became second or third wives; and very many were converted and married, and lived with considerable dignity and respect. We do not mean to suggest here that there were no cases of forcible kidnaping and abduction on both sides; merely that abduction as defined by the bill of 1949 assumed that any and every woman located in the home or under the control of a family or individual of the other community was eligible for recovery, regardless of any indications to the contrary.[8] Moreover, such a definition criminalized even the most humanitarian of responses on the part of Muslims and non-Muslims, and divested the women in question of any volition or choice in determining their lives.

Resistance to being recovered came not only from their abductors but from the women themselves (Menon and Bhasin 1998a). Many escaped from the centers to which they were brought and returned to their "captors," sometimes by the most extraordinary means. We were told by one Recovery Officer, in charge of recoveries from Lyallpur in West Punjab in early 1948, of a young girl he had recovered and sent to Lahore and then Jullundar: "She escaped from the camp—her menfolk dug a tunnel beneath the camp and retrieved her. If I were to do this job today, I would refuse. Why should I risk my life? But at that time, my objective was: how many girls have I recovered today?"[9]

The women often protested that their liaisons had been made freely and under no compulsion, and, indeed, we learned that many had taken advantage of the social turmoil to marry men of their choice from outside their community, something that would almost certainly have been disallowed in more normal times. Very many such "disputed" cases came up for arbitration at the special tribunal set up by India and Pakistan, as recounted by both Kamlabehn Patel and police officers in charge, and they readily admit that the resolution of these cases was beset with difficulties. Of those who were forcibly repatriated, an appreciable number simply refused to return to their natal families or husbands; some, in protest, refused to change out of the clothes they had been wearing when they were picked up by the social workers; and at least two Search Officers told us that, as far as they knew, not a single woman had come to the recovery centers of her own volition. "Who are you to meddle in our lives?" they shouted at the social workers when they were forced to go back, "What business is it of yours?" and "If you were unable to save us then, what right have you to compel us now?"[10]

Exactly how widespread this resistance was is difficult to ascertain, especially given the coercive powers of the police. But there was not a single social worker or police officer we spoke to who did not refer specifically to it; in fact, the act (renewed every year for six years) was allowed to lapse in 1956, when social workers and the police said they could no longer continue with Operation Recovery. As early as 1949, Rameshwari Nehru, honorary advisor to the government in the Ministry of Relief and Rehabilitation, resigned in protest against a policy that she believed worked against women. In a memorandum to the Minister of Relief and Rehabilitation, dated June 1949, she said:

> It is well known that a very large proportion of the women recovered in India were unwilling to go to Pakistan. Many of them, even after months of detention in our transit homes, were steadfast in their determination to remain with their new relations among whom they appeared to be happy and well settled . . . But I regret to say that their protests, their hunger strikes, their pathetic and heart rending cries of distress, widely witnessed by both workers and outsiders, were of no avail, for they were eventually sent away to Pakistan . . . We must admit that we have sent away these unwilling and helpless women to a future they can neither control nor choose. (Nehru n.d.)

She recommended that recoveries be discontinued altogether because she was "convinced that we have not achieved our purpose. . . . *By sending women away, we have brought about grief and dislocation of their accepted family life without in the least promoting human happiness.*" (Nehru n.d., emphasis added)

Secularity, Sexuality, and the State

The single most important point about the Abducted Persons (Recovery and Restoration) Bill was that it needed to be legislated at all, since the maximum number of recoveries had been made between 1947 and 1949, before the bill was introduced in Parliament. Why then was the Indian government so anxious to reclaim women, sometimes several years after their abduction? Why should the matter of national honor have been so closely bound up with the bodies of women, and with children born of "wrong" unions? The experience of Pakistan suggests that recovery there was neither so charged with significance nor as zealous in its effort to restore moral order. Indeed, informal discussions with those involved in this work there indicate that pressure from India, rather than their own social or political compulsions, was responsible for the majority of recoveries made.[11] There is also the possibility that the community stepped in and took over much of the daily work of rehabilitation, evidenced by findings that the level of destitution of women was appreciably lower in Pakistan. We were told that both the Muslim League and the All Pakistan Women's Association were active in arranging the marriage of all unattached women, so that "no woman left the camp single." Preliminary interviews conducted there also hint at relatively less preoccupation with the question of moral sanction and "acceptability," although this must remain only a speculation at this stage.

Notwithstanding these questions, some tentative hypotheses may be put forward. For India, a country that was still reeling from Partition and painfully reconciling itself to its altered status, reclaiming what was by right its "own" became imperative in order to establish its credentials as a responsible and civilized state, one that fulfilled its duties toward its citizens both in the matter of securing what was their due and in confirming itself as their protector. To some extent, this was mirrored in the refugees' own dependency in turning to the *sarkar* as its *mai-baap* (protector and provider) at this time of acute crisis.

But the notion of recovery itself as it came to be articulated cannot really be seen as having sprung full-blown in the post-Partition period, as a consequence of events that had taken place during and after the violence that accompanied the exchange of populations.

If we pause to look at what had been happening in the Punjab from the mid-nineteenth century onwards with the inception and consolidation of the Arya Samaj and the formation of a Punjabi Hindu consciousness, we might begin to discover some elements of its anxiety regarding Muslim and Christian inroads into Hinduness and the erosion of Hindu *dharma*, values and lifestyles through steady conversions to these two faiths by Hindus. With the creation of Pakistan, this anxiety found a new focus, for not only had it been unable to stem conversions to Islam it had actually lost one part of itself to the creation of a Muslim homeland. Just as earlier, the Shuddhi program of the Arya Samaj (even if it resulted in bringing only one convert back into the Hindu fold) served to remind the Hindu community that losing its members to Islam or Christianity was not irreversible, so now, recovery became a symbolically significant activity. Its eerie resonance in the current frenzy to recover sacred Hindu sites from the "usurping" Muslims is chilling. Recovering women who had been abducted and, moreover, forcibly converted, restoring them both to their own and the larger Hindu family, and ensuring that a generation of newly-born Hindu children was not lost to Islam through their repatriation to Pakistan with their mothers, can be seen as part of this concern. Because, in fact, such a recovery or return might not be voluntary, necessary legal measures had to be taken to accomplish the mission. In one sense, it would seem that the only answer to forcible conversion was forcible recovery.

We have explored elsewhere the particular anxiety surrounding the matter of the children of abducted women.[12] We have argued that the key to understanding this anxiety lies in the importance regarding the question of legitimate membership—of a family, a community, and, ultimately, a nation. The sanctity of all three lay in keeping the boundaries intact and in maintaining difference. Once nations become associated with ethnic purity, then women become the first Other within a community. As Rada Iveković (1993) argues, women come to represent the very principle of mixture. Inter-ethnic violence displays a preoccupation with women as harboring a dangerous potential for a dilution of the "pure," making their appropriation and control by their community and by the competing ethnic community appear imperative. This was also why the forced alliances resulting from abduction during Partition could neither be socially acknowledged nor legally sanctioned, and why the children born of them would forever be "illegitimate." And so the faked "family" had to be dismembered by physically removing the woman/wife/mother from its offending embrace and relocating her in the "real" one, where her sexuality could be suitably supervised.

The State, the Community and Gendered Citizenship

Unraveling the complexity of the question of citizenship, Helga Maria Hernes says:

> [It] refers to the bonds between stable and individual citizens as well as the bonds among individual citizens. These bonds are circumscribed by law ... by custom ... and by the material resources available to individual cit-

izens.... They are, in addition circumscribed by the political situation prevailing at any point in time. All the dimensions are gendered in a variety of ways, and states differ along all three dimensions: the nature of legal, social and material bonds among citizens; the nature of the institutions, which define and defend these bonds; and their capability of handling political crises. (Qtd. in Leech 1994, 81)

The historical and experiential material introduced in this chapter requires careful consideration of the contrasting—but not necessarily opposed—experience of citizenship by widowed and abducted women in such a moment of political crisis. In other discussions, we have elaborated the dynamic of gender, community and state in post-Partition India, and the importance of maintaining the purity of the "legitimate" religious community (Menon and Bhasin 1996, 1998a). Our concluding comments in this chapter explore how problematic the very notion of citizenship was with regard to both categories of women, and how it was "negotiated" by them, by the state, and by those responsible for their rehabilitation or recovery.

As with sexuality, the debates around citizenship, too, were explicit in the case of abducted women; implicit—or, shall we say, assumed—in the case of widows. Both were citizens of a secular democracy, but the exercise of the rights of such citizenship was far less contested where widows were concerned. The state as protector and provider (*mai-baap*) acted on behalf of both widows and abducted women, but with the latter it, in fact, *denied them the possibility of asserting their political and civil rights* through an act of Parliament, while ensuring that their civil rights were realized through the state's redistributive agencies (Leech 1994, 81). Because widows' political and civil rights were not in conflict with perceived community "rights" or claims, they were never put to the test in the same way as those of abducted women.

The extended debate on forcible recovery as violating the constitutional and fundamental rights of abducted women, as *citizens*, is evidence of this conflict;[13] the resistance by abducted women themselves further demonstrates their attempt to realize citizenship by acting independently and autonomously—of community, state *and* family. The attempt was thwarted through a consensus reached by all three on the desirability and necessity of women preserving community and national honor by subordinating their rights as individuals and citizens to the rights of the community and the will of the state. The freezing of boundaries, communal and national, calls for what Kristeva (1993) terms "sexual, nationalist and religious protectionism," reducing men and women, but especially women, to the "identification needs of their originary groups," imprisoning them in the "impregnable aloofness of a weird primal paradise: family, ethnicity, nation, race." The state cannot absent itself while these negotiations are taking place, for, as Kristeva continues:

> Beyond the *origins* that have assigned to us biological identity papers and a linguistic, religious, social, political, historical place, the freedom of contemporary individuals may be gauged according to their ability to choose their membership, while the democratic capability of a nation and social group is revealed by the right it affords individuals to exercise that choice. (1993, 16)

Free choice, freely exercised, is what neither nation nor community could allow the abducted woman in post-Partition India, so much so that it was legislated out.

With widows, on the contrary, the endeavor was to facilitate their entry into the social and economic mainstream of the country, as productive members of the citizenry, contributing to what Renuka Ray called the process of "nation-building." The oppressive bind of conventional widowhood was thus loosened sufficiently to enable women to emerge into, and assume, citizenship with all its rights and responsibilities. This category of citizenship simply collapsed in relation to the woman-out-of-place. The process of recovery, of putting abducted women back into place, was not conceived by the state as a relationship to women as *missing citizens* of the new state (if so, it would have endowed them with civil rights).[14] Rather, it chose to treat them as *missing members of religious and cultural communities,* on whose behalf choices had to be made. Widows were redefined as victims of a national disaster, requiring a direct form of intervention that did not end simply by restoring them to the communities to which they belonged. Instead, they were made viable as their own community, economically independent, and rehabilitated as citizens.

In both cases, the state was acting as custodian and guardian on behalf of missing or wronged men—in the case of widows, the men were permanently absent or missing; in abduction, it was the women who were "missing"—and the patriarchal bias of its intervention and ideology were evident in both, as is clear from much of the material quoted earlier. The post-Partition conjuncture was one of unusual flux and formative capacity, and made for some unprecedented relationships between women and the state; some of these continue, others have been closed off.

A comparison of the state's relationship with widows and abducted women sheds some light on the nature of this relationship and its implications for women. To begin with, it illuminates the workings of a state-in-transition as it negotiates both postcolonial independence and partition at the same time, and tries to put in place a relatively progressive political and social program. What is clear from our analysis is that, for women, the state functions in interaction with at least two other major institutions—community and family—and that, together, they constitute the contesting arenas for gender issues.

We have seen that the relationship between gender and state may be cooperative or conflictual; generally speaking, there can be cooperation on issues of welfare, and conflict on issues of rights, as is borne out by the experience of widows and abducted women. In the post-Partition period, the state itself was a complex confluence: redefining itself as secular, democratic and socialist, but operating in a politically charged atmosphere, keeping communal considerations in balance; incorporating a benign paternalism (or *mai-baap*ism) while simultaneously upholding patriarchal codes and practices; ensuring the realization of social rights, while withholding civil and political rights, even while it deliberated on fundamental rights and guarantees.

These tensions continue today—some might even say they have been accentuated—as communitarian politics are resurgent and the secular state more embattled. Women's democratic rights as citizens are often held in suspension, as the current debate on a uniform civil code has shown, and is once more cast in communal terms. A reexamination of the relationship between gender, communities and the state, post-Partition, may be useful in order to appreciate the process of identity formation, the complex nature of the state's involvement in this process, and what it means for women.

NOTES

We are truly indebted to Kalpana Ram for her close and insightful reading of this chapter and her thought-provoking comments on the issues discussed. It has benefited greatly from all her input. We have also received valuable feedback on variations of this chapter from Amrita Basu, Patricia Jeffery, Marty Chen, and Tanika Sarkar. The chapter itself is part of an ongoing study of women's negative experience of Partition, with a focus on Punjab.

1. For a detailed discussion of Partition historiography and our methodology, see Menon and Bhasin 1998a.

2. We make a distinction here between the Indian state and the government; the former a secular, democratic entity; the latter a government formed by the Congress Party, professedly secular but subject to the pulls and pressures of parties and communities.

3. *Hitavada,* a fortnightly publication from Nagpur, may be characterized as Liberal-nationalist during the 1930s. Clearly secular in its orientation, it gradually became more Congress-nationalist in the 1940s, by which time it had become a daily.

4. For a more elaborated discussion on this subject, see Menon and Bhasin 1998a, b.

80   Borders of Being

5. See, for instance, the report by the PUDR (1989) on refugee women workers in Delhi, which details the situation in the Union Territory of Delhi; and Latha Anantaraman, "In dependence," *The India Magazine* (August–September 1996). For a full-length discussion of social workers, see Menon and Bhasin 1998b.

6. In Delhi the executive authority was vested in the honorary director, who was free to develop her work as she chose. In Bombay the work was carried out by a women's committee of honorary members, who had executive powers and worked under the Rehabilitation Department of the state government. The same was true of Uttar Pradesh and West Bengal; only in East Punjab was the director of the women's section a regular salaried official of the state government. At the center Rameshwari Nehru, Begum Anis Kidwai, Mridula Sarabhai, Sucheta Kripalani, Mrs. John Mathai, Hannah Sen, Raksha Saran, and many others all worked in an honorary capacity, with executive authority.

7. Personal interview with a social worker in Karnal (Haryana).

8. See Devi 1995, for a most poignant account of a Hindu girl sheltered by a Muslim family in Noakhali in 1946.

9. Personal interview with a liaison officer assigned to Lyallpur (West Punjab) between 1948 and 1950.

10. As told to us by social workers in personal interviews.

11. We owe this information to Nighat Said Khan, researching the experience of women in Pakistan.

12. For a more detailed discussion on this, see Menon 1997.

13. Pandit Thakur Das Bhargava said: "Sir . . . yesterday when we were discussing clause 8 *viz.*, that detention should not be questioned in any court, I submitted that that provision is against the spirit of the Constitution. . . . I do submit that there is no reason why these girls, who are citizens of India, if they want to live here, should be forced to go away." He added: "I further submit that this (clause 8) is opposed to the fundamental rights guaranteed in the Constitution and is opposed to Section 491 of the Criminal Procedure Code. The writ of *habaeus corpus* is always open" (Constituent Assembly of India 1949).

14. We owe this formulation to Kalpana Ram.

REFERENCES

Basu, A. 1995. *Mridula Sarabhai: Rebel with a cause.* Delhi: Oxford University Press.
Constituent Assembly of India. 1948. *Debates,* vol. 3, no. 5, March. Delhi: Nehru Memorial Museum and Library.
———. 1949. *Legislative debates,* 15 December. Delhi: Nehru Memorial Museum and Library.
Devi, J. 1995. *The river churning.* Delhi: Kali for Women.
Hitavada. 22 May 1948. Nagpur, India.
Iveković, R. 1993. Women, nationalism and war: "Make love not war." *Hypatia* 8 (4): 113–26.
Keller, S. L. 1975. *Uprooting and social change: The role of refugees in development.* Delhi: Manohar Book Service.
Kristeva, J. 1993. *Nations without nationalism,* trans. L. S. Roudiez. New York: Columbia University Press.

Leech, M. 1994. Women, the state and citizenship: "Are women in the building or in a separate annex?" *Australian Feminist Studies* 19 (Autumn): 79–91.

Menon, R. 1997. Reproducing the legitimate community: Secularity, sexuality, and the state in postpartition India. In *Appropriating gender: Women's activism and politicized religion in South Asia*, ed. P. Jeffery and A. Basu, 15–32. New York: Routledge.

Menon, R., and K. Bhasin. 1996. Abducted women, the state and questions of honour. In *Embodied violence: Communalising women's sexuality in South Asia*, ed. K. Jayawardena and M. de Alwis, 1–31. New Delhi: Kali for Women.

———. 1998a. *Borders and boundaries: Women in India's partition.* New Delhi and New Brunswick, N.J.: Kali for Women and Rutgers University Press.

———. 1998b. Partition widows: The state as social rehabilitator. In *Widows in India: Social neglect and public action,* ed. M. A. Chen, 397–408. New Delhi: Sage.

Nehru, R. n.d. Private papers of Rameshwari Nehru. Delhi: Nehru Memorial Museum and Library.

PUDR [People's Union for Democratic Rights]. 1989. *Sadda hak, ethey rakh* (Our right—give it now). Report on refugee women workers in Delhi. Delhi: PUDR.

Rai, S. 1965. *Partition of the Punjab.* Bombay: Asia Publishing House.

CHAPTER 3

Rationalizing Fecund Bodies: Family Planning Policy and the Modern Indian Nation-State

Kalpana Ram

> At night . . . he would whisper to her about the dawning of a new world, Belle, a free country, Belle, above religion because secular, above class because socialist, above caste because enlightened, above hatred because loving, above tribe because unifying, above language because many-tongued, above colour because multi-coloured, above poverty because victorious over it, above ignorance because literate, above stupidity because brilliant, freedom, Belle, the freedom express, soon we will stand upon that platform and cheer the coming of the train.
>
> —Salman Rushdie

Reevaluations of Indian Modernity: Liberalism under Challenge

This chapter explores the Indian state's attempt to set up a specifically "modern" relationship to the reproductive bodies of its citizen-subjects. The discourse of demography and family planning is shaped by the broader forms of ethico-political legitimation that mark the particularity of the state. Partha Chatterjee singles out two features central to the self-definition of the Indian postcolonial state as it emerged from the anticolonial nationalism of the 1940s: first, the claim to representativeness that rested in the procedural forms of parliamentary government; and, second, the claim to representativeness that rested in "directing a program of economic development on behalf of the nation" (1994, 204). Family planning as state policy is shaped by both kinds of claims to legitimacy and is, in turn, integral to the state's representation of itself as modern and progressive.

Yet the basic terms of Indian modernity are now under critical scrutiny and challenge. In his novel *The Moor's Last Sigh* (1995) Salman Rushdie has his protagonist describe the early ideals of Indian modernity in a way that is designed at once to impress the contemporary reader with the lofty sweep of those ideals and simultaneously to strike the reader as verging on absurdity. Both qualities, the idealism that seeks to end the oppressions of caste and poverty as well as the absurdity of the ambitions, are made to spring from the same source—namely, the vertiginous attempt to soar "above" poverty but also above religion, class, tribe, and even language. These transcendent goals seem to find no moorings in the actual social fabric of India. Faith in modernity's promise threatens to turn into an unreflexive complacency ("above stupidity because brilliant").

Such a view of Indian modernity and nationalism is not confined to diasporic South Asian intellectuals such as Rushdie, whose location may be presumed to be more directly shaped by Western postmodernist perspectives. Within India a similar process of intellectual reevaluation marks the traversal of a political distance between the ideals of the first generation of Indian postcolonial intellectuals and those of the present. Veena Das, a leading sociologist, articulates the nature of this distance for many intellectuals in the social sciences:

> Unlike social scientists who came into the world of knowledge as part of the anti-colonial, nationalist enterprise, the new generation of social scientists in India have to live with a destruction of certainty as the only condition for the production of knowledge about Indian society. They cannot "represent" India as if India were absent and silent. They can only insert their voice within a plurality of voices within which agreement between prescriptive, normative, and even descriptive statements is not likely to be forthcoming. This, however, may be a more hopeful position than one in which a single authoritative truth, with claims to sovereignty, comes to reign over all intellectual discourses. (1995, 54)

Outside academic circles, the challenge to Indian modernity is, if anything, more intense and of greater consequence. The place of liberal secularism as a guiding principle for the exercise of state power is politically contested at present by both religious nationalists and left-liberal intellectuals. State policy in an area such as personal law therefore forms the focus for a whole range of critical positions on modernity, ranging from religious nationalist demands that the state adopt a uniform civil code and cease "pandering to Muslim minorities," to leftist critiques of the colonial legacies in state policies on religion, to feminist debates over the demand for a uniform civil code. Sections of the women's movement, in particular, are undertaking extremely nuanced adjudications of modernity, as they seek to reconcile the demands to respect "difference" among women—religious differences in particular—with the need to secure gender equity by providing all women with uniform access to a just set of personal laws (Hasan 1996; Sangari 1995; Working Group on Women's Rights n.d.).

In the area of family planning as state policy, however, the dominant brand of intellectual discourse stands out, I will argue, as a particularly stark example of the condition Gyanendra Pandey describes for Indian historiography:

> By attributing a "natural" quality to a particular unity, such as "India," and adopting its "official" archive as the primary source of historical knowledge pertaining to it, the historian adopts the view of the established state. (1991, 560)

In the area of family planning, the hegemony of "the view of the established state" entails the conflation of the state's particular vision of reproduction and fertility with modernity itself. Such an adoption of the state's viewpoint by planners, demographers, and policy makers is no coincidence. More than any other class of intellectuals, "planners are essentially concerned with serving the interests of the *state,* an entity which is 'relatively' . . . or 'potentially'. . . discrete from the interests of particular social classes—or from self-interested technocrats" (Robertson 1984, 94).

The hegemony of the planners' discourse is by no means uncontested or absolute. I will be unable, in this chapter, to give left and feminist critiques of family planning policy the attention they deserve, but the first half of this chapter is heavily informed by the tenor of these critiques,[1] while I have explored questions of modernity and the Indian women's health movement in another essay (see Ram 1998a). Yet, although such traditions of critique exist, we have yet to see the impact of recent debates over key aspects of modernity in the area of state policies on reproduction. There is little critique, in particular, of the way the state in India has framed notions of what it is to have a modern reproductive consciousness. In this chapter I set out to show why such a critique is important, not only in order to expand the horizons of what are considered permissible forms of reproductive consciousness but also because there are close links between discourses on fertility and broader discourses on state and citizenship. The women's health movement in India, for instance, driven as it is by an entirely legitimate focus on the contradiction between state family planning policies and women's health choices, does not address the broader contours of the state's discourse on reproductive rationality. Yet state-driven notions of reproductive rationality marginalize not only women but a whole range of identity formations as "minority identities." I devote the second half of the chapter to an extension of the debate in this direction.

Liberalism and Family Planning Policy: The Erosion of "Choice" and "Democratic Participation"

State family planning policy can be viewed as a particularly potent arena in which two quite distinct, even opposed, imperatives of the Indian state have been at work: those of liberalism and developmentalism. The values of liberalism have framed the discourse of family planning in India in certain important ways. First, they refer back to some of the primary values of the Indian state itself. The Constitution of the newly independent Indian nation-state takes on board the liberal definition of the private sphere as a sphere in which freedom to pursue one's interests and beliefs is guaranteed, a freedom checked only by the contending liberal principle of not infringing on the rights of other individuals. The Constitution tries to remain faithful to this founding vision, despite the conundrums created by its application in the Indian context.[2] Liberal values are invoked at two levels within family planning policy. Participatory democracy has been viewed as the necessary mediating procedure for the implementation of family planning, while, at the level of the individual "acceptor" of the policy, liberal values of informed consent and choice are perceived as desirable. We can see this both in the latest and in the very first of the five-year plans. The report of the Working Group of the eighth (and latest) five-year plan substantially invokes both these sets of liberal democratic values. The review process stresses the values of informed choice, community involvement and participation, active involvement by the elected representatives of the people in parliament, state legislature as well as in local government, and the special need to make "the weaker sections, including women, aware of their rights to demand the services to improve their health as well as their welfare" (Eighth Five Year Plan 1990, 17).

Nearly all the policy statements refer to the desirability of choice for the users of family planning policy. The preferred image of the policy for some time has been that of a "cafeteria" in which Indians figure as consumers of technological choices arrayed before them in impartial fashion. The recommendations of the Working Group for the latest five-year plan project a consumer who is kept well informed about the choices, and even the consequences of choices, in the cafeteria of contraceptive technology. "It is necessary to strengthen counseling about all the various methods, their benefits as well as contradictions and possible side effects" (1990, 18). If we look back at the first five-year plan, the draft form was circulated in 1951 with the assurance that "planning in a democratic State is a social process in which in some parts . . . every citizen should have the opportunity to participate" (cited in Raina 1988,

86 Borders of Being

9). The literature on family planning similarly commits itself to both aspects of liberalism. The key to shaping demographic behavior is considered to reside in access to knowledge, information, and services and the freedom to use them in any way (Basu 1992, 68).

I do not propose to view these commitments as purely formal or illusory. They have had their effects in a vigorous electorate and civil society and provide a set of genuine constraints that other imperatives such as developmentalism have to take into account, in a way that distinguishes the Indian state clearly from other states in Asia, where the adoption of liberal democratic values ranges from the tokenistic to outright rejection.

The Erosion of the Meaning of "Choice"

The divergence from liberal principles in the Indian case must be analyzed more subtly than is the case in states with little commitment to such principles. In India there is, instead, a process whereby the principles are both continually reiterated and equally constantly eroded, or in which the meaning of key terms is radically redefined and narrowed. We may clearly see this dual process at work in the operationalization of a key term such as "choice." I deliberately begin not with the spectacular example of the Emergency in 1976, when liberal democracy was suspended altogether and used to implement sterilization but, rather, with the more everyday, enduring, and persistent erosion of liberal values in family planning. The drama of the Emergency has obscured the fundamental continuities in state policy. As Soni puts it:

> The measures used in the Emergency were not in themselves new: the intensive "crash" programmes; the emphasis on sterilization as an easily administered method; the use of targets; payment of incentives and disincentives; sanctions against those who failed to comply with the government's wishes; and even, in some cases, forcible sterilization notwithstanding its illegality. What made 1976 different was the application of political muscle to the fertility control programme. (1984, 143)

The annual targets referred to by Soni are set by the Planning Commission in consultation with the Health Ministry and state governments and have been a feature of state policy since 1966. By their nature, they are aggregate goals for fertility reduction rather than goals set with an eye to the "consumer," or "user," of the contraceptive methods. Financial "incentives," too, were "the basic feature of the national program after 1965" (Vicziany 1982, 384).

When we examine the actual goods made available in the cafeteria of state-sponsored technology, the notion of informed choice has virtually no purchase. State policy has typically pushed only one method at any given time, usually in short and intensive phases. The first choice to be eliminated in state policy was a Gandhian advocacy of nontechnological methods (abstinence, rhythm, and withdrawal). Still somewhat influential immediately after Independence in the 1950s, this choice was quickly displaced by a general favoring of technological methods (Soni 1984, 149). For the most part we see a pattern not of several technological choices but of a single technology being pushed at any given time: either the intrauterine device (IUD) or sterilization or, more recently, a turn toward long-lasting hormonal implants.

The IUD was sponsored by the state in quite a strenuous fashion during the early phases of family planning policy in the early 1960s, yet it ceased to be promoted between 1974 and 1984 (see Soni 1984) and has only been fitfully promoted by the state since then. Sterilization has remained fairly constant as the state's preferred modality of "family planning" and now accounts for 70 to 80 percent of the contraceptive protection (Narayana and Kantner 1992, 106). Table 2 sets out the relative emphasis on sterilization as a means of achieving targets for the period 1970–89.

TABLE 2. Percentage of Couples Using Contraception, by Method, 1970–71 to 1989

Year	Sterilization	IUD	Other Methods	Total
1970–71	8.1	1.4	2.1	11.5
1971–72	9.7	1.4	2.4	13.5
1972–73	12.2	1.2	2.4	15.8
1973–74	12.2	1.1	3.0	16.3
1974–75	12.6	1.0	2.4	16.1
1975–76	14.2	1.1	3.4	18.7
1976–77	20.7	1.1	3.4	25.3
1977–78	20.1	0.9	3.0	24.0
1978–79	19.9	1.0	3.1	23.9
1979–80	19.9	1.0	2.7	23.6
1980–81	20.1	1.1	3.3	24.4
1981–82	20.7	1.2	3.8	25.7
1982–83	22.0	1.4	4.9	28.4
1983–84	23.7	2.3	6.8	32.7
1984–85	24.9	3.0	7.7	35.6
1985–86	26.5	3.9	8.3	38.7
1986–87	27.9	4.8	8.0	40.7
1987–88	28.9	5.5	5.7	40.1
1989 (Survey)	31.3	1.9	6.7	39.9

Source: Ministry of Health and Family Planning, Family Welfare Program in India, 1990; ORG 1990, Table 7.1 (qtd. in Narayana and Kantner 1992, 106).

Note: Contraceptives covered by the category "other methods" include condoms, jellies, foam tablets, and pills.

The table, however, dealing as it does in aggregates, does not capture just *who* is being sterilized. In fact, there has been a dramatic shift in terms of the sex of the bodies that are targeted as the object of sterilization policies. Up to the period of Emergency in 1976, male sterilization was four to five times more common than female sterilization, since the technology for cheap, mass female sterilizations was not available until the advent of mini-laparotomies and laparoscopic sterilizations in the early 1980s. The pivotal event for the shift was the Emergency state declared by Indira Gandhi between 1975 and 1977. A concerted push by the state in meeting targets of male sterilization was resisted by means of the electoral system—the Emergency and Mrs. Gandhi's Congress Party were electorally voted out. Male sterilizations have been regarded as electorally risky since then, and, once new forms of cheap female sterilization became technically possible, there has been an overwhelming shift toward women as the target of sterilization campaigns (Narayana and Kantner 1992, 108; Soni 1984, 151; Soonawala 1992, 83).

Such shifts in policy are marked not only by the sex of the targeted bodies but by the regional location of those bodies. The Emergency sterilizations, for instance, had been undertaken with particular ferocity in the northern states, where the Congress Party enjoyed a more undisputed electoral primacy than it did in the southern states. In addition, it was in the north of India where Mrs. Gandhi's son Sanjay Gandhi had carved out a particular sphere of influence in which he could pursue the sterilization targets he took as his personal agenda. Accordingly, it was in the north that the rejection of the Emergency was electorally registered in outstanding numbers (see later discussion). By contrast, the states of the south, while also experiencing the shift toward the targeting of women as the object of sterilization, never experienced the full impact of Emergency-style campaigns to sterilize men.

Equally revealing of the state's relationship to the bodies of citizens is the nature of the contraceptive technology preferred in state policy. The methods favored by the state for its citizens are the ones that allow the least amount of choice in terms of reversibility. Contraceptive technologies offering people greater choices in terms of preventing pregnancies and allowing reversibility have either been de-emphasized or have been denied an adequate infrastructure for meeting standards of health and safety. For example, of the contraceptives described as "conventional contraceptives" in documents issued by the Ministry of Family Welfare, which include condoms, diaphragms, jellies, foam tablets, and pills, only condoms have been promoted, and with varying reports of success. The Indian state, unlike other states, such as Bangladesh, has never seriously promoted the pill or made it widely available. According to the Rural Women's Social Education Centre (hereafter RUWSEC) in Tamil Nadu, the state and the medical establishment have been entirely negative in their attitudes toward the diaphragm (oral report, 17 August 1996). In recent interviews with doctors at public hospitals and in the Voluntary Health Service family planning clinics, moreover, I found that the diaphragm was simply regarded as superseded technology.

Abortion was made legal in 1971 under the Medical Termination of Pregnancy Act as a contraceptive measure. Contraceptive failure is included as a valid reason for seeking abortion. It has been noted in the literature that, although the utilization of this service has picked up, it has not reduced the number of illegal abortions (Soni 1984, 152). One reason why women may not avail themselves of the legal medical abortion facilities is that abortion itself is not made available as an independent choice. It is available, rather, through medical personnel who link it up with state-sponsored pressures to undergo sterilization. Doctors whom I interviewed in a public hospital in peri-urban Chennai, in Tamil Nadu, revealed that abortion was not made available except with strings attached. At the very least, the insertion of an IUD is required, and after a second child the abortion is virtually conditional on undergoing sterilization (field notes, August 1996).[3]

The preferences for particular contraceptive technologies expressed by state policy as well as by medical personnel are themselves revealing of an underlying distrust of liberal values. IUDs are adjudged a failure—not from the perspective of the women who use them but primarily from the point of view of population limitation. From the point of view of women, there is clear evidence that the health system is regarded as inadequate in providing women with the follow-up care required after insertion of IUDs (Srikantan, Balasubramian, and Nikam 1984, 160). The evidence of women's lack of satisfaction with contraceptive side effects is striking. In contrast to other countries, where around half of IUD acceptors may complain of discomfort in the first month of use, 70 percent of Indian women did so (Narayana and Kantner 1992, 110). A microstudy of contraceptive use in a Delhi slum reports that women were reluctant to continue because of bleeding, pain, discharge, as well as fear of the operation, while there was a general unhappiness with follow-up services (IPP VIII, n.d.). Other case studies report that women have been fitted with IUDs without their knowledge following hospital delivery of their first child. The women discovered the insertion only after developing problems with bleeding a few months later, and they had the IUDs removed (Ravindran 1993). Doctors now claim to be satisfied that the new IUD being promoted by the government—the copper-T—overcomes the design deficiencies of the earlier "Loop" (fieldwork interviews between author and a doctor in a public hospital at Chengalpattu Public Hospital, August 1996). It is clear, however, that the problems lie not with the design of the technology alone but with the attitudes of the state and medical personnel. In August 1996 in a Tamil Nadu village I encountered a woman who had had a copper-T inserted without her knowledge at a government hospital in Chennai. During her periods, she felt a protrusion and attempted to pull out the object, experiencing agonizing pain. She went to a different doctor, who removed the remaining parts of the IUD but failed to inform her that this meant she could now become pregnant. She conceived a child shortly after and experienced an extremely difficult and painful pregnancy and delivery, since the uterus had barely healed from the previous laceration.

Yet it is not these kinds of problems that figure in the concerns of the family planners and policy makers. Problems with IUDs are most commonly discussed under a rubric known as "the problem of discontinuance." In other words, the problem is not that the woman experiences pain or discomfort, but that she discontinues using the IUD and therefore cannot be relied upon to carry out the goals of population policy. Failure to match the liberal values of offering safe choices to women and men is not the primary reason for shifts in state-sponsored contraceptive technology.

Statements made by the director of Bangladesh's fertility research program indicate that the recent turn toward subdermal implants are also connected to state distrust of its citizen-subjects. Initiating trials for subdermal implants of hormonal contraceptives known as Norplant in 1985, the director, Dr. Hanum Akhtar, had this to say:

> It has been found by researchers that contraceptive pills containing progestin and more commonly used other reversible methods necessitated continuous motivations involvement [sic] by the user. In a country like Bangladesh this fact is more true than in the developed world. It is therefore necessary to introduce methods in Bangladesh which can continue to be effective for long periods without continuous motivation by Family Planning workers. Norplant is perhaps the most effective method which is likely to prove successful here. (Cited in Indian Health Activists n.d., 1)

The third five-year plan in Bangladesh justified the use of Norplant in the following terms:

> [This] long lasting method has the potential advantage of not requiring day to day use and therefore may be particularly suitable for our semi-literate population. (Cited in Indian Health Activists n.d., 1)

The female consumer in the cafeteria of state discourse is someone who cannot be trusted. After all, the choosing subject may initially figure as an "acceptor" of the IUD but then discontinue using it. Or she may fail to adduce the internal "motivation" necessary for a daily dose of oral contraceptives such as the pill or to insert a diaphragm at the right time.

Class and gender inequities find renewed expression through this distrust. Narayana and Kantner comment on the "conviction among many professionals and lay persons [in India] that the requirements of the pill regimen were beyond the powers of mind and discipline of 'illiterate Indian housewives'" (1992, 111).

The construction of women as incapable of planning and rationality becomes all the more consequential when applied to poor women. Such constructions turn into real obstacles placed in the way of attempts by nongovernment organizations, for example, to widen the range of choices available to poor women. RUWSEC, a nongovernment organization working with urban and rural poor women in Chennai (Tamil Nadu) and rural areas near Chennai, held a day-long workshop in mid-1996 to publicize the results of its work.[4] They described in vivid detail the opposition from the medical establishment and the government to their attempts to introduce the use of diaphragms to urban poor women in three areas of Chennai. The authorities gave the following reasons for their opposition: poor women did not have the facilities to clean and store the diaphragm hygienically; they were culturally too inhibited to successfully insert the diaphragm; and, last, it was beyond their capacity to insert the contraceptive successfully at the right time. The nongovernment organization went ahead and educated the women in the method while awaiting an arrival of supplies (diaphragms are difficult, if not impossible, to obtain within India). Ninety-eight women used the diaphragm and six months after use reported no pregnancies. They were delighted with the lack of side effects and, although five had also used other methods, were glad that there was no need to resort to a doctor for use or removal. Negotiating obstacles such as the lack of privacy was hardly, they pointed out to the researchers, a new skill for them to learn.

Where such dedicated efforts by nongovernment groups are not available, the result of official attitudes and policies is a drastic foreshortening of choices for the poor, reinforcing the contours of class as well as gender inequality. While urban, middle-class feminists are critical of the lack of mandatory information regarding the side effects of the pill (Raghuram and Rahman 1996) and of the lack of education on sex or sexual health in government schools,[5] these preoccupations themselves seem a luxury when compared to those of the rural poor, who seldom encounter alternatives to sterilization or, at best, to the IUD. The data for India as a whole, reported by Narayana and Kantner (1992, 107), indicates that the rural poor do not know of any alternatives to sterilization and abortion. Such statistics are not to be explained away by reference to the ignorance of the poor. Poor women, too, have shown themselves to be interested in limiting their number of children. The point may be best illustrated with reference to the state of Tamil Nadu. The data for Tamil Nadu corroborates the all-India data cited by Narayana and Kantner—the rural poor, for the most part, know only of the different forms of sterilization. A study by Sundari Ravindran (1993) compares two groups of poor women in Tamil Nadu, one located in a peri-urban fishing community, and the other among agricultural Dalits (the "Scheduled Castes," in terms of government discourse). All respondents (numbering 1,307) knew of the different forms of sterilization and of little else. All had heard of tubectomies and laparoscopic sterilizations known to them simply as the "operation." Less than 5 percent had heard of the IUD, and only one had heard of the pill. Eighty-five percent were aware of legal abortion facilities, and all knew an illegal abortionist.

Yet Tamil Nadu is also the state that currently brings a gleam to the eye of demographers and planners, since the state has witnessed a slump in fertility rates over the last decade, moving from 3.5 in 1979 to 2.2 in 1991 (TV Antony 1992). This result seems to have been achieved—in contrast with the state of Kerala, which has long stood as a model of holistic development predicated on a mass communist mobilization (Jeffrey 1992)—without any significant improvement in the key indications of "development," such as alleviation of poverty, and without a decline in infant mortality rates. The result has already triggered a renewed regionalist complacency among state ministers.[6] The prospect their response offers (particularly in the context of structural adjustment programs and a greater reliance on a privatized market economy than in the past)—of fueling an even more single-minded concentration on population control—has alarmed feminist activists and scholars. Several have undertaken a closer investigation into the links between fertility decline and female status in Tamil Nadu (Ravindran n.d.; Swaminathan 1996). Ravindran's wide-ranging study of all districts in Tamil Nadu uses focused group interview techniques rather than a purely statistical method. The results are too complex to be summarized, but I will pull out the details relevant to my point about choices for the poor. The study found that rural women are demanding more access to modes of birth control. In contradiction to state government declarations, however, the fall in fertility is not due to the superior status of women in Tamil Nadu. Although an improvement in female status—such as a rise in rates of female education—can be glimpsed in certain areas, there has also been a marked deterioration in female status in the rising rate of dowry and an associated rise in violence against women (cf. Robinson, this volume, on women's "status" and fertility). Such a deterioration in female status can also, it would seem, be linked with a greater desire on the part of women to limit the number of children. The author of this particular study (Ravindran n.d., 36) concludes that it is women themselves who are at the forefront of a conscious move toward fertility decline.[7]

Yet for all their desire for contraception—which sometimes meant women undertook measures without consent from their in-laws or husbands—female sterilization was the only method that was known to all and the most commonly used. The sources of this information were mainly government health functionaries, family planning outreach workers, government posters, newspapers, and the radio. It was the government nurse or primary school teacher (usually a woman) who had taken batches of women to the local primary health center or government hospital for sterilizations and IUD insertion. None of these recruiters had either informed the women or made available any other form of contraception. In the same study (Ravindran n.d.), all the men knew of the condom and where to obtain it, but there was little evidence of its use. Induced abortions were used as a means of spacing births, because the side effects of the IUD were feared.

Class differences show up not only between urban and rural locations but within the rural population. In the study mentioned earlier, those women whose ability to provide a meal for the family at the end of the day depends on their being fit for doing agricultural labor were more affected than others by the nonavailability of choices. My own fieldwork among agricultural laboring women testifies to their fear at the prospect of sterilization. They believed it would make them less able to work and to breastfeed and nurture their babies.

The Redefinition of "Motivation"

The transformations in the meanings of the term "motivation" are one telling gauge of the general tenor of family planning discourse. The term no longer refers, as in popular understanding, to a psychological state of mind internal to the subject. In family planning discourse, "motivation" is located externally. "Motivators" are typically health workers (family welfare health assistants, village health guides, auxiliary nurse midwives) employed at state-run family welfare centers and primary health centers in urban and rural areas. It is impossible to be sure, however, that even these motivators are equipped with the requisite degree of motivation. They themselves require external motivation by the application of targets, transfer disincentives, and additional monetary payments set by the state. The chain of externally directed motivators quite undermines the liberal notion of a choosing subject. This is reflected in common usage. Village women report perceiving family planning personnel as people who are there to recruit a "case" (Ravindran 1993, 2511; see also Narayana and Kantner 1992, 90ff.; Rao 1994a).

There is evidently a profound tension within family planning policy. On the one hand, there is a desire to enshrine the values of choice and agency. On the other hand, the actual implementation of the policy too often testifies to a *want* of choice and, indeed, to a distrust of precisely those technologies that rely on the active participation of users. Usually, only one technology is promoted. And this single technology is consistently the same one: time and time again, the method promoted by the state proves to be the nonreversible method of sterilization. Poor and rural citizens are not trusted to exercise choice in a manner consistent with the goals of the state. The result is that, as far as the poor are concerned, the family planning program has virtually become identified with sterilization. Methods that require continuous decision making, such as the pill, are viewed as suitable for middle-class educated elites. Those devices, on the other hand, that are inserted and removed by medical personnel, such as the copper-T IUD, are favored for the poor and for less-educated women.

The Undermining of Democratic Electoral Participation in Family Planning Policy

A similar process of erosion characterizes the adoption of democratic electoral participation in the implementation and design of policy. The apotheosis of this erosion was the period of the Emergency, between June 1975 and January 1977. It was then that the suspension of civil liberties and electoral processes was most directly and dramatically experienced in the realm of family planning. The figures for sterilization—predominantly of *men*—rose dramatically. The Shah Commission, which was appointed in retrospect, after the resounding electoral defeat of Mrs. Gandhi by the Janata Party, brought out its report in 1978. According to the report, the number of sterilizations rose from 1.3 million in 1974–75 to 2.6 million in 1975–76. It then rose again, dramatically, to 8.1 million in 1976–77. The populous belt of Uttar Pradesh is one of the northern states where the policy was implemented with zeal. In the year before the Emergency, 1974–75, the state had failed to achieve its state-set "target" of 175,000. In dramatic contrast, in the first year of the Emergency alone, the number of sterilizations rose to 837,000 (Shah Commission of Inquiry 1978).

The change in the relative powers of the central government and the state governments was of particular importance to population policy and its implementation. Under the Indian Constitution, health and family planning are the domain of the states; the states are responsible for administering and implementing the programs. The Center, however, keeps control over finances and undertakes planning, research, evaluation, and training for the program as well as makes key decisions relating to the introduction of new contraceptive technology. Through five-year plans the Center determines overall program policy regarding the establishment of clinics, the introduction of new schemes and patterns of staffing, pricing, and expenditure (Soni 1984, 144). The states simply administer and implement the program. Until the Emergency, this division of powers was not often enforced. There were no official sanctions against a state that did not pursue the implementation of Central policy with zeal (Soni 1984). In 1976 the Constitution was amended to equip the Center with greater powers. States were given permission to pass legislation, in conformity with central government requirements, introducing compulsory sterilization. Civil service regulations were amended to ensure that central government employees adopted the small family norm.

> Political pressures on all government departments, and at every level of administration to recruit or face disciplinary action, non-payment of salary and even suspension, turned family planning into a crusade of political tyranny. For the rest of the population too, the pressures were stringent if arbitrary: a variety of licenses and permits, school admissions, rural credit, fertilizer supplies, food rations and many other economic processes superseded legal changes during what was in effect a phase of compulsory sterilization, since the severity of the economic alternative to sterilization in many instances left the individual with no real choice. (Soni 1984, 142)

The high drama of the events of the period has served to obscure questions that should have been raised about the formation and implementation of family planning policy in "normal" periods of electoral democracy in India. The dramatic electoral rejection of sterilization campaigns and of the Emergency that permitted them to occur did occasion a good deal of debate in the aftermath. Yet the parameters within which the debates were conducted do not fundamentally challenge the "view of the established state."[8] A classic example occurs in a population policy workshop conducted in 1978, whose proceedings were published in 1984 (Gandotra and Das 1984). Compulsion by the state, of the direct and punitive kind associated with the Emergency, is placed under question. "Free choice," however, is not understood as the freedom for citizen-subjects to choose goals out of line with state policy. Instead, the state retains a monopoly over agency, except that it now utilizes "development" instead of coercion to achieve its goals of population control. The only "option" that remains to be exercised by citizen-subjects is whether they will participate in the "Voluntary Acceptance of Family Planning." The editors of the volume, Gandotra and Das, express a common view when they make even such limited forms of agency, as indicated by a term such as "voluntary acceptance," conditional on the achievement of material and cultural modernization.

> The most important question today is whether in a country where more than 70 per cent of the people are illiterate, where more than 80 per cent of the people live in villages with very inadequate facilities for sanitation, hygiene, medical care or pure water supply, where superstition, old beliefs as well as fanatic and dogmatic leaders and interested politicians rule unhindered, can we hope to fully achieve "Voluntary Acceptance of Family Planning"? (Gandotra and Das 1984, ix)

None of the commentators on population policy openly discredit liberal democratic values per se. Instead, the state is presented as progressive both in its liberal democratic values and in its early commitment to family planning. *Both* are important credentials as markers of progress in this discourse:

> India, not yet the world's largest country, is on its way to becoming so. . . . Size is undeniably important but of greater significance is what India represents in the world "community" of nations and what it might be in the future. However troubled and divided—and despite occasional lapses into nondemocratic ways—India stands out among less developed nations of substantial size as one that is attempting to modernize itself, socially and economically, without sacrificing its commitment to democratic processes. . . . A nation, it might be said, with steadier and nobler aspirations for itself and its people than most post colonial societies. (Narayana and Kantner 1992, 1)

The historical fact that the Indian state was one of the first nation-states to adopt family planning as official state policy in 1951 is another important feature of this state-identified nationalist discourse on family planning. According to the vice president of the Family Planning Association of India, it is a clear indication that the Indian state "was certainly ahead of its time" (Soonawala 1992, 77).

Yet, just as family planning and liberal democracy are markers of the progressiveness of the Indian state, so also the failure of the electorate to adopt family planning becomes a marker of the backwardness of the electorate and a sign that it is not worthy of participating in an electoral democracy either. Failure to adopt family planning is linked to particular forms of identity formation that are threatening not only to family planning but to the unity of the nation:

> In India caste, religion and class are exploited as instruments of political mobilization. Electoral politics thus keeps the cauldron of cultural antagonism bubbling. (Narayana and Kantner 1992, 5)

Elsewhere Narayana and Kantner refer to the politics of caste and religion as "a sack full of writhing cobras . . . threaten[ing] to break through a dangerously threadbare social fabric" (1992, ix).

Another set of commentators on population policy, Pai Panandiker and Umashankar, begin more cautiously. They suggest that India's "diversity" and "federal democratic political system" have "deeply conditioned" the success or failure of population policies. As their account develops, however, it becomes clear that diversity figures to them almost exclusively as a problem. The policy's chances of success are threatened precisely by this diversity. India's multiplicity of languages is an obstacle to official communication and to national consensus around the program (Pai Panandiker and Umashankar 1994, 93). Regional differences raise the specter of secessionist mobilizations and undermine national unity. Religious leadership, which they see as responsible for "propaganda" (97), undermines the influence of a secular leadership committed to "education." Even the emergence of lower-caste political leaders, themselves beneficiaries of the idealism of the nation-state in its early adoption of affirmative "reservation" policies, permits the influence of the wrong kinds of identities and frustrates the attempts of the nation-state to modernize and secure general welfare:

> The backward castes, as a group, have observed the political power of numbers and are suspicious of proposals for controlling population growth. Brought up in a rural agricultural milieu where large families are respected, and where at least two sons are desired, members of these castes are highly suspicious of the perceptions of urban elites drawn from socially and economically advanced sectors of the population. One of the chief ministers of a state from a backward caste has nine children, and is reported to have said that he had this large family because he opposed the family planning program of the Congress Government. (98)

Gender is not included in Narayana and Kantner's list of "writhing cobras" (1992). Gender identities are not among the list of identities regarded by Pai Panandiker and Umashankar (1994) as problematic for population policy—presumably because they have not figured as a major determinant of electoral politics in India. Where gender *has* emerged as a basis for political mobilization, as with the urban women's movement, we find it incurring censure phrased in identical terms. When the president of the Family Planning Association of India addressed the International Planned Parenthood Federation's Family Planning Congress in New Delhi in 1992, she found the urban women's movements guilty of sectional and unrepresentative politics.

> The so-called pro-feminist groups, through their empty contraceptive policies, are in reality working against the welfare of their fellow women. In India injectible contraceptives were ready to be introduced into the national programme about five years ago, but a stay was ordered by the Supreme Court because certain women's groups claimed that injectibles were being forced on women. And there are certain individuals, very vocal, very well funded, though in a minority, who are able to affect the judgement of the majority by having a ban placed on certain hormonal contraceptives. There are certain constraints within a democracy; because of the freedoms that it gives, minorities are able to push their views forward, sometimes to the detriment of the majority. (Soonawala 1992, 85)

A characteristic move on the part of all these commentators is to make an implicit and perhaps unconscious distinction between liberal democracy as a concept (which is highly valued) and its actual functioning in the Indian polity. Liberal democracy is good, but the politics of caste, religion, language, class, and gender are bad and inappropriate for a proper democracy. Yet for all those who regard electoral politics in India as an obstacle to the implementation of a desirable family planning policy, the events of the Emergency should give pause. For it was precisely the curbing of electoral politics and the strengthening of the central government at the expense of all other sources of agency that led directly to the "excesses" (as all agree to call them) of the forced-sterilization campaigns.

The approval of electoral politics in principle—while decrying its actual functioning—is at times only a hairsbreadth removed from the outright disapproval of both practice and principle. Electoral politics is then seen as undesirable *in itself,* since it is divisive, competitive, and politicizes the issue of population:

Each identity-bound group, whether religious or ethnic, caste or linguistic, feels that its safety lies in numbers and percentages; the moment its demographic leverage decreases, its importance and influence in government suffer, and its vital interests are at stake. This anxiety over numbers is the central problem of the Indian family planning program. (Pai Panandiker and Umashankar 1994, 103)

Such a perception is certainly taken very seriously in India. One of the measures retained from Indira Gandhi's Emergency period (1975–77) is the freezing of representation in parliament at the population figures of 1971 up until the year 2000.

Gyanendra Pandey has argued that Indian nationalism has become more intolerant to diversity than at any time since Independence:

"Unity in Diversity" is no longer the rallying cry of Indian nationalism. On the contrary, all that belongs to any minority other than the ruling class, all that is challenging, singular, local—not to say, all difference—appears threatening, intrusive, even "foreign" to this nationalism. (1991, 559)

If, as he argues, historiography has been active in reinforcing such notions of "a natural Indian unity and an Indian nationalist essence," then the discourse of planners and demographers is even more closely identified with the production of such a view of nation, nationhood, and citizenship. The attitudes of citizens toward their reproductive bodies has, in this discourse, become a crucial indication of whether they belong to the "progressive," modern culture that characterizes the worthy participant of liberal democracy or whether they belong to a premodern backward culture. For those who distrust liberal democracy itself, the electoral system elicits the worst possible combination of the modern and the premodern. The rational policy maker is confronted with collectivities of caste and religion behaving like electoral-minded individuals. They become disruptive, competitive, and self-interested "vote banks."

In the next section I examine one element of the process by which citizenship became invested in India with a particular kind of identity formation.

Developmentalism and Modernity in the Indian Postcolonial State

Following the path-breaking work of Partha Chatterjee on Indian nationalism (1986, 1994), I suggest that in order to understand the foundational discourses of the postcolonial state, we need to depart from the premises emanating either from within Western political theory or from purely "indigenous" sources and to examine, instead, the way in which nationalism in India fashioned an inevitably contradictory *combination* of Western political philosophy with the imperatives of anticolonialism. At the very least, the shaping power of this anticolonialism imparted to the leaders of the nationalist movement a communitarian orientation, a vision of society as a "whole," which radically tempered the individualist premises of liberalism.

This communitarian concern consolidated around what, following the work of Escobar, may be termed not simply "development, but a *discourse* of 'developmentalism'" (1995, 5ff.). Escobar's work, in part due to its empirical focus on the period after World War II, portrays developmentalism as a discourse emanating almost exclusively from Western or Western-dominated locations, such as the World Bank, the United Nations, and North American and British universities. His representations of developmentalism have been criticized for encouraging an unnecessarily homogenized and North American–centered construction (Grillo 1997). Consideration of India certainly provides an instructive contrast (but cf. also the case of China, Anagnost 1997). In India, crucial elements of the developmentalist discourse were elaborated much earlier than the time Escobar's narrative begins, not by Western experts at all but by Third World nationalists in the course of anticolonial struggle. Satish Deshpande traces the centrality of "the economy" in the imagined "nation" of the Indian nationalist struggle to the "Swadeshi" movement of the last quarter of the nineteenth and early years of the twentieth century. In that era, Indian nationalism was confronted with "the glamour of the imported commodity and the mystique of western technology" (1993, 18), not simply as so many isolated goods but as "implying certain social and moral responsibilities" (1993, 20). The ruin of the Indian handlooms by the textile industry of Lancashire had come to stand for the failure of the British colonial state to recognize these responsibilities. Deshpande traces two varied nationalist responses to this predicament, both mediated by the commodity form: on the one hand, we have Gandhi's emphasis on a nonmodern economy based on moral rather than commodity relations; and, on the other hand, we have Nehru's model of socialist planning and development economics. Chatterjee, for his part, also locates developmentalism within the central thrust of anticolonial critique. By the 1940s, he argues, the main critique of colonial rule was an economic one: colonial rule was regarded as a historical fetter on the nation's development, exploitatively creating a backward economy. Self-government was therefore legitimate because it was the historically necessary form of national development (Chatterjee 1994, 203). Accordingly, the postcolonial nation sought its distinctive content in "a new mechanism of developmental administration . . . working for the universal goals of the nation" (205). The indistinguishability of much of the postcolonial state's framework from that of the rejected and superseded colonial state made this developmental welfare bureaucracy all the more crucial as a location of newness and legitimacy.

Rationally "Planning" the Nation-Family

The discourses on population control and family planning have elaborated the centrality of a disembodied rationality and planning that is applied directly on a body that is conceived only as the passive carrier of a discrete biological fertility. How did rationality come to occupy this regulative role in governmentality, and what are its peculiarly colonial and postcolonial ramifications?

In his account of a particular form of rationality associated with the evolution of the modern state between the sixteenth and eighteenth centuries, Foucault (1991 [1978]) traces the partial displacement of an older model of the state. He finds that the definition of a good ruler in the older model of "sovereignty" is one who produces good subjects, while good subjects are in turn defined, in purely circular fashion, as those who submit to the will and authority of the sovereign. By contrast, the emergent model of the state, that of governmentality, is one that requires the government of people and things to increase the wealth of the population. For this to occur, political economy has to emerge as a separate sphere. Henceforth, to the extent that this model is able to impress itself successfully, governance must be justified through principles of rationality rather than with reference to natural or divine laws. The key point of interest to us is the centrality that Foucault assigns to the category of "population" in this new order of things. Population emerges "as a datum, as a field of intervention, and as an objective of governmental techniques" (1991 [1978], 102).

In the colonial context, the state similarly undertook such rationalizing classifications of "the population" in India, aggregating and typifying them into so many generic descriptions of castes, tribes, and religions. Crucial modifications need to be made to Foucault's account, however, when viewed from the perspective of the colonies. While India was constituted as a population and as an object of knowledge for administrative purposes, it was not constituted as a population whose wealth was to increase as a result of such rationalizing processes. Indeed, the very swiftness with which nationalists were able to draw lessons from experiences such as the ruin of the Indian handloom industry stemmed from this difference. The two dimensions of "governmentality," which coincided and provided a support for one another in the European experience, failed to coincide for the population of the colonies.

In the colonial context, therefore, governmentality took on fresh connotations. Caste and religion were not only forms of classification—they were also the features that were singled out by the colonial state as the essence of the Indian social structure and the source of its conflict-ridden divisiveness. The term *communalism*, still used to characterize religious conflict in India, has its origins in such colonial constructions (Pandey 1992). Such understandings also persist in the discourses of Indian political science, demography, and family planning, in which—as we saw earlier in this chapter—caste, region, and religion emerge as so many examples of the particular and the sectional in contrast to the rational purposes of the nation-state and its intellectuals. If, argues Chatterjee, Western theorists, such as Hegel, located the concrete expression of a more generalized rationality in the bureaucracy as "the universal class" and in the monarch "as the immediately existent will of the state," then Indian nationalists sought to locate this rationality in the head of state, and in a development bureaucracy (1994, 205).

The Indian state and the bureaucracy, in particular, assumed that the rationality of the development bureaucracy was concentrated above all in the function of *planning*. The discourse of planning elaborates and puts into operation the notion of a rational and general will, which is the premise of development. This is a consciousness that fixes priorities between long- and short-term goals and makes possible a *conscious choice* between alternative paths.

> [Planning] was a bureaucratic function, to be operated at a level above the particular interests of civil society, and institutionalized as such as a domain of policy-making outside the normal processes of representative politics and of execution through a developmental administration. But as a concrete bureaucratic function, it was in planning above all that the postcolonial state would claim its legitimacy as a single will and consciousness—the will of the nation—pursuing a task that was both universal and rational: the well-being of the people as a whole. (Chatterjee 1994, 205)

My examination of the early adoption of family planning as state policy leads me to argue for an even greater elaboration of rationality as an attribute of the new nation-subject than even Chatterjee's formulation would lead one to suspect. We find in the arguments that surround population control (from before the time of independence, and certainly by the time of the first five-year plan) a projection by nationalists of the faculty of rational planning. This is attributed not only to the Indian state but also to the potential citizens of new India. Even more radically, the nationalism requires, and indeed assumes, that citizens will practice this faculty not only in the public sphere of citizenship but in virtually every area of their lives, including the spheres of sexuality and reproduction.

The genesis of the argument for family planning is embedded within a broader argument for population control, which in turn is fed by several streams of argumentation. The economic critique of colonialism called forth the valorization of rational planning as the solution to colonial underdevelopment. At least one way in which the new nation was imagined was as an economic unit in which productivity is determined simultaneously by both an increase in production and by minimizing costs, that is, decreasing the population.

The early ramifications of the process by which the faculty of rationality was derived from economic planning but then projected onto the bodies of Indians are perfectly illustrated in a text published in the year before independence by Dwarkanath Ghosh.[9] *Pressure of Population and Economic Efficiency in India* (Ghosh 1946) underscores simultaneously the central importance of population in shaping the new nation's options and the dream quality of Ghosh's faith in a new rational consciousness on the part of Indians that will allow population goals to be adopted as everyone's personal choice. The preface states:

> Great events have happened in this country. We have entered the penultimate stage of our political development, and acquired wide powers of shaping our future. In the construction of this future the size and growth of our population will play a large part.

The book is itself meant to be an exemplum of the new rationality: "I have, moreover, endeavoured to be as objective as possible, to state the facts, analyse them and draw the conclusions which the analysis suggests." Nowhere is rationality needed more urgently than on the "population question." The precarious purchase of this rationality on Indian subjects is acknowledged, however, even in the anticipatory moments before Independence:

> As far as possible, emotions have been kept at bay; there is no economic question in which they intrude so easily and obscure reasoning as that of population. . . . Let the people of this country be population-conscious, realize its supreme importance and understand the infinite ways in which it influences their life. They will then someday agree on its solution. To-day reasoning is opposed by emotion, and conclusions carefully arrived at are opposed by unexamined prejudices. The first step in the solution of our

population question is to get out of this stage of obscurantism, and if this small book makes any contribution to this result, my labours would be amply rewarded. (Ghosh 1946, preface)

What is significant here is that, despite these fears, Ghosh is addressing not the nationalist leadership but the potential subjects *of* planning. Ghosh imagines the newly emergent Indian citizen of postindependent India as an "intelligent layman" who can be persuaded by being exposed to facts and to an analysis that simply draws the logical conclusions. In other words, the citizen-subject of independent India, who is the object of state policies, is also—ideally, at any rate—as rational as the state itself and will take on him- or herself the tasks of planning and control over his or her own body. The rationality of the intelligent layman turns out to also be a primarily economic rationale. The "facts" through which the new nation is to be imagined by the emergent citizens are economic ones:

> We, as a nation, are badly handicapped in the race of life by our mortality conditions. From the economic point of view, the manner of our growth involves an immense waste of national resources and productive capacity. First, we nurse, feed, clothe, house, and train every batch of newly born population only to lose 45% of them before they reach the age of 15 at which they can make any contribution to national income. (Ghosh 1946, 22)

In this scenario, in which human life and death become translated into economic resources and costs, Ghosh considers whether industrialization, rationally planned to encourage coordination as well as minimizing dependency on foreign capital (93), will be sufficient to offset the increase in population attendant on welfare and health improvements (72). He finds it insufficient in the absence of population measures, and the book culminates in an argument for contraceptive technology to be widely distributed.

The triumph of such a developmentalist liberalism seemed complete by the time of the first five-year plan (1951–56). The plan came out unambiguously and confidently in favor of a state-sponsored family planning policy, involving provision of facilities for sterilization and giving advice on contraception.

Yet there were other competing visions of the new nation that had to be marginalized in order for this to happen. I cannot give Gandhi's framework the treatment it deserves in this chapter, yet it is important to mark the fact that Gandhi provides the resources for quite an alternative conceptualization of the emergence of Indian subjecthood in the new nation-state. Here the emergent subject is a moral subject, rather than the bourgeois citizen-subject of political theory. Where the bourgeois citizen-subject is eligible for certain rights and civic responsibilities on the basis of rationality, Gandhi exhorts Indians to claim their subjecthood through a quest for moral truths. In articles published in the journal *Young India* from 1913 onward, right through to *Key to Health,* the book written in jail in 1942, Gandhi seeks to unlock the potential for a great nation through a regimen of bodily self-discipline (Alter 1996). His stance on birth control derives from this quest. *Ahimsa* (nonviolence), *satya* (truth), and the quest for self-restraint dictate a view of the body as a site to exercise moral rather than technological regulation. *Brahmacharya,* or the vow of sexual abstinence, was principally a mode of self-regulation. Yet it also allowed the regulation of births in a way that not only avoided the reliance on modern industrial technology but also encouraged men in particular to relinquish their selfish subjugation of women in keeping with the moral virtue of *aparigraha,* or nonpossession.

Gandhi's views on the matter were much publicized in India after a meeting with Margaret Sanger, who had been invited to address the All-India Women's Conference (AIWC) in 1935 at which resolutions approving birth control for health and welfare reasons were eventually accepted. Gandhi's larger vision, within which his views on birth control were embedded, was in the event subsumed by one that stressed developmentalism and liberal democratic values. Yet his legacy is being reviewed all over again as the limits of liberalism explode in postcolonial India[10]—while emancipatory discourses such as contemporary feminism must be said to share at least a common orientation with Gandhi insofar as they place emancipatory subjecthood (here of women) at the center, rather than at the periphery, of policies such as birth control.[11]

The Five-Year Plan and the Family Plan

The five-year plan had to mediate between the terms provided by a liberal democratic constitution and the terms provided by developmentalism. Population control evidently owes more to the imperatives of the latter than of the former, both in the arguments leading up to its adoption and in the actual implementation of the policy in subsequent years. The first plan, however, attempted to bridge the gulf. It tried to derive *family planning* from *population control*. More accurately, it simply assumed a coincidence between the welfare of the nation and the welfare of the family. The rationale for the adoption of state-sponsored family planning is given in the plan as a happy coincidence of what is necessary and desirable for both nation and family:

(a) The reduction of the birthrate to the extent necessary to stabilize the population at a level consistent with the requirements of the national economy.
(b) Family limitations or spacing of children is necessary and desirable in order to secure better health for the mother and better care and upbringing of children. (First Five-Year Plan, cited in Raina 1988, 10)

Rationality is imputed not only to the state planners but also to the individuals who must take up the task of planning their families. The subcommittee of the Planning Commission (leading up to the first five-year plan) makes its recommendation in the following terms:

> Family limitation is necessary and desirable in the interest of the family. It is necessary and desirable that the members of every family comprising the nation take all suitable and practicable steps for securing that the occurrence of a birth in the family is properly spaced in time and limited in number, so as to safeguard the health of the mother and child and enable an adequate share of the resources of the family being applied effectively to the care and upbringing of children. (Cited in Raina 1988, 6)

Just as the nation-state must embody universal rationality on behalf of the welfare of the nation, so the family members must come to take on the attributes of rationality in order to plan the welfare of the whole family.

Even more strikingly, both sets of rational planners are motivated by a concern for the welfare of the underprivileged members within their domain. The nation-state emerged from the anticolonial struggle with a strong brief for giving equality a substantive content: reservations and affirmative action policies for lower castes, for which provisions were made in the Constitution itself; agrarian land reform for the peasants; maternal health programs for women and children; and constitutional protection for the religious rights of minority religions. The family emerges in the discourse of family planning as endowed with exactly the same faculty and goals of exercising rational planning in protecting the welfare of *its* "weaker sections," its minorities—namely, women and children. The family, no less than the nation, is an economic unit. The "family plan," therefore, treats the family as an economic unity, with its resources to be assessed and allocated through the application of a single rational will. This rational will is exercised in terms of choices that conceptualize time in the same way that the five-year plan conceptualizes the time of the nation: in terms of "proper spacing" of output/births as well as limits placed on total costs. In the process, the welfare of all is secured but, more particularly, the welfare of the underprivileged members—minorities, mothers, and infants—is improved in accordance with the logic of developmentalism.

We see here a mixed relation between state and family. On the one hand, there is a relation of homology, in which the state takes care of "the weaker sections" through planning, just as women and children are taken care of through family planning. In this scenario, the rational planner in the family is implicitly masculine, and, indeed, those elements of family planning policy that minimize women's agency elaborate precisely such a masculinism. Menon and Bhasin's striking exploration (this volume) of the newly independent state's attempt to recover and rehabilitate women perceived as "out of place" when they can no longer be located in their "proper" family structure is another example of this homology between state and patriarchal authority.

On the other hand, coexisting with this tendency and in tension with it is the break that the Indian state attempts to effect with this patriarchal model of sovereignty by imputing to the family (implicitly, at least, to all adult members of the family) the same rationality and locating it in the same empty, homogeneous time as that which the nation-state inhabits. Both the state and this imaginary family inhabit a time that is measurable in terms of planned intervals ("spacing"). Both the state and family exercise their rational agency over the reproductive bodies that fall within their respective units of political economy.

The uniqueness of this second tendency, even if it exists primarily at an imaginary level, comes into clearer relief if we compare it with modern Western political theory. In the West, natural law theorists such as Hobbes and Locke attempt to effect a break with the classical model of political authority, in which the family occupies the central place in economic as well as political relations. This model, handed down since Aristotle (Bobbio 1993, 13; but also cf. Foucault 1991 [1978], 99) and predicated on precapitalist relations of production, is the one that Hobbes and Locke, in their different ways, depart from. They posit, instead, a new realm of civil society that is characterized by free and autonomous individuals consenting to states of affairs and entering into contracts. The family is not part of this recharacterization of political life. Instead, the theorists drive a sharp wedge between this civil society and the family, which is now located in the state of nature. Henceforth, the political life of the state is legitimized by principles entirely different to the principles that legitimize the power of "a Father over his Children, a Master over his Servant, a Husband over his Wife, and a Lord over his Slave" (Locke, cited by Bobbio 1993, 17). As feminist theorists, such as Pateman (1989), have pointed out, such a carving out of spheres has effectively left women without recourse to democratic rights in the realm of the family and, equally, has made it anomalous to be both a woman and a citizen. Whatever the differences between "conservatives" like Hobbes and "liberals" like Locke, both concur that principles of rationality and contract cannot possibly extend to the family.

In India, by contrast, the "Nehruvian" imagining of the nation attributes the same rational capacities to the family as it assumes for the state. Why did the leadership of the newly emergent state feel impelled to expand the exercise of rationality from the state to the family in such an extraordinary fashion? In my account, this tendency emerges as no mere fanciful wish. Rather, it is one of the few ways in which the contradictory imperatives of liberal democratic discourse and developmentalist discourse could be reconciled, if only, as I have stressed, in imaginary terms.

Remove this imaginary creature, the superrational subject of family planning, and we are left with two scenarios, both of which are unpleasant to contemplate. In the first, we have a developmental agenda that is really concerned only with population control, rather than with either participatory democracy or the provision of safe contraceptive choices to individuals. The events of the Emergency, but also the general tenor of the implementation of policy, amply testify to the ease with which such a scenario can emerge. Or, in the second scenario, we have a more scrupulous adherence to liberal democratic values, but, in the process, the state becomes unable to implement its developmental interventions. As we have seen, intellectuals adopting "the view of the established state" proffer precisely such an assessment of the fortunes of family planning. It is presented as a victim to the way in which groups have manipulated the democratic ideals of the Indian state.

The superrational subject of family planning allows state policy formulation to proceed as if neither of these undesirable scenarios need apply to India. Individuals in the new India will come to *choose freely* for themselves goals that synchronize with the developmental goals of the nation, because both are impelled by the same rational subjectivity. In this sense, the rational subject is a kind of wish-fulfilling dream formation for the state, reconciling otherwise contradictory imperatives.

A comparison between India and China illuminates the broader postcolonial politics of this "dreaming." In both cases, the state initially adopted rationally planned economic development as the socialist alternative, not only to its capitalist "other" (Anagnost 1997, 122; but see Sigley, this volume) but to specifically colonialist forms of capitalism. In both cases "reproduction becomes the locus for the imposition of a planning rationality that will demonstrate the superiority of socialism" (Anagnost 1997, 122). In India, however, the adoption of the socialist model was diluted in the economy by the presence of private enterprise and in politics by the presence of liberal doctrines. In both countries the relation between state and population was shaped by the politics of mass mobilization before the Congress and the Communist Party of China came to power. Such a history led to a construction of "the people" as already equipped with the requisite attributes for full political sovereignty. In India, with its adoption of a more liberal-democratic formulation of politics, this took, as we have seen, the form of attributing a rationally choosing and planning subjectivity to its citizens, who will freely and independently take up the same projects as the state. On this basis, the socialist faith in planned development and the liberal principle of electoral participation were artificially conjoined. In China, Mao's faith in the people led him initially to eschew any version of population control, characterizing eugenics as a "tool of imperialism" (Anagnost 1995, 29), until the famines of 1959 to 1962 and the first national census results convinced him and other leaders otherwise. It took another twenty years for mandatory population control measures to be pursued, when surveys indicated a disproportionate number of women of childbearing age (Handwerker 1995, 360)—striking testimony to Foucault's suggestion that statistics, population, and governmentality are intimately linked. By the 1970s, "overpopulation" came to be recognized as a threat to national development; and, in 1979, China instituted the world's first compulsory one-child policy.

In both India and China, a further dimension of the postcolonial predicament is this: despite the desire to impute a certain self-sufficiency to the people, the project of state-driven modernity simultaneously comes up against the fact that the people are also characterized by lack or backwardness. In India, they are retarded by the forces of religion and caste; in China, in the language of socialism, they are held back by "feudal" practices. Here a difference between India and China shows up in the degree to which the state undertakes to refashion the population to measure up to the project of modernity. In China, the one-child policy is enforced through rewards (job promotion, bonus money, better housing, educational facilities) and punishments (fines, job transfers, demotions) as well as a massive ideological campaign combined with unprecedented efforts at governmentality entailing "the management of every aspect of ordinary life, including registration of marriages, births, deaths, adoption, residence" and the use of state collectives and street committees (Handwerker 1995, 362). In India, on the other hand, we have seen that state authoritarianism has to contend with competing political principles. In India, therefore, the tensions in the postcolonial dream formation show up in the contradictory character of state policy, as it explicitly disavows the excesses of Emergency, only to have the repressed content reemerge in other forms.

The report of the Working Group of the latest five-year plan (Eighth Five-Year Plan 1990) is a classic instance of this contradictory policy. The report recommends that incentives be disallowed at the individual level either to acceptors or to family planning program workers or to government employees. The next recommendation simply shifts the jurisdiction of state control, from control over the individual to control over the "community." Recommendation 4.8(d) states that funds for community rural development—which includes fundamental resources such as water and sanitation in this list—should be allocated to "communities having achieved certain levels of family planning practice and maternal and child health" (1990, 17).

Recently, the Ministry of Health and Family Welfare released the *Manual on Target Free Approach in Family Welfare Programme* (1996), recommending a shift away from targets toward an approach driven by the demand for quality services. The document is currently being debated by health activists and women's groups, who welcome the shift but are renegotiating certain familiar patterns: the rationale for the change in policy is understood in terms of the technical incapacity of the previous approach to reduce birthrates, rather than in terms of its inability to meet the needs of the people. The new patterns of monitoring and evaluation are still to be implemented from the top, and, although auxiliary nurse midwives are asked to work closely with other field-level personnel, no role is allocated to local women themselves in evaluating or monitoring the program (Sen 1996). The example of China, where local women *are* drawn into becoming "birth workers" but only in order to better effect a local surveillance of state policy (Handwerker 1995), further alerts us to the fact that women's involvement or lack of involvement cannot be made into the sole criterion of real change in this respect but must be contextualized through a wider appraisal of the field of power.

Conclusion

Western feminist philosophical critiques of Reason, such as Lloyd's *Man of Reason* (1984), find that the exclusions wrought by the operation of Reason find their key Other in the construction of femininity as the inferior binary of Reason. In postcolonial societies such as India, reason and rationality—in the specific and somewhat narrow sense that these terms have acquired within modernity—are not associated with an independent and indigenous philosophical tradition but, rather, with the colonial and postcolonial state's function as the main interpreter and harbinger of modernity. I have argued that a certain view of rationality underlies and links the consciousness attributed by the state first to itself, as the planner of the nation, and then to its subjects, both as citizens and as carriers of a reproductive consciousness that is specifically modern. It is important to stress that this combination of reason and developmental modernity excludes far more than just femininity. Those whose reproductive consciousness can be shown to be affected by the supposedly "premodern"—by religion, by caste, by patriarchy (in its specifically premodern form), by language and ethnicity, even by poverty itself—become marked as "irrational." It is important to bear in mind that the same coercive strategies applied since the Emergency in relation to poor women were pursued in the sterilization of poor men before the Emergency.[12]

Anthropological accounts of fertility are increasingly highlighting the complexity of reproductive behavior and consciousness—not only is fertility inextricably "situated" by the power relations and dynamics of social location, but it is marked by "the ambiguity, spontaneity, and improvisation, the bungling, changing-of-mind, and full-scale about-faces that characterize most peoples' lives, reproductive and otherwise" (Greenhalgh 1995, 22). State-sponsored technologies, such as sterilization, are therefore particularly starkly at odds with human consciousness, even before we add the enormous uncertainties faced by the poor in terms of the survival of their existing children.

Despite this growing anthropological challenge to the assumptions of demographers and planners (see also Carter 1995; Robertson 1984; Robinson, this volume), this body of work remains separate from debates on citizenship and political theory. Yet the two domains of demography and citizenship are integrally linked in India by notions of rationality and modernization. Since rationality is supposed to be a marker of the citizen-subject who can identify with the state's vision of the needs of the nation as a whole, the bearer of a premodern reproductive consciousness becomes the Other of citizenship, marked as sectarian, sectional, irresponsible. Given the impossibility of finding Indians who measure up to the stringent identity of citizenship, it is small wonder that the discourse on minorities multiplies the number of minorities almost as rapidly as the "breeding" attributed to the minorities themselves.

In the context of current mobilization against Muslim "minorities" in the name of the democratic rights of the Hindu majority, the contribution of population and family planning discourses to the construction of minority status needs to be taken particularly seriously. The liberal state is accused by religious nationalists of "pandering" to a Muslim minority that, in not submitting to the reform of its personal law, has shown itself to be unwilling to be suitably modern. It is no coincidence that accusations of identical phrasing are directed toward the Indian state for not being coercive *enough* in relation to making family planning compulsory. The two accusations fuse easily, as in anti-Muslim propaganda: those who do not inhabit a suitably modern family (equipped with lifelong monogamy, nuclear family, educated husband and wife) and who will not have their personal laws reformed by the state to produce such a family are the main perpetrators of overbreeding. Since they simultaneously violate the requirements of rationality, modernity, and citizenship, they do not deserve the freedoms and civil liberties bestowed by a liberal democratic state.

Yet the threat from religious nationalism should not lead us to overlook the dangers of embracing a version of secular modernity that is excessively narrow in its interpretation both of reason and of citizenship. I have not attempted in this chapter to venture into the question of how we might reconceptualize citizenship in the light of these criticisms.[13] What my examination of family planning as state policy does indicate is that ideals of modern reproductive consciousness and of modern citizenship, interlinked as we have found them to be, exclude far too much of social life, with its complexities of class, gender, and caste—as well as the varied forms of embodied existence that attend such forms of diversity.

NOTES

1. I have been unable, given the scope of this chapter, to incorporate one of the key elements of left critiques of population policies: the pressures placed on the Indian state by international agencies such as the World Bank, United Nations' advisory missions, United States Agency for International Development, etc. Current debates on this set of issues focus on the impact of structural adjustment programs for health care. On family planning and the impact of the 1993 World Development report, see essays by Rao and others in *Social Scientist* 22 (9–12) (Rao 1994b).

2. A clear example of such a conundrum is the way in which the liberal components of protecting individual rights requires the Constitution to separate the practice of "Hinduism" (guaranteed under the right to pursue religious belief) from the maintenance of caste inequalities (an infringement of the rights of others). Thus, temples are open to all castes, unless a religious group can show that it needs to exclude others not as a result of their caste position but because of its pursuit of its own distinctive religious character, appealing to the right to manage its own affairs free of interference (Galanter 1989, 176).

3. In an independent analysis on Tamil Nadu's recent demographic "successes" in bringing down fertility rates, Padmini Swaminathan observes: "Our very limited interaction with NGOs active in this field in Tamil Nadu reveal that a large number of abortions take place outside the formal system since very often the state through its family planning outlets tries to impose its own morality on women seeking abortions" (1996, 13).

4. Seminar on "Users' Perspective on Acceptability of Norplant and Diaphragm," 17 August 1996, Mahabalipuram, Tamil Nadu, organized by RUWSEC.

5. The curriculum devised by the National Council for Education, Research and Training provides only for talks on the small family norm and population control, not sex education.

6. TV Antony (1992) has been attributing the fertility decline to the superior sta-

tus of women in the south, thanks to the Dravidian kinship system and the efforts of the early leadership in the regional nationalist Dravidian movement.

7. Such a conscious desire for reproductive control is itself not the unambiguous sign of progress it is interpreted to be in discourses of developmentalism. Taken in the wider context of a deterioration in certain dimensions of female status, such control over births may be exercised on a gender-selective basis, with particularly grievous consequences for girl babies. The phenomenon of female feticide has been a growing problem in Indian cities and small towns from the mid-1970s onward, associated particularly with the rapid proliferation of amniocentisis technology (Menon 1996). Certain parts of rural Tamil Nadu have become notorious for female infanticide.

8. For a review and critique of the "mainstream of thinking on the Indian Emergency" in relation to family planning, see Vicziany 1982, esp. pt. 1.

9. I am not investigating here the colonial prehistory of the possibility of this text, but a fuller examination of this kind would evidently need to inquire into the ways in which the colonial state itself established the precedents for a conceptualization of India in terms of numerical aggregates, enumerating communities in terms of fixed attributes, through the process of census taking beginning in 1891. The classic account of census taking in colonial India remains Cohn's account (1987), but see also Barrier 1981. Equally important in the colonial politicization of population as an electoral issue was the move to set aside special electorates for Muslims as a minority. It was a move that was opposed by nationalists but which continues to resonate strongly in contemporary Indian politics, as in the charge that the Indian state "panders" to the Muslim minority.

10. Discussions on the twin legacies of Gandhi and Nehru for postcolonial India are one of the features of intellectual stocktaking that is occurring in contemporary India. See, for example, essays by Parekh, Rao, Chatterjee, and Nandy (Parekh and Pantham 1987).

11. In an essay first presented to the conference "Rethinking Indian Modernity: The Political Economy of Indian Sexuality" in Chennai, Anandhi (1998) has traced other lineages of the present-day women's health movement in the language and efforts of women such as First Secretary Kamaladevi Chattopadhyay of AIWC, who was instrumental in making the AIWC adopt resolutions in favor of birth control clinics from the 1930s onward. She also emphasizes the path-breaking discourse of the leader of the Self-Respect Movement in Tamil Nadu, Periyar E. V. Ramasamy, who argued that contraception was essential not for women's health or the national economy but "for women to be free and autonomous." She argues that his concept of female autonomy included not only education and employment but sexual freedom.

12. For a detailed account of the implementation of state-sponsored vasectomies before the Emergency, see Vicziany 1982, pt. 2.

13. Western feminists, such as Genevieve Lloyd (1984), have examined the exclusion of the feminine from Western philosophy in the name of Reason; while other writers, such as Anne Phillips (1993), have argued that it may be possible to envision a politics in which identities of gender and other forms of difference are transformed, rather than transcended, in the public sphere. In my own work I have been concerned to do justice to the varied ways of experiencing one's reproductive embodiment that are available in a country like India and which are in tension with the discourses of rationalized bodies (see Ram 1994, 1998b, c).

REFERENCES

Alter, J. 1996. Gandhi's body, Gandhi's truth: Nonviolence and the biomoral imperative of public health. *Journal of Asian Studies* 55 (2): 301–22.

Anagnost, A. 1995. A surfeit of bodies: Population and the rationality of the state in post-Mao China. In *Conceiving the new world order: The global politics of reproduction*, ed. F. D. Ginsburg and R. Rapp, 22–41. Berkeley: University of California Press.

———. 1997. *National past-times: Narrative, representation, and power in modern China*. Durham and London: Duke University Press.

Anandhi, S. 1998. Reproductive bodies and regulated sexuality: Birth control debates in early twentieth century Tamilnadu. In *A question of silence? The sexual economies of modern India*, ed. M. E. John and J. Nair, 139–66. New Delhi: Kali for Women.

Barrier, N. G. 1981. *The census in British India: New perspectives*. New Delhi: Manohar.

Basu, A. M. 1992. *Culture, the status of women, and demographic behaviour*. Oxford: Clarendon Press.

Bobbio, N. 1993. *Thomas Hobbes and the natural law tradition*. Chicago and London: University of Chicago Press.

Carter, A. 1995. Agency and fertility: For an ethnography of practice. In *Situating fertility: Anthropology and demographic inquiry*, ed. S. Greenhalgh, 55–85. Cambridge: Cambridge University Press.

Chatterjee, P. 1986. *Nationalist thought and the colonial world: A derivative discourse?* London: Zed Books for the United Nations University.

———. 1994. *The nation and its fragments: Colonial and postcolonial histories*. Delhi: Oxford University Press.

Cohn, B. 1987. The census, social structure and objectification in South Asia. In *An anthropologist among the historians and other essays*, ed. B. S. Cohn, 224–54. Delhi: Oxford University Press.

Das, V. 1995. The anthropological discourse on India: Reason and its Other. In *Critical events: An anthropological perspective on contemporary India*, ed. V. Das, 24–54. Delhi: Oxford University Press.

Deshpande, S. 1993. Imagined economies. *Journal of Arts and Ideas* 25–26:5–35.

Eighth Five Year Plan. 1990. *Population projections and family planning: Report of the Working Group*. New Delhi: Planning Commission.

Escobar, A. 1995. *Encountering development: The making and unmaking of the Third World*. Princeton, N.J.: Princeton University Press.

Foucault, M. 1991 [1978]. Governmentality. In *The Foucault effect: Studies in governmentality*, ed. G. Burchell, C. Gordon, and P. Miller, 87–104. London: Harvester Wheatsheaf.

Galanter, M. 1989. *Law and society in modern India*. Delhi: Oxford University Press.

Gandotra, M. M., and N. Das. 1984. *Population policy in India: With special reference to infant mortality and fertility*. Bombay: Blackie and Son Publishers.

Ghosh, D. 1946. *Pressure of population and economic efficiency in India*. Bombay: Oxford University Press.

Greenhalgh, S. 1995. Anthropology theorizes reproduction: Integrating practice, political economic, and feminist perspectives. In *Situating fertility: Anthropology and demographic inquiry*, ed. S. Greenhalgh, 3–28. Cambridge and New York: Cambridge University Press.

Grillo, R. D. 1997. Discourses of development: The view from anthropology. In *Discourses of development: Anthropological perspectives,* ed. R. D. Grillo and R. L. Stirrat, 1–33. Oxford: Berg.
Handwerker, L. 1995. The hen that can't lay an egg (*"Bu xia dan de mu ji"*): Conceptions of female infertility in modern China. In *Deviant bodies: Critical perspectives on difference in science and popular culture,* ed. J. Terry and J. Urla, 358–86. Bloomington and Indianapolis: Indiana University Press.
Hasan, Z. 1996. Uniformity versus equality: Gender, minority identity and the debate on the uniform civil code. Paper given at "Communications with/in Asia," Twentieth Anniversary Conference of the Asian Studies Association of Australia, La Trobe University, Melbourne, 8–11 July.
Indian Health Activists. 1992[?]. *Report: Norplant—an account of its use in Bangladesh,* roneoed pamphlet.
IPP VIII [Indian Population Project VIII]. N.d. Summary of the findings of surveys on fertility, contraception and health and family welfare service delivery system for Delhi's urban slums (*Jhuggi-Jhompri bustees*). New Delhi: Government of India/UNICEF.
Jeffrey, R. 1992. *Politics, women and well-being: How Kerala became "a model."* Basingstoke: Macmillan.
Lloyd, G. 1984. *The man of reason: "Male" and "female" in Western philosophy.* London: Methuen.
Menon, N. 1996. The impossibility of "justice": Female foeticide and feminist discourse on abortion. In *Social reform, sexuality and the state,* ed. P. Uberoi, 369–92. New Delhi: Sage Publications.
Ministry of Health and Family Welfare. 1996. *Manual on target free approach in family welfare programme.* New Delhi: Ministry of Health, Government of India.
Narayana, G., and J. F. Kantner. 1992. *Doing the needful: The dilemma of India's population policy.* Boulder: Westview Press.
Pai Panandiker, V. A., and P. K. Umashankar. 1994. Fertility control and politics in India. In *The new politics of population: Conflict and consensus in family planning,* ed. J. L. Finkle and C. A. McIntosh, 89–104. New York: Population Council.
Pandey, G. 1991. In defence of the fragment: Writing about Hindu-Muslim riots in India today. *Economic and Political Weekly* 26 (11–12): 559–72.
———. 1992. *The construction of communalism in colonial north India.* Delhi: Oxford University Press.
Parekh, B., and T. Pantham, eds. 1987. *Political discourse: Explorations in Indian and Western political thought.* New Delhi: Sage Publications.
Pateman, C. 1989. *The disorder of women: Democracy, feminism and political theory.* Cambridge: Polity Press.
Phillips, A. 1993. *Democracy and difference.* Cambridge: Polity Press.
Raghuram, S., and A. Rahman. 1996. Charting the reproductive rights agenda. In *Rethinking population,* ed. S. Raghuram and A. Rahman, 1–7. Proceedings of a consultation on women's health and rights. Technical Report series, 1.4. Bangalore: Hivos Regional Office South Asia; and New York: Center for Reproductive Law and Policy.
Raina, B. L. 1988. *Population policy.* Delhi: BR Publishing Corporation.
Ram, K. 1994. Medical management and giving birth: Responses of coastal women in

Tamil Nadu. *Motherhood, fatherhood and fertility. Reproductive health matters*, special issue 4:20–26.

———. 1998a. Nāshariram nādhi, "my body is mine": The urban women's health movement in India and its negotiations of modernity. *Migrating feminisms: The Asia/Pacific region. Women's Studies International Forum*, special issue 21 (6): 617–31.

———. 1998b. Maternity and the story of enlightenment in the colonies: Tamil coastal women, south India. In *Maternities and modernities: Colonial and postcolonial experiences in Asia and the Pacific*, ed. K. Ram and M. Jolly, 114–43. Cambridge: Cambridge University Press.

———. 1998c. Uneven modernities and ambivalent sexualities: Women's constructions of puberty in coastal Kanyakumari, Tamilnadu. In *A question of silence? The sexual economies of modern India*, ed. M. E. John and J. Nair, 269–303. New Delhi: Kali for Women.

Rao, M. 1994a. Voices from the wilderness. *Voices* 1 (2): 3–9.

———. 1994b. The writing on the wall: Structural adjustment programme and the World Development Report 1993—implications for family planning in India. *Social Scientist* 22 (9–12): 56–78.

Ravindran, T. K. S. 1993. Users' perspectives on fertility regulation methods. *Economic and Political Weekly* 28 (46–47): 2508–12.

———. N.d. Factors contributing to fertility transition in Tamil Nadu: A qualitative investigation (in conjunction with UNDP project on "Strategies and Financing for Human Resource Development").

Robertson, A. F. 1984. *People and the state: An anthropology of planned development*. Cambridge: Cambridge University Press.

Rushdie, S. 1995. *The Moor's last sigh*. London: Jonathan Cape.

Sangari, K. 1995. Politics of diversity: Religious communities and multiple patriarchies (pts. 1–2). *Economic and Political Weekly* 30 (51): 3287–310; (52): 3381–89.

Sen, G. 1996. Review of *Manual on target free approach in family welfare programme*, by Ministry of Health and Family Welfare; May (draft response). Bangalore: Indian Institute of Management.

Shah Commission of Inquiry. 1978. *Third and final report*. New Delhi: Ministry of Home Affairs.

Soni, V. 1984. The development and current organisation of the family planning programme. In *India's demography: Essays on the contemporary population*, ed. T. Dyson and N. Crook, 141–57. Atlantic Highlands, N.J.: Humanities Press.

Soonawala, R. P. 1992. Family planning: The Indian experience. In *Family planning: Meeting challenges—promoting choices*, ed. P. Senanayake and R. L. Kleinman, 77–87. Proceedings of the IPPF Family Planning Congress. Lancaster and New York: Parthenon Publishing Group.

Srikantan, K. S., K. Balasubramian, and S. Nikam. 1984. The performance of India's family planning programme. In *India's demography: Essays on the contemporary population*, ed. T. Dyson and N. Crook, 159–74. Atlantic Highlands, N.J.: Humanities Press.

Swaminathan, P. 1996. The failures of success? An analysis of Tamilnadu's recent demographic experience. Working Paper no. 144. Madras: Madras Institute of Development Studies.

TV Antony. 1992. The family planning programme—lessons from Tamil Nadu's experience. *Indian Journal of Social Science* 5 (3): n.p.

Vicziany, M. 1982. Coercion in a soft state: The family-planning program of India. Pt. 1: The myth of voluntarism; pt. 2: The sources of coercion. *Pacific Affairs* 55 (3): 373–402; (4): 557–92.

Working Group on Women's Rights. N.d. *Civil codes and personal laws: Reversing the option.* New Delhi: Working Group on Women's Rights.

CHAPTER 4

Keep It in the Family: Government, Marriage, and Sex in Contemporary China

Gary Sigley

Problematizing the Family as a Site of Government

It has been popular among various accounts of the family in the first three decades of the People's Republic of China to perceive the traditional Confucian family as a major obstacle for Communist Party policy (such as in Kazuko 1989 [1978]; Orleans 1972; Yang 1959). If we take the "traditional Confucian family" to imply rigid feudal patriarchy and fierce opposition to all the trappings that go along with a modern discourse on the family, then this may indeed be the case. The Marriage Law of 1950 puts the "traditional family" well within its sights when it explicitly calls for equality between husband and wife, the abolition of arranged marriages, and equal rights to divorce. Campaign after campaign is incessantly waged against "feudal" family vestiges in both urban and rural areas. It thus appears at first glance that the Communist Party of China (CPC) has made a concerted effort to "liberate" the family, and in particular women, from the shackles of feudalism and patriarchy.

Yet when we investigate the matter more closely this apparently stern opposition between traditional Confucian and radical Communist family systems begins to become increasingly unstable. There is certainly a great deal of concern in the present period with the continuing persistence of "feudal remnants" within the modern Chinese family, such as the reemergence of female infanticide and the abduction and selling of women and children. But there is also equal concern with the deterioration of family relations between children and parents and between husband and wife. Conventional values concerning the veneration of elders and the role of virtuous mothers and wives are then redeployed in an attempt to rectify these problems.

It is precisely this discourse of "liberation" from the shackles of feudal remnants that needs to be addressed here. Rather than propounding a radical view of the family and the means of its transformation, Chinese authorities have remained, in large part, staunchly "conservative." Apart from periods of excessive communalization such as occurred during the Great Leap Forward (1958), rather than attempting to abolish the "natural" realm of the family (as much of the anticommunist propaganda of the time assumed), the People's Government has deployed and developed numerous methods for enlisting family members into various governmental programs that take the family unit as the point of departure. "Liberation" refers as much to "enlistment" as it does to "freedom."

The fields of hygiene, health, reproduction, juvenile delinquency, and so on have, in some way or another, been caught up in this governmental discourse on the family. No less than bourgeois Western political discourse, the family is understood as the "basic cell of society" in which practices of marriage, sexual relations, child rearing, and social welfare take place. If only the family can be managed well, then social stability and prosperity will inevitably follow. It has been the government's concern therefore to enlist family members, particularly mothers, in these various normative programs in order to reshape familial conduct.

In some ways this mimics the classical relationship between Confucian government and the family—the family is incapable of conducting itself correctly and thus requires both moral guidance and physical intervention. It is this relationship and its strategic operation on the part of the various participants (that is, the Confucian elite and the "common people") that in some ways sets the ground for the way in which the problem of the population, reproduction and, indeed, the family is constructed. Two broad kinds of relationship between state and popular culture may be distinguished in this instance. Either a cultural and social elite attempts to set up a rigid distinction between their values (political, esthetic, sexual, economic) and those of the "common people"; or these elites attempt to "mold" the conduct of the "common people" in more favorable directions. Both of these options have operated in China at some time or another, but it is more the attempts to shape popular culture in its image that has the strongest tendencies. Much of Confucian discourse deals with educating (*jiaohua*) the common people so as to universalize social propriety and rites (*li*)—"there is nobody that cannot receive instruction"[1] runs a famous Confucian maxim. This perception of cultural practices also extends to the Chinese conceptual division between a "cultured" civilization and a "barbarous" one—culture as defined in terms of certain "techniques of living."[2]

Patricia Ebrey (1991, 153–54), for instance, refers to the efforts of scholars and government officials to promote the neo-Confucian Song dynasty philosopher Zhu Xi's (1130–1200) famous work *Family Rituals*. There was a persistent concern on the part of the elite to transform the practices of the masses and impose their own Confucian esthetics of conduct. As Ebrey notes, "many scholars and officials retained the belief, already common in the Sung, that promulgating models for ritual performance was not simply a symbolic gesture but was one of the most effective means of promoting good behavior among the common people" (1991, 155). Scholars regularly made distinctions between *li* (authentic rituals) and *su* (vulgar familial traditions) and sought to promote the moral transformative qualities of *li* while demeaning the degenerative practices of *su* (1991, 10–11).[3]

The problematization of familial conduct is thus not new. There have, of course, been a number of significant shifts in the relation between government and the family, most notably the high level of technical intervention into everyday practice, the nuclearization of the family in most urban areas and the dissemination of many of the larger family's functions to the socialist work-unit (Davis and Harrell 1993, 1–2; Kane 1987, 137; Peng Xizhe 1989, 36). What I am arguing here is that Chinese government of the family, marriage and reproduction is an amalgamation of various forms of knowledge and practice, some of which have distinct historical antecedents within China and others that bear the indelible marks of importation. This approach involves an equal refutation of "the new" replacing "the old" and "the old" haunting "the new." What it does entail is acknowledging that these governmental practices have unique and often innovative histories that deserve highly specific historiographic or, to use a term more in vogue, genealogical attention.[4]

This study draws upon a range of textual sources, and, while it attempts to give as wide a coverage as possible, it cannot attempt to speak of marriage, family, and sex as uniform phenomena. There is a great deal of variation within China according to region, class, ethnicity, and gender. Most of the discussion here focuses on official (or at least semiofficial) pronouncements found in academic writing and popular publications (advice literature). The latter constitute the main body of textual evidence and are readily available at most corner newsstands and bookstores (especially in urban centers). I have endeavored to understand the statements manifest in these texts from the perspective of governmental reasoning—that is, the way in which various governmental agents (which includes any institution or discourse concerned with managing the conduct of others) have conceived of the object to be governed (in this case that of the heterosexual married couple, but also to a lesser extent the premarital subject).

In this chapter I thus analyze this diverse array of knowledges and techniques centered on the Chinese family. In particular, concern will focus on the family as a site for regulating reproduction and pleasure. We will soon see how the management of birth has in some ways meant actually encouraging marital sex, at least insofar as sex and procreation are rendered as distinct practices. I will also endeavor to trace how a distinct intellectual perception of the family within Chinese sociological discourse has serious ramifications for the moral management of the family. In so doing, we will be in a more favorable position from which to gauge the importance of mothers and wives as relays within the Chinese governmental nexus. This ensemble of forms of knowledge and areas of problematization can be schematically divided into a number of distinct yet interconnected topics. These are: a unique sociology of the family, marriage as a means of policing the family, an economy of sexual pleasure, and a concern with mothers and wives as relays for governmental programs, topics that this chapter addresses sequentially.

Speaking of the Family

Before we do so, I first pose a question: When we speak of the "traditional" and "modern" family are we speaking of the same thing? Is the family an always-already preexistent entity that in China finally succumbs to the rigors of government?[5] In order to appreciate the significance of this way of understanding the family, some conceptual and methodological bearings on what is meant by "the family" is necessary. In particular we need to examine the various ways in which the idea of the family has become constituted as a site of government.

Jacques Donzelot's (1979) *The Policing of Families* goes some way toward clarifying this problem. Donzelot argues that the family is the product of a modern history, the result of an intersection of various governmental programs. This modern family is contrasted to the form of social organization under the ancien régime. Unlike conventional histories of the family, Donzelot does not describe the way in which government comes to act upon the pregiven family unit, but rather how governmental reasoning comes to formulate and construct the family as an object and technique of government itself. The family is "*reconstructed* as an intimate environment through the action of social policy" (Minson 1985, 183).

It is at this point, sometime in the eighteenth and nineteenth centuries, that the family emerges as a key component in the shifting balance between "public" and "private." Under Western liberal reasoning the family is "private" insofar as it is hidden from the direct glare of the state and allowed to run its "natural" course. It is "public" insofar as Western liberal reasoning, often in the guise of philanthropy and hygienist movements, isolates key family members and enlists them in various campaigns to address the "failure" of the family unit. *Hybridization* is the term used to describe this coming together of private and public functions. Thus, while the family is separated from social and political life, new ways of governing its relations reconstitute and reconstruct the family.

The family is, therefore, both an end and means of government. It is, as Donzelot suggests, a mechanism rather than an institution:

> The family became a *target;* by taking account of their complaints, they could be made agents for conveying the norms of the state into the private sphere. (Donzelot 1979, 58)

That is, the family becomes an object of a series of normative campaigns seeking to construct a well-regulated and harmonious family for the sake of itself, and it is also invested with the task of creating wider social harmony and national productivity. The Chinese case does not closely follow the events Donzelot describes. The categories of "public" and "private" do not operate in the same social, economic, and political circumstances. Whereas Donzelot talks of the liberal vision of the family in terms of the "premodern" family (how to govern the family without recourse to the regulation of everyday practice), the Chinese case suggests how the family can be even more tightly and effectively regulated.

These disparities aside it is possible, nonetheless, to at least tentatively note the connection between the moral philanthropic and hygienist movements of nineteenth-century Europe and the influence these had on Chinese governmental perceptions of the family. The moral and physical quality of the population as a concern of government in the West comes to prominence within the work of late-nineteenth-century Chinese intellectuals such as Yan Fu and Kang Youwei (see Hsiao Kung-Chuan 1975; Pusey 1983). During the first decades of the twentieth century the family begins to emerge as a focal point for efforts to save the Chinese from racial degeneration. Movements in both the Nationalist regime and Communist-controlled areas have as their objects the moral and physical well-being of the population. These are in part derived from conventional Chinese accounts of cultivating correct moral conduct and the exigencies of war and insurrection, but are also influenced by similar movements in the West (cf. Dikötter 1995, 1998).[6]

Hence, it is ironic to note that certain aspects of Chinese Marxist strategies to rectify the moral and physical purity of the family after 1949 may have partial foundations in nineteenth-century Protestantism and the early-twentieth-century eugenics movements.[7] Forms of governmental calculation and reasoning have particular, peculiar histories. For China, the family has a modern history in which the biopolitical connections with the population and nation are of paramount significance.

A Sociology of the Family: "The Cell of Society"

Much has already been said about the way in which the Chinese family unit has been linked to issues of productivity (Bray 1997; Davin 1976; Jacka 1997; Kane 1987). Yet, although there is an emphasis on gearing the family toward productive goals, the family is not perceived as a production unit in the strict economic sense, but rather, as Liu Zheng (1980, 16) points out, as a communal living unit (*shenghuo danwei*). In fact the relationship between economic and social responsibilities is a distinctive feature of Chinese governance of the family (hence the various laws in China and Singapore regarding the financial responsibilities of children to their parents).[8]

This communal living unit is not necessarily a harmonious one. On the contrary, Chinese governmental discourse on the family perceives it as almost always on the brink of collapse. The various social relations between husband and wife, parents and children, and spouse and in-laws are a virtual tinderbox waiting to ignite the volatile precariousness of the family structure. These sentiments are not necessarily openly expressed by the authorities (who do not wish to give the impression that they lack control). But the sheer quantity of text and media devoted to promoting familial harmony is testimony, I think, to the imminent possibility of familial chaos. Thus, the family must not be allowed to follow its "natural" course and must be thoroughly divested of all patriarchal and feudal relics. In a word, the family must be "civilized."

In this sense, the family is taken as the starting point—the cell of society—for effective government (Liang Zhongtang et al. 1985, 274). Good government can only be achieved through fostering a harmonious and productive family. Like the conventional Confucian perspective, it is held that correct government of the family will bring about social stability. "Civilizing" the family, enhancing family morals, establishing a "civilized family life" are all part of the process of the construction of "socialist spiritual civilization":

> The classics state: "Establish the family, govern the country and there will be peace under heaven." This highlights the dialectical relationship between the government of the family and the government of the country. The family is the cell of society, it is the basic unit that makes up society. The functions, quality and level of stability of the family have serious implications for the development of the country and society. It is difficult to

imagine that a society with low levels of familial civilization can create a civilized and prosperous "utopia." It is thus worth noting the importance modern domestic economy [*jiazhengxue*] has for the construction of socialist spiritual civilization. (Ren Jianying 1993, 13; my trans.)

In a text on household management, Liu Guangren argues that it is of paramount importance to know the family in detail, because it is the basic social unit for socialization and reproduction:

The family is the most basic environment for human life. It is the long-term locus of human activities and individuals. No matter whether one speaks in terms of physiological or psychological development; the study and accumulation of life skills intimately both depend on the family. . . . If the existence of the family—a collective social body—is stable, then this in turn can provide a stable basis for the rest of society. (1992, 3; my trans.)

The role of government is therefore to ensure that conditions are created that foster a harmonious family life. These conditions must in turn have a direct relation with the interests of the population at large. For instance, Liang Zhongtang (1985, 319) refers to the need to "adjust" relations within the family, particularly "abnormal" families, so they accord with accepted standards that are conducive to improving the stock of the population. Family management and social development should be harmonious. Thus, if on a national level authorities perceive that China is facing a crisis of overpopulation, then families should willingly respond to the call to have only one child.

These examples demonstrate the important position of the family within Chinese governmental discourse. As Donzelot (1979) suggests in relation to developments in Europe, family members are also resources for national targets of government: in China no less than the West good government means "getting the family right."

But what form of reasoning informs this governmental discourse about the nature of the "ideal" family? It is here that our discussion on Chinese sociological perceptions of the family comes into effect. One of the clearest indications from the Chinese intelligentsia vis-à-vis the premises establishing what constitutes a family comes from the eminent Chinese sociologist Pan Yunkang. In his book on the sociology of the family Pan Yunkang (1986, 35) asks rhetorically, "What actually constitutes a family?" He begins to answer this by stating that the family is first a social unit based on marriage and consanguinity. Hence, in order for the family to be social it must have at least two members—one person cannot constitute a family (Pan Yunkang 1986, 35). Marriage, furthermore, is the basic foundation for any family and is, as Pan Yunkang argues, the determining factor in what constitutes a family. The next most important factors are the blood relations between family members and their level of economic interdependence. A further factor is the legal recognition of the family through marriage and household registration.

Pan Yunkang (1986) is also at pains to point out, however, that a *hu* (household) does not necessarily correlate to a *jiating* (family). He draws out this point not by referring to the Chinese case but to foreign examples and, in so doing, highlights the central elements of concern for Chinese governance of the family:

> In foreign countries in recent years the phenomena of divorce and family breakdown have become rather serious, sexual liberation has become popular, and sex lives have become chaotic. Hence, there has been the appearance of many abnormal families. Actually, in the strict definition of the term, these so-called abnormal families can only be referred to as households, and not as families. For instance, celibates (*dushenzhuyizhe*) who live by themselves are not prevented from informally getting married and having casual sexual relations with members of the opposite sex. How can this kind of single bachelor system (*danshenzhi*) that does not have a formal and stable partner, and that does not involve marrying another person or establishing blood relations, be called a family? The same can be said for homosexual couples and groups of young males and females living together—they also cannot constitute a family, but only households. Yet, even a household needs to go through some process of household registration before it can gain recognition in the eyes of the law. However, there are some abnormal families, such as unmarried male and female couples who cohabitate without undertaking any legal formalities whatsoever. These abnormal families are not even households, let alone families. (Pan Yunkang 1986, 37–38; my trans.)

In posing a rhetorical question of our own, we might ask, "Why does Pan Yunkang find the thought of cohabitation of unregistered and unmarried individuals so abhorrent and abominable?" Part of the answer lies in the perception of the historical evolution of the family and the development of the practices of marriage, registration, and sexual conduct. In true Marxist fashion, Pan and his associates regard the family as an historical entity that, like other parts of society, is bounding along on its inexorable journey toward utopia. In the earliest stages of human existence, there were no boundaries for sexual conduct between sisters and brothers, parents and children. Hence, there were no families. With the development of human society, two important events occurred that effected the emergence of the family. First, there was the elimination of sexual relations between parents and children; and, second, the elimination of sexual relations between brothers and sisters and other close relatives.[9]

Pan Yunkang (1986, 38–39) even goes so far as to suggest that the elimination of interbreeding and the resulting improvement in the human stock had a profound effect on the intellectual and physical capabilities of humans and in turn spurred on the development of the forces of production to even greater heights. The evolution of the family increasingly restricts sexual relations between close relatives (hence, the obsessive fear of rural villages reverting to primitive barbarism by engaging in intrafamily marriage).

Drawing from the work of Engels and Morgan, Pan Yunkang (1986, 38–39) and Zhou Xizhang (1982, 44) argue that such steps helped to improve the physical and intellectual quality of human beings.[10] A similar line of thought can be found in a late 1980s handbook for the self-conduct of women:

> From an overall perspective, the heterosexual relationship in human society developed slowly—it was determined by the forces of production. Cross-breeding amongst close relatives is the product of an extremely low level of the productive forces. In order to strengthen the ability to struggle with nature, people lived in a primeval communal mode. They did not differentiate between elders and juniors and practiced cross-breeding. With the development of stone tools there was a step forward in development. The use of fire had also begun. These required the mastering of certain skills and in this respect people of older years were stronger than the younger members. And in this way the differentiation between senior and junior generations began to gradually form. Moreover, in the extended process of production and living, people gradually realized that the offspring of the sexual union of brothers and sisters were physically weak and not beneficial for the raising of tribal production and strengthening tribal fighting strength. Hence, the concept of restricting marriage of close relatives gradually developed. (Yang Lingling 1989, 145; my trans.)

Marriage is thus both a social and biological necessity, because it ensures that procreation will occur within the healthy "eugenic" confines of the family rather than among strangers or relatives, as in primitive times (Chen Qingliang 1992, 69–70). The family is thus a locus of problems that reflect directly on the health and well-being (mental and physical) of the population. Its importance does not diminish as time progresses; it merely becomes smaller, more nuclear, and the central mechanism for socialization and the regulation of reproduction (Wang Enfeng and Liu Xianming 1989, 4). Many of these problems are closely associated with the practices of sex and reproduction, which among other factors are the keys to ensuring familial and social harmony.

Marriage and the Policing of Families

The first thing to note, before discussing specific government measures in utilizing marriage and the family as technologies in themselves, is the importance placed upon marriage in China—marriage is almost universal (Peng Xizhe 1991, 116).[11] The 1950 Marriage Law is thus significant on two major accounts. First, it is significant in its attempt to break previous power arrangements (that is, feudal and arranged marriages) and in its offer of greater autonomy to women in the choice of marriage partner (Kane 1987, 19).[12] This autonomy is increasingly the object of governmental concern for several reasons, one of which is to empower women to take charge of their own bodies and reproductive capabilities.

Second, this legislation represents the first time that marriages were made official by the state. That is, the state now has a direct interest in regulating the specific form and constitution of marriage. De facto marriage did not legally exist in China before the new regulations—marriage was a matter arranged by the respective families of the bride and groom. Marriage did have a public aspect insofar as a marriage could be legally dissolved or nullified, but the legitimation of the government authorities was always post facto. Nor was there any registration of marriage required in the Nationalist Civil Code of 1931 (Cartier 1996b, 229; Meijer 1971, 178).

It was under the auspices of the communist movement that marriage became a crucial mechanism for governing the health and well-being of the population. Chen Shaoyu presents the Chinese Marxist case for marriage registration in the following terms:

> From the time of the Government of the Soviet Areas until the present Government of the People's Republic, it has been a government of the people themselves.... It has no other interests but those of the people and it does not interfere in matters in which the people do not want it to interfere. Therefore the People's Government cannot keep aloof from that great event of marriage in the life of a man and a woman which also *affects the health of the whole people, the happiness of the family, the health of the whole nation and the reconstruction of the State.* And not only can the Government

not keep aloof, it must show greater concern in these matters than even the marrying parties themselves and their relatives do, and it has to assume an even more serious responsibility. (Meijer 1971, 179; my emph.)

Marriage is, therefore, a very public affair that impinges on the health and prosperity of the whole nation.[13] By rendering the act of marriage as a public act, it was then possible to use the process of registration to highlight the imperative of health and hygiene. The concern with health in marriage registration in the early years of the People's Republic was erratic, and regulations differed from province to province and municipality to municipality. As early as 1950, directives were issued by the central authorities that stated clearly that marriage registration is the concrete materialization of the marriage law and called for close cooperation between the marriage registration organs and the Women's Federation (DCAPRC 1989, 88–89). Yet it was not until June 1955 that the general procedures for marriage registration were promulgated by the central government through the Ministry of the Interior.

The preamble to the Procedures for Marriage Registration states that the purpose of marriage registration, among other things, is to ensure the health of future generations by restricting marriage between close relatives and sufferers of certain diseases (DCAPRC 1989, 90).[14] The health examination seeks to trace the medical history of both families, to check for hereditary illnesses and whether or not the couple constitute close relatives. The health examination also examines the reproductive organs, checks for venereal diseases, and informs newly wedded couples of family planning practices and obligations. Young couples are also informed about basic sexual knowledge and physiology and the importance of having healthy, eugenically blessed offspring (Yan Shi et al. 1991, 225).

Nonetheless, the premarriage health examination was not mandatory. In fact, it seems quite paradoxical that the health checkup component of registering marriage should be viewed as noncompulsory, especially in light of some of the other more "interventionist" strategies used by authorities to regulate the health and reproductive conduct of the population. Huang San (1986, 252) notes that in the years after liberation, in order to implement the Marriage Law of 1950 effectively, the premarital checkup, which included an examination of the genitals, was widespread. Many people objected to these checkups, and they were suspended in 1954, just before the promulgation of the Procedures of Marriage Registration in 1955. Hence, one possible explanation is the fear that such an examination would promote fear and misunderstanding among the population and be susceptible to abuse and corruption.[15]

Despite these efforts to separate the health checkup and marriage registration the tendency to link the two was very strong. This was further exacerbated by the implementation of the family planning program in the 1970s and its expansion and increased eugenic content in the 1980s. In the 1980s many local governments reimplemented premarital checkups, such as Shanghai (1980), Beijing (1981), Hefei (1981), and Ha'erbin (1984). In terms of the increased eugenic content, the calls to limit reproduction and strengthen marriage registration have often been described in ways that stress increasing the health and quality of the population—"controlling the quantity and increasing the quality."

More important for our interests here are the concerted efforts to separate marriage and childbirth. First, in terms of the "later, longer, and fewer" (*wan xi shao*)[16] campaign of the 1970s, couples were asked to delay birth after marriage. This represents a significant break with the traditional attitude that marriage is almost universally followed, shortly after, by the birth of a child (Kane 1987, 88). Children were to be replaced by productivity in other areas. In rural areas that might mean encouraging peasants to raise more domestic animals as an alternative to having children—"More Pigs, Less Kids" is the slogan for one recent campaign. In urban areas it would enable young couples to pursue further education and raise their level of maturity before having children, and hence they would be in a much better position to raise "good-quality" children.

Thus, armed with a technological vocabulary centered around social management and planning, Chinese Marxism explicitly links economic and social planning with human reproduction (see also Ram, this volume).[17] The crisis of the population and its perceived impact on the development of the economy intensifies the need for Chinese governmental authorities to cut to the very core of reproduction. Hence, when the reassessment of the state of Chinese social and economic development takes place, after the rise of Deng and the fall of the ultra-left, the "later, longer, and fewer" family planning campaign of the 1970s is deemed severely inadequate. Therefore, it is not surprising that the one-child policy that emerged in the late 1970s and early 1980s is reckoned to be as important a priority as production in any state enterprise because of the perceived direct relationship population growth has with national prosperity and productivity (Croll 1985, 211).[18]

The authorities thus accepted the desire of couples to marry and would do little to discourage this practice other than by raising the age of marriage. They did, nonetheless, insist that people begin to rethink what marriage meant—it was definitely not a sign to start producing children en masse. In 1980 the new marriage law raised the ages of marriage by two years, from twenty to twenty-two years for men and eighteen to twenty years for women. Since the introduction of the new marriage law, family planning campaigns have stressed that these new ages do not mean that people are obliged to marry once they reach that age or that marriage means childbirth. On the contrary, late marriage and childbirth should be encouraged for reasons of maternal health and family planning. For instance, a directive issued from the central government on 3 October 1980 attempts to clarify this position by stating that the separation of marriage and childbearing requires the intensification of educating the masses about the use of contraceptives and family planning knowledge (DCAPRC 1989, 48).

The act of marriage has thus become a valuable governmental technology in the policing of reproductive conduct in modern China. It has enabled governmental authorities to harness the biological capacity of newly wedded couples to produce healthy offspring. It has also served as a platform from which to problematize certain undesirable acts, such as early marriage and childbirth. The act of registration by no means guarantees that all couples will comply with the wishes of family planning authorities. Indeed, the "failure" of marriage is a perpetual problem for the policing of Chinese families. Nonetheless, it has made a significant impact in reweaving the social fabric of Chinese reproductive and familial conduct.

Sex and the Economy of Pleasure

All of this is part and parcel of the larger program to manage the reproductive regularities. But what is the relationship between reproduction and sexual conduct? Ask any Chinese family planning cadre, and its members might respond by stating that reproduction involves sex, but sex does not necessarily equate with reproduction. This is the linchpin of Chinese efforts to encourage family planning.

How does this differ from the biopolitics of sexuality, population and family described for Europe by Foucault? In volume one of *The History of Sexuality* Foucault (1978) describes a contrast between two forms of government—alliance and sexuality. The system of alliance refers to the transference of names and the inheritance of property within the economic and political context of the ancien régime. Hence, the system of alliance is intimately tied to the process of law and the maintenance of definite social statuses. The deployment of sexuality as a mode for regulating the conduct of sexual partners stems from the system of alliances. Sexuality does not replace alliance but, rather, is superimposed upon it. It has as its object not the circulation of wealth and property but the circulation and proliferation of bodies. This is the beginning of biopolitics.[19]

An important reason for outlining the emergence of sexuality as a mode of governance is to challenge the assumption that modern society is characterized by sexual repression. Foucault terms this the "repressive hypothesis." This proposition argues that sexuality is a core aspect of self-realization, and only speaking openly and frankly about it will ensure liberation. Foucault demonstrates that sexuality and the techniques that surround it (therapy, confession, self-scrutiny) constitute the deployment of a new mode of individualization centered around the health and conduct of the population at large. This confessional mode of governance is contrasted with an Eastern regime of apprenticeship in the giving and receiving of sexual pleasures (*ars erotica*). Whereas the truth of sex in Western society revolves around the infamy of what is permitted and forbidden, in certain other societies the truth of sex is located in the principle of pleasure passed from master to disciple (Foucault 1978, 57–58).[20] As Foucault queried in an interview shortly after the publication of *The History of Sexuality*:

> How is it that in a society like ours, sexuality is not simply a means of reproducing the species, the family, and the individual? Not simply a means to obtain pleasure and enjoyment? How has sexuality come to be considered the privileged place where our deepest "truth" is read and exposed? (Cited in Miller 1994, 293)

In order to illuminate this point further we need to refer to Foucault's (1993 [1980], 203) distinction between a perpetually internalizing hermeneutic self and a mnemonic self. The hermeneutic self that Foucault talks of is rooted in the Christian problematization of desire. It is a self in which one takes up a specific position to oneself in which the measurement of conduct is internalized in an ongoing moral struggle with the self. By contrast the mnemonic self is "less permanently self-reflexive" (Minson 1996). The mnemonic self operates by drawing from a diverse array of cultural practices—"techniques of living." As Ian Hunter (1993, 128) suggests, the operation of an internalizing self within a given culture or historical period does not mean that the conscious or unconscious self has been revealed. Rather, it highlights the contingent nature of ethical self-conduct within a given social formation. In the Chinese case, it suggests that the apparent subversion of the individual to the interests of the collective does not represent a denial of the population's sense of self but points to a particular construction of selfhood.

The key point here is the deployment of sexuality as a mode of individualization and governing bodies. Recent Chinese history has been characterized by two discourses on sexual pleasure—the sexual austerity of the Mao period (1949–78), in which there was a distinct absence of discourse on pleasure, and the recent confinement of sexual pleasure to the married heterosexual couple.

Both of these discourses on sex are related to the emergence of a distinct Chinese biopolitics insofar as they delineate normal and pathological modes of sexual conduct. Indeed, the concern with obscuring sex from public view, veiling it in secrecy, and the second mode of sexual discourse stem from the same governmental program. That is, whereas the first mode denies discussion of pleasure, the second mode concedes that pleasure is important but on one condition: that the pleasure of sex be confined to the institution of marriage and the family.

Apropos of sexual austerity, Pan Suiming (1995b, 53) argues that China does not have a strong discourse on bodily ascetics (*routi jinyuzhuyi*) that parallels Western experience.[21] Rather, China is dominated by a spiritual ascetics (*jingshen jinyuzhuyi*) that derives from the Manchu adaptation during the Qing dynasty of Song neo-Confucianism (Pan Suiming 1995a, 27–28). For Pan Suiming (1995b, 56) this represents a sexual "revolution" that moves from education to control, from advocacy to prevention, and from restriction to suppression.

Is Pan here expounding a Chinese version of the repressive hypothesis? No, at least not in terms that ascribe self-realization from sexual liberation. A similar point is made by Li Yinhe (1996) insofar as she argues that "sexuality" is not a "problem" in Chinese society. In light of this, Ann Anagnost (1995, 26–27) suggests, and in many ways I concur, that Foucault's concern with *sexuality* in Western societies as a pivotal focus of political, economic, and social interventions can be replaced in China with *population* and *reproduction*. Hence, sexuality, in the sense that Foucault uses the term, is absent as a means of self-problematization in China. This is not to suggest that sexuality is not problematized. Rather, the dissemination of sexual knowledge and practice is governed in a more mechanistic manner, that is, in terms of pleasure and "getting it right," rather than an interrogation of the self. The techniques of sex no longer reside in the secret wisdom of the master but in the authority of the medical establishment, especially as it is linked to reproduction. Hence, here we have a biopolitics without the secret lever of sexuality.

This flies in the face of Frank Dikötter's (1995, 185) claims that "official discourse has not considered each person's particular and unique preferences to be significant and has refused to confer any rights to pleasure upon individuals." On the contrary, the ubiquitous marriage and sex guides readily available in contemporary China instruct couples to have satisfying sex lives and enjoin women in particular not to be passive about fulfilling their desires. These manuals openly refute Dikötter's claim that "sex has not been disassociated from procreation" or at least suggest that both messages coexist. This would seem to indicate a tension between a strongly medicalized discourse, on the one hand,

and a more fluid official discourse on the importance of maintaining familial harmony and balance, on the other (with links to indigenous knowledges about *yin* and *yang*). Thus, while certain sections of the medical establishment may have severed pleasure from procreation, family planning authorities have argued for quite some time that you can stop people from having children, but you cannot stop them from having sex.[22] Indeed, sex is regarded as a vital component in ensuring emotional and physical well-being:

> People often regard the suppression of sexual desire and victory over the flesh as an ideal for a healthy personality—it signifies high aspirations and a strong spirit. However, in reality a perfect, healthy and strong personality must be one that has ample sexual satisfaction. (Quan Yazhi 1993, 129; my trans.)

Chinese subjects are thus encouraged to engage in an economy of sex but not in its liberation. Indeed, sexual liberation is anathema to many Chinese commentators on the family and sexual conduct. For instance, Chen Yiyun (1994, 88), a prominent scholar on the family and women in the People's Republic, warns of brazenly following Western trends. One of the key problems for Chinese authorities on morality and ethics is sexually liberating the body from feudal patriarchy and, at the same time, keeping the "excessive" tendencies of capitalist Western forms of sexual conduct at bay. Whereas in the past, they assert, Chinese women were oppressed by feudal sexual bondage, now they face the threat of contamination from Western "sexual liberation" and "sexual freedom." Yang Lingling (1989) admits that liberation and freedom sound very attractive but on closer scrutiny can be seen to be fundamentally harmful to both the individual and society at large. Hence, Chinese interlocutors hold that, while modern sexual conduct must incorporate equality between the sexes and that it is good that the "mysterious" or "solemn" nature of sex has been eroded and one can now conduct a reasoned and scientific discussion about sex, sex in the final analysis is a family concern and sexual freedom should not lead to sexual liaisons beyond the confines of marriage and the family.

> Thus it is possible to note that when compared to feudal thought, "sexual freedom" contains elements of rationality, such as the destruction of the mystery of sex, the popularization of sexual knowledge, the emphasis on harmonizing the sexual life of husband and wife, and so on. However, under certain conditions these problems have adopted distorted forms and have gone to the extremes. This then condones the licentious pursuit of

sensual pleasures without the guidance of any social regulations, responsibilities or obligations. (Yang Lingling 1989, 138; my trans.)

Hence, sexual liberation becomes mere individualistic hedonism. Sexual conduct under these conditions leads to a number of undesirable outcomes, such as an increase in divorce, incest, young mothers, the commodification of sex, juvenile crime, increase in venereal disease, and pornography (Chen Yiyun 1994; Yang Lingling 1989, 139–42). "Getting the family right" means confining sexual conduct to married heterosexual couples. Sexual conduct must be properly regulated within the family to ensure harmony (cf. Handwerker 1995). To do otherwise is to threaten the very social fabric.[23]

The Dissemination of an Economy of Pleasure in Popular Marriage Manuals

Part of the process of fostering harmony within the family means informing people about the reproductive processes of the body. Indeed, in both rural and urban areas, there is a proliferation and dissemination of material—handbooks, traveling exhibitions and education units, movies and stage productions—geared toward informing the public about the reproductive processes, the importance of family planning, and the use of various contraceptives. As Ruan Fangfu (1988) notes in *Xing zhishi shouce* (The Sexual Knowledge Handbook), there are many valid reasons for promoting sex education. The main purpose, however, is to avoid misunderstandings about sexual activity, make people more aware about their own bodies and avoid problems relating to sexual conduct in the family and marriage situation.[24] While hesitant to say that this or that form of sexual conduct is innately abnormal, Ruan Fangfu, an eminent sexologist, nonetheless argues that, because general social feeling sways in a particular direction, it is best to avoid uncertainty by discouraging socially unacceptable behavior, such as homosexuality. Hence, the family must provide a harmonious and stable environment to educate children properly about sexual norms and hygiene (Ruan Fangfu 1988, 193).

This practical application and know-how of sex runs alongside the discourse on the economy of pleasure. This has not always been the case. As Harriet Evans (1995) has argued, the current proliferation of popular magazines on the family and marriage represents a significant development of the last two decades. Indeed, in the early 1980s government authorities were particularly alarmed at the rapid increase in publications dealing with sexual conduct. One statement from the Central Department of Propaganda (1981) issued in March 1981 noted that the campaign on sex education among young people was progressing well. The campaign, it stated, involved the publication of handbooks and information guides on the physiology of sex, reproduction, and sexual hygiene. It was concerned, however, with the enthusiasm some publishing houses had expressed in running off many more copies than they considered necessary. But what was particularly alarming from their point of view was the inclusion of detail on methods of copulation and accompanying diagrams. This information, they argued, was not desirable for the health of young people, because it put dangerous thoughts in their minds.

The notable absence of explicit material on sexual technique is a considerable blemish on the traditional *ars erotica*.[25] Nonetheless, the same cannot be said for the role that pleasure takes within the discourse on sexual conduct. Many of the popular family and women's magazines, which are generally published by the local or provincial Women's Federation, frequently carry articles on the importance of pleasure in the sexual lives of married couples. These publications carry titles that clearly indicate the significance of marriage and family, such as *Marriage and Family; Dating, Marriage, Family; Family Friend;* and the Chinese Eugenic Society's own publication *Happy Families*.

Of equal interest here are the "question-and-answer guides," "hotline" publications, and marriage manuals.[26] These texts address a popular audience and are formatted in a characteristically Chinese question-and-answer format. It is within the answers provided by these sources of textual authority and expertise that we can gauge the attempts by Chinese governmental discourse to regulate sexual conduct within the family. In the majority of these cases, it is the family, and especially the relationship between husband and wife, that is the central source of concern. Having surveyed the marital relations literature, we should not neglect the large number of inquiries regarding premarital sex and trial marriages. In what follows I will briefly deal with premarital sex, trial marriages, and regulating the sexual conduct of married couples.

First, responses to questions regarding premarital sex are invariably formulated around promoting chastity and the sanctity of marriage, but in circumstances that are not necessarily "conservative" but strategic. For instance, one caller explained that she and her boyfriend were deeply in love and had agreed to marry in a year's time. The boyfriend requested, however, that they first have sex. She was not willing to do so but was afraid of disappointing her boyfriend. Indeed, her boyfriend told her that her refusal to do so was an indication that she did not trust or truly love him. The respondent explained that her intended course of action was admirable and that she should under no circumstances relent to her boyfriend's requests. The respondent argued that the consequences of sex were more serious for women than for men, especially in Chinese society, where most men expected future brides to be virginal. Women would suffer from unwanted pregnancies and the threat of actually losing somebody they really loved because they had been promiscuous in a previous relationship. For the male, by contrast, this was not much of a concern (Wang Xingjuan, Xu Xiuyu, and Wang Ling 1995, 46–47).

In another hotline the question "Shall I tell my fiancé that I have already lost my virginity?" was posed. The anonymous caller was concerned that her boyfriend would reject her upon discovering she was no longer a virgin or that his parents would object to their marriage if they too discovered it. The response is similar to the previous one and begins by scolding the woman for already finding herself in such a situation. She is told that women should separate "dating" (*lianai*) and "marriage." Women should use the process of dating to find a suitable partner and not jump straight into a full relationship. Her problem now, it is suggested, is deciding whether or not to risk telling her boyfriend, who may either stay with her or leave her upon hearing the news (Hu Jin and Zhao Pinghe 1996, 3).

Men are often understood within these texts as possessing uncontrollable sexual desires, and women in the process of courtship must resist their demands for sex (Ding Juan et al. 1995, 39). In their study of similar advice literature published in the 1980s, Emily Honig and Gail Hershatter note that, although both young men and women are constantly warned about "the dangers of unrestrained sexual activity," it invariably falls on the shoulders of young women to "channel and control the sexual desires of young men as well as their own and to defer acting on those desires until they reached the socially appropriate age for courtship and marriage" (1988, 53). The strategic importance of balancing this form of "animalism" with "social convention" is caught up in the deployment of social etiquette aimed at discouraging abnormal sexual conduct:

> Avoiding premarital pregnancy depends on the spiritual [*xinling*] establishment of a moral and ethical foundation. The greatest difference between humans and animals lies in the human capacity for thought—[humans] can use the process of thought and reason to regulate their own conduct. (Ren Wen and Yin Ming 1993, 39; my trans.)

The authors explain that young couples not yet married should temper themselves and resist the temptation to let their passions fly; they should take careful note of what they wear, how late they stay out, and not engage in vulgar and dirty talk (1993, 39). Girls are further encouraged to monitor the actions of their boyfriends carefully and not let them get wrong impressions: "If he wants to kiss you, let him, but not for too long" and "if he holds you, make sure his hands do not stray to the breasts and buttocks" (1993, 40). Thus, males are expected to "restrict" (*yangyi*) their sexual impulses, while women are encouraged to be sober and carefully monitor their emotional responses (Chi Guifa and Gu Zhiwei 1994, 65).

In the case of trial marriages, one caller explained that he had requested his girlfriend to live with him. He believed that doing so would enable them to see if they could function as a couple, both sexually and spiritually. He argued that they could avoid the pitfalls of many couples who do not adequately understand each other and blunder into marriage only to suffer serious consequences later on. His girlfriend was, in his opinion, too conservative and would not agree. The response is framed in protecting the interests of the woman involved and pointing out that China is still a deeply feudal society in which men expect prospective brides to be virgins and that in the case of trial marriages it is the women who inevitably suffer (Wang Xingjuan, Xu Xiuyu and Wang Ling 1995, 48–50). Women who live in trial marriages or with their partners, without the intention of marriage, invariably reduce their future marriage prospects. Trial marriages, the respondents argue, undermine the authority of marriage precisely in their claims to be "trial"—the commitments to working through problems, sexual and economic, are not as secure as partners within a married relationship (Yue Ping et al. 1995, 2–3; Zhang Xiyu et al. 1993, 104).

Thus, premarital sex and trial marriages are expressly discouraged by the official Chinese discourse on the family. Premarital sex and trial marriages are approached in these texts from two major fronts. In one sense they are not regarded as necessarily immoral in their own right. It is the Chinese social context in which men have high expectations of prospective brides that forces women to be strategic and protect their integrity. Yet, they are told, men have the sexual drives of animals and will attempt to seduce and lead astray a woman's virtue at every turn. In this case women must take charge of the situation by closely monitoring their own personal conduct and the conduct of their partners.

Sexual conduct must therefore be confined to the sanctity of marriage. Indeed, as I have already noted, many of the marriage manuals hold that a successful marriage depends on a harmonious and satisfying sex life of both partners.[27] It is here that the economy of pleasure is at its most vigorous. Women are not expected to merely serve the desires of their husbands. As one sex manual explains, many Chinese women have been forced into a situation in which their own sexual desires come second to those of men and are tied to the "four step dance—foreplay, insertion, intercourse, and ejaculation" (Ma Xiaonian 1995, 74). In order to overcome this obstacle and establish sexual equality between husband and wife, a great deal of emphasis has been placed on separating the traditional perception of marriage followed closely by childbirth. Sex means more than just procreation: it is also an important component of ensuring a harmonious family life. Indeed, there are numerous cases in which a distinction is made between love (*qingai*) and *sexual love* (*xingai*):

> The modern family has not only love [*qingai*] but sexual love [*xingai*] as well; sexual love is not only concerned with having children, but more so with achieving the sexual happiness and pleasure of both partners. (Han Lei 1993, 4; my trans.)

These two aspects must be intimately united and not separated, as they are in feudal and modern Western attitudes toward sex. According to these texts, feudal practices provide no freedom in matters of sex, especially for women, while Western sex entails sex for its own sake without consolidation of the mutual bonds of love and affection between partners. When one young university student wrote to a popular health magazine seeking help in dealing with her sexual impulses toward her boyfriend, the respondent answered by instructing her to differentiate rigorously between sexual love (*xingai*) and lust (*xingyu*). Lust is base and animalistic and means losing control of self-restraint, the writer told her. Sexual love, on the other hand, is built upon a certain amount of animalistic attraction, but more so on emotional sentiment (Zhong Jiaoshou 1995, 25). What distinguishes humans from animals is precisely the ability to divorce sex from procreation and utilize sexual love (*xingai*) to strengthen love (*qingai*) (Wang Wei and Gao Yulan 1992, 110; Yu Jing 1992, 218).

Married couples should, therefore, take active roles in their sexual lives. The feudal influence of female passivity and perception of sex as inherently immoral must be eliminated (Zhu Junlun 1993, 31). Women are encouraged to enjoy sex and find suitable means to realize sexual satisfaction and are criticized for harboring feudal attitudes:

> Some women, especially those of low cultural education, regard married sex lives as base and ignoble because they harbor feudal thoughts. As a result they suppress their own sexual desires and never take the initiative in sex and even when their husbands request it [sex] they are not enthusiastic partners [*bujiji*]. (Li Xingchun and Wang Lirun 1988, 105; my trans.)

Husbands are expected to be "sex guides" for their wives, considering that women are assumed to be more most ignorant when it comes to sex, especially in terms of separating procreation and sexual pleasure (Dong Jian 1995, 22; Wu Yishi and Wu Ling 1995, 133). But, quite often, husbands are also criticized for harboring feudal attitudes toward sex as well. For instance, one caller was concerned about his newly wedded wife, who, he believed, was too interested in sex often took the initiative and asked him to do things he could not bring himself to do. The response was to suggest that he was "constricted by traditional thinking" (Wang Xingjuan, Xu Xiuyu, and Wang Ling 1995, 35–36). This form of thought, the respondent argued, held that women should have no sexual desires and are merely instruments for the sexual satisfaction of men. The wife in this case is said to be upholding her rights to sexual equality within the marriage; her conduct suggests her deep affection for the husband and recognition of the importance of sex within marriage:

> That your demands for sex are not very strong suggests that you may have a physiological problem. Or perhaps because your wife is so assertive you are placed in a passive [*beidong*] position in which you feel uncomfortable and this influences your interest [in sex]. Perhaps you feel that because you are the husband you should reserve the right to take the initiative and your wife's assertiveness has violated your sexual rights. You do not understand that a harmonious sex life requires the combined efforts of both parties. That old view of the male as the only one able to take the initiative and that women can only be passive, cold, and obedient is an old-fashioned traditional concept. (1995, 35–36; my trans.)

The caller is told that he should understand that marriage means learning—including about sex. He should, it concluded, learn from his wife.

On a similar note another caller noted that his wife demanded more sex than he felt he could offer. He also complained that his wife had some strange practices, such as having sex during the day, placing a large mirror next to the bed, and requesting oral sex. The respondent argued that the husband should have more sympathy for his wife and realize that different people and sexes have different ways of achieving pleasure (1995, 85). Here the hapless husbands are chastised for being the ignorant ones and scolded for referring to women who take the initiative (*zhudong*) as manifesting "tigressism" (*mulaohuzhuyi*). Indeed, women are encouraged to be more assertive right from the wedding night in order to establish the foundations for a harmonious sex life with their partners (Ren Wen and Yin Ming 1993, 76). Husbands are also instructed to take more concern of the sexual needs of their partners, especially in relation to orgasm. They should work toward a sex life in which both partners are satisfied. This means husbands must take the effort to understand the sexual psychology and physiology of their wives (Dong Ren 1990, 276; Zheng Xiaoyang and Chen Yuhan 1995, 130).

Married couples are not called upon to question their sexuality or to link sexual liberation to some form of self-realization. They are encouraged to divorce sex from procreation and invest their sexual lives with pleasure. Women are instructed to overcome passivity, just as men are told to treat their wives as sexual partners rather than sexual objects. This agenda appears as a stark contrast to earlier Chinese philosophies of sex, especially that which developed during the Qing dynasty. Of interest here is the way in which reproduction and pleasure have been disarticulated. Nonetheless, the discourse on pleasure in China seems tame and confined in comparison to those found in Western societies. But, as this chapter has demonstrated, this particular way of ascribing the natural domain of sex to the family is best understood in terms of the sociology of the family deployed in the Chinese context. This particular sociology also makes apparent the importance of eugenics in Chinese family planning and the way in which much of this is ascribed to the domain of the family.

Virtuous Wives and Good Mothers

But who is going to manage sex within the family? Upon whom should the burden of responsibility for the moral and physical monitoring of family members fall? The answer, it seems to me, in a Chinese context is that women, and in particular married women and mothers, must take charge of sex within the family. As we have seen, women must be aware of their own physiological processes and how to control them and must also be aware of the desires of their husbands and how to satisfy and temper them. Hence, much of the call for the emancipation of women in China has meant not casting off the shackles of marriage and the family but, rather, reconfiguring the lines of power within the family so that women become the primary conduits for governmental programming. In this case the state-family relationship is restabilized with the mother as the main relay for adjusting certain reproductive and sexual practices. Thus, even though family planning authorities have stressed that family planning is the responsibility of both husband and wife, the responsibility tends to fall on the shoulders of women. As Lisa Handwerker (1995, 366) notes, it is invariably women who take the blame for both infertility and for being too fertile. There is a disproportionate amount of statistical revelation focusing on the reproductive practices of women when compared to those of men. Thus, both the female body and its physiological processes and the familial position occupied by women in the family are open to governmental scrutiny and intervention.

The "father" of the Chinese nation, Sun Yat-sen, regarded the dispersed nature of Chinese clan and family life as the greatest obstacle to the formation of a strong and vibrant Chinese nationalism. China, he remarked, was like a plate of loose sand. In order for the state to draw the female body into its governmental agenda, the back of the clan had to be broken, but in a way that still allowed the family to remain as an operative governmental category. In this connection, Tani Barlow notes:

> The newly minted Maoist family formation . . . made the body of a woman a realm of the state at the same time as it opened the state to inflection by kin discourses and kin categories. The entry point was reproductive science. Woman-work *ganbu* (cadres; particularly nurses, who were known as "Nightingales" in honor of Florence Nightingale) brought to political activity the powerful new scientific knowledge of sanitation, physiology, and scientific midwifery. Texts drilled village women in reproductive physiology ("it's just like your farm animals") and dispensed information on bodily functions like the menstrual cycle and hygiene (don't borrow pads, don't drink cold water, stay away from dirty menstrual blood, which carries diseases, don't have intercourse during your period, visit the doctor for irregularities, etc.). (1994, 272–73)

Barlow outlines here the shift from the traditional "nongendered" distinction between females based on rank and social position to the specifically gendered distinction based on the material ground of scientific physiology. This shift coincides with the emergence of innovative ways of conceiving of birth, death, and illness (as Barlow hints but does not discuss in any detail). The connection between the health of the population, in this case of women, is intimately tied to the welfare and prosperity of the nation and race (*minzu*). It is in this way that the reproductive conduct of the family and the welfare of the nation are united. The population has thus been imbued with a different sense of utility. It is no longer something to be merely taxed, corveed, punished, and led by moral example. The population is now seen as a visible mass of bodies that require appropriate intervention in order to increase their physical well-being and in turn strengthen the nation.

Throughout the 1950s debate raged within China as to the status women were to assume in society and the family. On the one hand, women were encouraged to become involved in production. For instance, the Dependents' Organization that emerged during the 1950s attempted to "liberate" women through production by offering them a chance to leave the strict confines of the family and experience productive labor (Davin 1976, 59–61). The object of such organizations was to promote a harmonious home atmosphere to assist the menfolk in focusing on production. On the other hand, women were encouraged to regard housework as a celebrated and productive activity—"housework is glorious" (Davin 1976, 108). Hence, the "five goods" movement of the mid-1950s argued that women should run the home thriftily, unite family and neighbors, lead the old, care for the young, and teach the children.

Although these virtues were disrupted by the Great Leap Forward and criticized as part of the revisionist package during the Cultural Revolution, they still form the central elements of current opinion on the role of wives as family managers. For instance, Yang Lingling instructs women how to be good housewives; a woman, she informs the reader, can only be complete when she is both a wife and a mother and is encouraged to "dialectically" work out the relationship between work and the family (1989, 164). Women must learn how to "scientifically manage the family, to mobilize the enthusiasm of other family members in order to become masters of 'the art of managing family members'."[28] The husband and wife relationship is the basis of the family, so it must be managed well—a woman needs to support her husband, so he can go forth and be successful (1989, 165).

Women thus need to be in possession of a great deal of "know-how" about the family, of how best to manage family relations, of how to encourage their husbands, of how to deal with in-laws. It is the relations among family members, particularly between husband and wife, that must be governed most carefully in order to ensure harmony and productivity (Honig and Hershatter 1988, 179). Sex in governmental literature and campaigns is by all means a family affair. Much of the burden is placed on the shoulders of women. They are instructed to manage both the concern with reproduction and the economy of pleasure. They are confronted with the formidable task of relaying governmental programs from the macro level of the population to the micro level of the family.

Conclusion

In this chapter I have traced key components in the governmentalization of the Chinese family, noting a variety of ways in which the family has been reconstituted as an object of governmental scrutiny and intervention. The interests of Chinese governmental reasoning in isolating family members have invariably been caught up in the discourse on the current state of the population which has had a serious impact upon the status of women in Chinese society, as they are most often held responsible for problems with excessive reproduction. This has meant deploying governmental technologies that are often seen by Western (and indeed many Chinese) observers as serious encroachments on the reproductive rights of women.

But we have also noted the concomitant development of a discourse on the economy of pleasure in recent times. Not content merely to divorce sex from reproduction, Chinese governmental reasoning has been at pains to ensure that sexual conduct, particularly the sexual conduct of women, is confined to the institution of marriage. This, it seems to me, stems in large part from the foundational status the family assumes in Chinese Marxist sociological and historical understanding. The family, in this view, is the teleological endpoint of familial evolution. It has played a key role in the development of the productive forces and continues to function as a regulatory mechanism in the "quality" of the population. Hence, it comes as no surprise that, although the family has gained much autonomy from the apparent "retreat of the state" since 1978, it has in the case of marriage and reproduction intensified as the key link in governing the reproductive regularities of the population. Women have endured the brunt of this intensification.

One notable aspect of Chinese discourse on the family is the way in which sexuality functions as a means of problematizing familial relations. Rather than seeing sexuality as a means of self-interiorization, sexual conduct in these texts are linked to a discourse of balance and to the dissemination of "techniques of existence" (which are fundamental to maintenance of this balance). This includes the dissemination of a whole body of literature on the know-how of sex and an economy of pleasure. Sex, like the consumption of food and the wearing of clothing, is part and parcel of harmonizing individual and familial life. But the nature of these practices (sex, food, and clothing) and their significance to the individual are arranged according to various socially constructed categories (class, gender, and ethnicity). In the case of sex, know-how—that is, knowing about the nature and significance of sex in human life—is not a call to sexual liberation. On the contrary, sex must remain strictly within the bounds of matrimony. It cannot be permitted under any circumstances to extend beyond the confines of the married relationship. To do so risks inciting physical and, more important, social and moral decay. Of course, we know that this is wishful thinking and that sexual activity constantly inhabits ground outside of the married relationship. The point here is to understand both why and how Chinese governmental authorities invest so much energy in trying to disseminate this ideal.

In this connection, Kay Ann Johnson has noted that "woman's sexuality and reproductive capacity appear to be simultaneously the source of her greatest value to the male group and the primary source of her power to disrupt it"

(1983, 17). Hence, in the popular advice literature we have seen that much attention has been focused on instructing young women to manage and control the sexual advances of their courtiers. Newly wedded wives must also be adept at satisfying the sexual needs of their husbands while also staying clear of the dangers of extramarital affairs.

We have also seen that husbands are not exempt from injunctions. They are also instructed to pay attention to the sexual desires of their wives. The texts clearly note that women have sexual desires and the ability to experience sexual pleasure. Men and women, however, experience their sexuality in naturalized forms, which posits a fundamental biological and psychological distinction between the sexes. If we take K. Johnson's statement seriously, we can assume that the instructions given to both men and women in these texts are geared toward maintaining control over the sexuality of women (and this may entail satisfying their sexual "needs" so as to prevent them from seeking "relief" elsewhere). Sexual pleasure, for both husband and wife, thus plays an important role in the maintenance of familial harmony.

What are the strategic and theoretical implications of this for the way we think about the brutality of aspects of Chinese government, particularly those directed at women and their reproductive capacities? How do we reconcile "brutality" with "pleasure"? Forced abortion and sterilization are especially abhorrent, and it is correct to direct our outrage toward those institutions involved. It is clear that, if the state is not directly involved (which it resolutely claims not to be), then it is at the very least to be held responsible. By the same token, we should recognize the efforts made by the state (and at the moment there is not much scope for nonstate activity in China) to advance the cause of "sexual equality," no matter how distasteful the actual way this is done may appear. We need to critique this program of (dis)information but acknowledge simultaneously that we are dealing with much more than just "the state" in this instance. The state is not a totality. It is made up of diverse factions and forces. Chinese culture is not a totality but is constituted by diverse traditions and practices.

Indeed, there is no simple solution to the problems of population and sexuality in contemporary Chinese politics. Despite twenty years of economic growth, poverty in rural China is still a serious fact of everyday life. Many intellectuals and government officials view the source of poverty as chronic overpopulation. They argue that, confronted with low levels of education (cultural and political) and well-entrenched feudal practices (such as favoring male offspring), they have no choice but to regard family planning as a purely administrative measure that pays little attention to the rights of the individual. We have seen from this analysis that the problems are as much historical as they are contemporary. Strategies for resistance and overcoming excessive state intrusions into everyday life must take into account the historical nature of the context within which a specific problem is located. We should highlight the historical and contingent nature of Chinese government. We should ask ourselves what makes such practices knowable, calculating, and amenable to governmental intervention. In so doing, we hope to be in a better position to make use of this particular mode of reasoning in defining localized strategies of resistance.

NOTES

I am indebted to my dissertation supervisors and examiners, and the editors and reviewers for this volume, in assisting in refining this chapter.

1. *you jiao wu lei.*
2. The debate over Chinese "culturalism" is highly controversial. The basic gist of the culturalist argument states that traditional Chinese forms of identity were based on adherence to certain cultural and social practices (hence the reference to "techniques of living") rather than racial or nationalist forms of collectivity. This culturalism is in turn eroded and eventually replaced by forms of "Chinese-ness" that are directly linked to "nation and race." For more on this, see the various contributions to Unger 1996; and Tu Wei-ming 1994.
3. One way in which government authorities attempted to redirect the conduct of the common people was to take an active part in popular festivals and religious ceremonies. James Watson (Johnson, Nathan, and Rawski 1985) in a study of the Mazu cult (a popular cult in southern China, particularly Taiwan, Fujian, and Guangdong) describes how authorities made use of the popularity of the local cult and transformed it through government patronage so as to ensure heterodox tendencies were kept in check. A more recent example can be found in the attempts of government authorities to exert influence over the direction and activities of the *qigong* (meditative and breathing exercises) craze that swept across China during the 1980s (see Chen 1995).
4. The socialist work unit is a case in point. As Henderson and Cohen sagaciously note, "On paper, the regulations of the *danwei* [the socialist work unit] create a rigid and comprehensive system of life and work. In practice, though still awesome in scope, this new form of Communist organization has blended closely with older, traditional styles of organizational behavior in China" (1984, 9). The work unit is at once revolutionary and traditional. They note that the *danwei* is not organized on family or kinship ties: "Rather, the work unit has been created and administered by the state to orchestrate more closely life and work in Chinese communities" (1984, 27). These prerogatives mesh closely with concerns with productivity and planning. The work unit made possible a vast array of relations that were beyond the immediate grasp of the family, enterprise, and government (horizontal and vertical relations with other units, organizations, programs, etc.). As David Bray (1997, 40) explains in his work on the readaptation of traditional architectural modes to modern settings, the spatial configuration of the work unit is far more conducive to "collective" modes of subjectivity.
5. Or in the case of Western liberal thought the family is at last liberated from the burden of over-government.

6. In terms of the exigencies of war Kane (1987, 16) notes that for the strategic agenda of the CPC war of resistance against Japan the "family" meant the "big family," the clan or semiextended family, and not the small conjugal unit. The move toward nuclearization does not occur until much later. This is especially the case in terms of family planning when in the 1970s educational materials were designed specifically for young couples and not the larger family unit. By this time most urban couples have developed a sufficient level of literacy to form the primary focus of this kind of governmental material. Literate capacities are an important part of the formative work of governance.

7. Indeed, some contemporary Chinese commentators have noted the recent revitalization of fascist-inspired terminology that was originally in vogue in the 1930s in China. Chinese intellectuals who lived during that period connected talk of "spiritual and physical civilization" with the eugenics movement and were surprised to see it once again plastered across the Chinese media during the course of the 1980s (private discussions with Chinese writer Sang Ye).

8. Whereas mainland Chinese authorities avoid mention of the word *Confucian*, the Singaporean government has been very explicit in its praise for various "Confucian values" concerning the family, civility, and education (see Hill and Lian Kwen Fee 1995).

9. It is worthwhile noticing the importance of Lewis Henry Morgan in establishing the theoretical preconditions for this kind of history. Morgan's classic work *Ancient Society*, first published in 1877, was admired by Marx and used extensively in Engels's history of the family; hence, it is not surprising that he is considered as one of the most revolutionary contributors to the disciplines of history, anthropology, and sociology by many Chinese scholars. This may help explain the particular "conservative" position on the family within orthodox Chinese Marxism.

10. On the connection between familial evolutionism, "civilization," and the work of Engels and Morgan, see Cartier 1996a, 491.

11. The rise in the number of unmarried urban youngsters in their late twenties has been regarded as a potential source of social instability. Authorities believe that efforts must be made to get them married—this will help "calm" them down. Hence, various associations such as the Women's Federation, the Youth League, and private agencies are very active in finding partners for unmarried young adults.

12. Of course, like many other state initiatives set in place after 1949, marriage laws had a trial run in the liberated areas. Meijer (1971, 177) notes that the obligation to register marriage in the liberated areas was generally conceived in the various Marriage Regulations as an obligation of both a moral and legal kind but not a condition for the very existence of the marriage—except in the case of divorce, in which it was definitely required.

13. The original intention of the new marriage law was that, once marriages ceased to be feudal, there would be little ground or need for divorce, because the new marriages existed on the basis of the socialist principles of equality and willingness (Kane 1987, 19).

14. The new Procedures of Marriage Registration adapted to the new Marriage Law in 1980 state the same purposes (DCAPRC 1989, 100).

15. Indeed, this is precisely what happened in Tiexi District of Shenyang City in September 1963. The Health Ministry issued a directive condemning the practice of the marriage registration procedures in that district, which required a virginity check for women that was witnessed and signed by the prospective male groom. The directive

states that it is not necessary to check the reproductive organs, the only concern is with the diseases syphilis, tuberculosis, mental illness, and leprosy (DCAPRC 1989, 95). This was followed by another directive in October stating that such practices humiliate women and that the masses are not used to the idea of a health check for marriage. Moreover, if not done correctly, a lot of problems could emerge. The directive further noted that the health check is not compulsory and that, if a couple should desire one, then they reserve the right to go to a hospital of their choice. Refusing the health check is not adequate grounds to deny registration of the marriage (DCAPRC 1989, 97). The intent of this directive seems to have largely been ignored by consequent policy initiatives. More recently, in the city of Wuhan women found to be "nonvirgins" during the course of the premarriage health examination face a fine of between one hundred and two hundred yuan. They must also compile a self-criticism and if found pregnant must pay a fine of an extra one hundred yuan for each month that has passed between conception and the checkup (*China News Digest* 1996a). Needless to say, the practice has caused much controversy, with both sides of the debate claiming moral authority. In defense of the policy the director of the Marriage Department at the Wuhan Bureau of Civil Affairs argued that it was necessary in order to combat the rising tide of immorality. In addition to the fining of nonvirgins the Marriage Register in the same city is also fining couples up to two thousand yuan for living together without a marriage certificate and has the authority to order them to separate (*China News Digest* 1996b).

16. Later childbirth, longer spaces between pregnancy, and fewer children.

17. This link is clearly demonstrated in Engels's "two forms of production" theory, which was widely disseminated in the first few years after 1978. See Liu Zheng 1980, 7.

18. The one-child policy was first implemented on a trial basis in Sichuan Province in 1979, from which it spread rapidly to the rest of China. The policy dictated that the vast majority of Chinese citizens should only have one child and that there should be social and economic incentives (longer maternal leave; subsidized education, health, and housing) and disincentives (fines, social stigma of being a *hei haizi* (black child) in order to achieve that goal. The policy has also gone through alternating periods of "enforcement" and "coercion" and periods of relative leniency. Most of the specific measures are formulated at the provincial or municipal level, and hence there is a degree of disparity about the exact conditions under which families can give birth to a second child (Peng Xizhe 1991, 16). Generally speaking, a second child is allowed when the first child is physically or mentally handicapped, the family lives in a remote mountain region, or they belong to one of China's many minorities. Hence, while the policy exemplifies the totalizing momentum of "governmentality" in China, it is by no means totalitarian. The policy has been neither centrally directed nor inflexibly applied. I have discussed the one-child policy in terms of governmental strategies for managing the population previously. See Sigley 1996.

19. See Minson 1985, 29–37, for an extended discussion on the relationship between alliance and sexuality as deployed within Foucault's work.

20. Charlotte Furth (1994) brings to our attention that these oriental *ars erotica* are highly male centered, and in many cases little is said of pleasure but more of "life preserving" and "attaining immortality."

21. Only in Buddhism does a similar concern with "the flesh" appear. But, as Pan Suiming (1995a, 29) notes, this has never hindered Chinese people from holding a healthy skepticism toward the chastity of Buddhist nuns and monks. The author has

published a selected translation of Pan Suiming's *Zhongguo xing xianzhuang* (The state of sex in China) and translations of other work on the family and sex that are referred to here in a special edition of *Chinese Sociology and Anthropology* (Sigley 1998).

22. I would like to thank an anonymous reviewer for forcefully noting this coexistence of views. This also makes an interesting contrast with Mohandas Karmachand Gandhi's views on birth control and sex produced under conditions of colonial hegemony. Like many Chinese discussions on sex and procreation, Gandhi emphasizes the importance of correct moral conduct in conditioning the self. Whereas contemporary Chinese discourse on sex and procreation separates pleasure from conception, Gandhi's adopts a position of pure abstinence. See Alter 1996, for discussion regarding the "biomoral imperative" in Gandhi's work on self-restraint and public health.

23. This concern with understanding and governing the sexual conduct of citizens is further expressed in the recent survey of twenty thousand subjects in China on the question of sexual activity and attitudes toward sex (Liu Dalin 1992). This is another instance in which different forms of knowledge and practices of knowledge (i.e., sexology and statistics) are deployed in order to "know" the population. The important question here is not so much what the results reveal—although this is undoubtedly significant—but more so how governmental agencies interpret and act upon those results, what technological means they deploy to direct undesirable practice in more favorable directions, and, indeed, how much the results and methodology themselves are caught up in the wider governmental ethos that I have been attempting to outline. What matters are the procedures through which the problems of sex, marriage, and the family are problematized and interconnected. For instance, in the survey sex becomes the prime object of governmental scrutiny, but only insofar as it is assumed that the proper place for sex is in the family and between lawfully wedded couples of the opposite sex. Indeed, it is assumed that the family is the only and prime place for lawful and socially condonable sexual relations—anything other than this is considered "abnormal" (*fanchangde*). Statistics are useful in this sense in materializing such abnormalities and making them amenable to governmental intervention. Sections of this work have been translated by Linda Javin (1994).

24. The numerous cases of young couples, especially in rural areas, unaware of how to copulate and conceive children is testimony to the importance of this point.

25. This is not to suggest that there is absolutely no discussion on sexual technique. On the contrary, there is a great deal of emphasis on the role of foreplay and the need to satisfy the requirements of both partners. What is lacking is the graphic detail on different sexual positions that can be found in most similar publications in Western societies. There has also been a burgeoning interest in the classic Taoist sex manuals with the recent publication of many modern annotations and commentaries.

26. These manuals differ, for instance, from similar texts in other cultural contexts, such as those described by Corbin (1995), which were compiled by French medical practitioners in the eighteenth and nineteenth centuries. These texts also stress that sex is to be enjoyed within the context of the married relationship, but they are far more assertive about the need for men to engage in spermal economy (1995, 135) and do not by any means encourage excessive intercourse. By contrast, there is little discussion of the adverse effects of excessive sexual activity in the contemporary Chinese texts—if there is, it is usually confined to the practice of masturbation.

27. In fact, the necessity for a harmonious sex life is often cited as one of the draw-

backs of voluntary life alone (*dushenzhuyi*). People who choose not to marry or have any partners are deficient in their sexual requirements and do not, as a consequence, live as long as people within married relationships (Ding Juan et al. 1995, 10).

28. Kane (1987) notes an interesting point vis-à-vis recruiting family members into governmental programs. She refers briefly to the importance of the mother-in-law and comments on the "amount of effort the present Chinese government has put into educational materials designed to counter her 'feudal' influences and enlist her in the battles to reform the family" (1987, 7). We can see other "tensions" in programs to venerate elders and yet also challenge their "feudal" tendencies. Davin (1976, 41–42, 125–56) also talks of the importance of mother-in-laws in liberated areas in getting mothers involved in production. Traditionally, mothers-in-law could "sit back and supervise"; now they had to take an active role in caring for children and doing housework.

REFERENCES

Alter, J. 1996. Gandhi's body, Gandhi's truth: Nonviolence and the biomoral imperative of public health. *Journal of Asian Studies* 55 (2): 301–22.

Anagnost, A. 1995. A surfeit of bodies: Population and the rationality of the state in post-Mao China. In *Conceiving the new world order: The global politics of reproduction,* ed. F. D. Ginsburg and R. Rapp, 22–41. Berkeley: University of California Press.

Barlow, T. E. 1994. Theorizing woman: *Funü, guojia, jiating* (Chinese woman, Chinese state, Chinese family). In *Body, subject and power in China,* ed. A. Zito and T. E. Barlow, 253–89. Chicago: University of Chicago Press.

Bray, D. 1997. Space, politics and labour: Towards a spatial genealogy of the Chinese work-unit. *Asian Studies Review* 20 (3): 35–43.

Cartier, M. 1996a. China: The family as a relay of government. In *A history of the family,* vol. 1: *Distant worlds, ancient worlds* (trans. of *Histoire de la famille,* by S. Hanbury Tenison, R. Morris, and A. Wilson), ed. A. Burguière et al., 491–522. Cambridge: Polity Press.

———. 1996b. The long march of the Chinese family. In *A history of the family,* vol. 2: *The impact of modernity* (trans. of *Histoire de la famille,* by S. Hanbury Tenison), ed. A. Burguière et al., 216–41. Cambridge: Polity Press.

Central Department of Propaganda. 1981. Guanyu shidang kongzhi xing zhishi tushu chuban de tongzhi (A notice on the correct way to control the publication of material on sex education). *Guojia chubanju wenjian* 211.

Chen, N. C. 1995. Urban spaces and experiences of *qigong*. In *Urban spaces in contemporary China: The potential for autonomy and community in post-Mao China,* ed. D. S. Davis et al., 347–61. Cambridge: Cambridge University Press.

Chen Qingliang, ed. 1992. *Saohuang—shensheng de shiming* (The elimination of pornography—a sacred quest). Beijing: Zhonggong zhongyang chubanshe.

Chen Yiyun. 1994. *Rang xing kexue zoujin jiating* (Bringing sexology to the family). Beijing: Hongqi chubanshe.

Chi Guifa, and Gu Zhiwei, eds. 1994. *Xinhun shenghuo daquan* (The compendium for newly married life). Zhengzhou: Henan kexue jishu chubanshe.

China News Digest. 1996a. Newsletter, <http://www.cnd.org>, accessed 11 May 1996.

———. 1996b. Newsletter, <http://www.cnd.org>, accessed 19 May 1996.

Corbin, A. 1995. *Time, desire and horror: Towards a history of the senses.* London: Polity Press.
Croll, E. 1985. Introduction: Fertility norms and family size in China. In *China's one-child family policy,* ed. E. Croll, D. Davin, and P. Kane, 1–36. Basingstoke: Macmillan.
Davin, D. 1976. *Woman-work: Women and the party in revolutionary China.* Oxford: Clarendon Press.
Davis, D., and S. Harrell, eds. 1993. *Chinese families in the post-Mao era.* Berkeley: University of California Press.
DCAPRC [Department of Civil Administration under the Ministry of Civil Administration of the People's Republic of China (Zhonghua renmin gongheguo minzhengbu minzhengsi)], ed. 1989. *Hunyin gongzuo shouci* (The marriage work manual). Beijing: Qunzhong chubanshe.
Dikötter, F. 1995. *Sex, culture and modernity in China: Medical science and the construction of sexual identities in the early Republican period.* Honolulu: University of Hawaii Press.
———. 1998. *Imperfect conceptions: Medical knowledge, birth defects, and eugenics in China.* London: Hurst and Co.
Ding Juan et al., eds. 1995. *Funü rexian 100 wen* (One hundred questions from the women's hotline). Beijing: Haitun chubanshe.
Dong Jian. 1995. Nüxing xing xinli tanmi (The sexual psychology of women). *Jiating zhi you* 12:22–24.
Dong Ren, ed. 1990. *Fuqi xingfu baba* (Eighty-eight points for happiness for married couples). Ha'erbin: Beifang wenyi chubanshe.
Donzelot, J. 1979. *The policing of families.* London: Pantheon Books.
Ebrey, P. 1991. *Confucianism and family rituals in Imperial China: A social history of writing about rites.* Princeton, N.J.: Princeton University Press.
Evans, H. 1995. Defining difference: The "scientific" construction of sexuality and gender in the People's Republic of China. *Signs* 20 (21): 357–94.
Foucault, M. 1978. *The history of sexuality,* vol. 1. London: Penguin.
———. 1993 [1980]. About the beginning of the hermeneutics of the self. *Political Theory* 21 (2): 198–227.
Furth, C. 1994. Rethinking van Gulik: Sexuality and reproduction in traditional Chinese medicine. In *Engendering China: Women, culture, and the state,* ed. C. K. Gilmartin et al., 125–46. Cambridge, Mass.: Harvard University Press.
Han Lei, ed. 1993. *Xing zhishi congshu—xing hexie* (The sex knowledge series—sexual harmony). Wulumuqi: Xinjiang weiwu'er zizhiqu xingxue xuehui.
Handwerker, L. 1995. The hen that can't lay an egg (*"Bu xia dan de mu ji"*): Conceptions of female infertility in modern China. In *Deviant bodies: Critical perspectives on difference in science and popular culture,* ed. J. Terry and J. Urla, 358–86. Bloomington and Indianapolis: Indiana University Press.
Henderson, G., and M. S. Cohen. 1984. *The Chinese hospital: A socialist work unit.* New Haven: Yale University Press.
Hill, M., and Lian Kwen Fee. 1995. *The politics of nation building and citizenship in Singapore.* London: Routledge.
Honig, E., and G. Hershatter. 1988. *Personal voices: Chinese women in the 1980s.* Stanford: Stanford University Press.

Hsiao Kung-Chuan. 1975. *A modern China and a new world: K'ang Yu-Wei, reformer and utopian, 1858–1927*. Seattle: University of Washington Press.
Hu Jin, and Zhao Pinghe, eds. 1996. *Funü ertong xinli zixun 100 lie* (One hundred questions from women and children). Shanghai: Xuelin chubanshe.
Huang San, ed. 1986. *Dangdai zhongguo de weisheng shiye—xia* (Hygienic work in modern China—volume 2). Beijing: Zhongguo shehui kexue chubanshe.
Hunter, I. 1993. Subjectivity and government. *Economy and Society* 22 (1): 123–24.
Jacka, T. 1997. *Women's work in rural China: Change and continuity in an era of reform*. Cambridge: Cambridge University Press.
Javin, L., ed. 1994. Sex. *Chinese Sociology and Anthropology* 27 (2): 3–9.
Johnson, D., A. Nathan, and E. Rawski, eds. 1985. *Popular culture in late Imperial China*. Berkeley: University of California Press.
Johnson, K. A. 1983. *Women, the family, and peasant revolution in China*. Chicago: University of Chicago Press.
Kane, P. 1987. *The second billion: Population and family planning in China*. Ringwood, Vic.: Penguin.
Kazuko, O. 1989 [1978]. *Chinese women in a century of revolution, 1850–1950* (trans. of *Chugoku joseishi* by K. Bernhardt et al., ed. J. Fogel). Stanford: Stanford University Press.
Li Xingchun, and Wang Lirun. 1988. *Fuqi hexie quanshu* (A complete guide to harmony for married couples). Tianjin: Nongcun duwu chubanshe.
Li Yinhe. 1996. *Zhongguo nüxing de xing yu ai* (Sex, love and Chinese women). Hong Kong: Oxford University Press.
Liang Zhongtang. 1985. Yanjia renkou lilun kongzhi renkou zengzhang. In *Renkou suzhi lun* (On population quality), ed. Liang Zhongtang et al., 10–20. Taiyuan: Shanxi renmin chubanshe.
Liang Zhongtang et al. 1985. *Renkou suzhi lun* (On population quality). Taiyuan: Shanxi renmin chubanshe.
Liu Dalin, ed. 1992. *Zhongguo dangdai xing wenhua* (Sexual behavior in modern China). Shanghai: Shanghai sanlian shudian.
Liu Guangren. 1992. *Hukou guanlixue* (Household management studies). Beijing: Zhongguo jiancha chubanshe.
Liu Zheng. 1980. Xiang renkou ziran zengzhanglü wei ling jinjun (Toward the realization of goal-zero rate of natural increase in the population). *Sichuan daxue xuebao* 2 (3): 10–17.
Ma Xiaonian, ed. 1995. *Nüxing zixun* (Questions on sex for women). Beijing: Kexue chubanshe.
Meijer, M. J. 1971. *Marriage law and policy in the Chinese People's Republic*. Hong Kong: Hong Kong University Press.
Miller, J. 1994. *The passion of Michel Foucault*. London: Flamingo.
Minson, J. 1985. *Genealogies of morals: Nietzsche, Foucault, Donzelot and the eccentricity of ethics*. Basingstoke: Macmillan.
———. 1996. Ascetics and the demands of participation. MS.
Orleans, L. 1972. *Every fifth child: The population of China*. Stanford: Stanford University Press.
Pan Suiming. 1995a. *Zhongguo xing xianzhuang* (The state of sex in China). Beijing: Guangming ribao chubanshe.

———. 1995b. Xing wenhua: Zenyang zoudao jintian (Sexual culture: How it developed into its present state). *Dongfang zazhi* 4 (1): 50–58.
Pan Yunkang. 1986. *Jiating shehuixue* (A sociology of the family). Chongqing: Chongqing chubanshe.
Peng Xizhe. 1989. Major determinants of China's fertility transition. *China Quarterly* 117 (March): 1–37.
———. 1991. *Demographic transition in China: Fertility trends since the 1950s*. Oxford: Clarendon Press.
Pusey, J. R. 1983. *China and Charles Darwin*. Cambridge, Mass.: Harvard University Press.
Quan Yazhi, ed. 1993. *Rang mei zai xing shenghuo zhong dangyang* (Let your sex life ripple with beauty). Beijing: Huaxia chubanshe.
Ren Jianying. 1993. *Dakai xingfu zhi men de yaoshi* (The key to opening the door to happiness). Shanghai: Lixin kuaiji chubanshe.
Ren Wen, and Yin Ming, eds. 1993. *Xinhun fufu bidu* (Essential reading for newly wedded couples). Beijing: Jindun chubanshe.
Ruan Fangfu, ed. 1988. *Xing zhishi shouce* (The sexual knowledge handbook). Beijing: Kexue jishu wenxian chubanshe.
Sigley, G. 1996. Governing Chinese bodies: The significance of studies in governmentality for the analysis of birth control in China. *Economy and Society* 25 (4): 457–82.
———, ed. 1998. Getting it right: Marriage, sex and pleasure. *Chinese Sociology and Anthropology* 31 (1): 3–13.
Tu Wei-ming, ed. 1994. *The living tree: The changing meaning of being Chinese today*. Stanford: Stanford University Press.
Unger, J., ed. 1996. *Chinese nationalism*. Contemporary China Papers series. Armonk, N.Y.: M. E. Sharpe.
Wang Enfeng, and Liu Xianming. 1989. Renkou, jiating yu weilai shehui (Population, family and the society of the future). *Renkou yu yousheng* 4:28.
Wang Wei, and Gao Yulan. 1992. *Xing lunlixue* (Sexual ethics). Beijing: Renmin chubanshe.
Wang Xingjuan, Xu Xiuyu, and Wang Ling, eds. 1995. *Rang xing shenghuo meiman hexie* (Let your sex life be happy and harmonious). Beijing: Haitun chubanshe.
Wu Yishi, and Wu Ling. 1995. *Xinhun zhi shi* (The teacher for newlyweds). Chengdu: Sichuan renmin chubanshe.
Yan Shi et al., eds. 1991. *Ruhe yu minzheng jiguan da jiaodao* (How to deal with administrative organs). Beijing: Falü chubanshe.
Yang, C. K. 1959. *Chinese communist society: The family and the village*. Cambridge, Mass.: MIT Press.
Yang Lingling. 1989. *Xiandai nüxing xiuyang mantan* (Self-cultivation for the modern woman). Beijing: Xueyuan chubanshe.
Yu Jing, ed. 1992. *Xinhun daquan* (The compendium for newlyweds). Beijing: Nongcun duwu chubanshe.
Yue Ping et al. 1995. *Hemu shenghuo zai tongyi kongjian* (Living together in harmony). Beijing: Haitun chubanshe.
Zhang Xiyu et al. 1993. *Funü shenghuo daquan* (The complete guide for a woman's life). Zhengzhou: Henan kexue jishu chubanshe.

Zheng Xiaoyang, and Chen Yuhan. 1995. *Xinhun yixue zhinan* (A medical guide for newlyweds). Beijing: Renmin junyi chubanshe.

Zhong Jiaoshou. 1995. Xing'ai yu xingyu (Sexual affection and sexual lust). *Jiating yisheng* 129:24–25.

Zhou Xizhang. 1982. Cong renkou zhiliang fangmian tan liangzhong shengchan xiang shiying de guilü (On the law of mutual conditioning of two types of production from the perspective of population quality). *Renkou yanjiu* 1 (2): 44–49.

Zhu Junlun. 1993. *Xinhun bidu, fuqi bibei* (Essential reading for newlyweds and married couples). Chengdu: Chengdu keji daxue chubanshe.

CHAPTER 5

Doing God's Work: Citizenship, Gender, and Sexuality in the Philippines

Anne-Marie Hilsdon

From the 1970s politics and religion have come even closer together in the Philippines. After Vatican II many Catholic nuns and priests began to work closely with poor communities in political programs of self-determination to increase and restore their citizenship in areas of education, employment, and health. This coincided with a war in which the government and military pitted itself against the communist New People's Army (NPA). The Christian churches (of which 85 percent of the Filipino population are members), particularly the progressive Catholic Church, practicing liberation theology,[1] emerged as major protagonists. They were involved in the political struggles of the poor for more equitable distribution of resources, and they also protected poor civilians from the military, whose efforts to defeat the communist guerrilla New People's Army resulted in evacuation, destruction of property, arrest, detention, torture, and killing.

Catholic nuns played an important part in this struggle. In so doing, they renegotiated their status both as citizens and as clerics. New models of citizen-subjects vied with other models—predictably, those of the conservative state but also those of national liberation and liberation theology. This chapter deals with the formation of the nun as Filipino citizen—as woman and cleric.

The New Social Movements: National and International Connections

New social movements that emerged in the Philippines from the 1960s offered new trajectories for citizens. Such revitalization movements included the progressive (politically left) Catholic Church, the women's movement, and the movement for national liberation. Deploying the several discourses of liberation theology, feminism, and Marxism, these new social movements have reinvented notions of "nation" both as a system of cultural representation and as shared experiences of imagined community and identities (Anderson 1991). This might be compared with other Asian nations (see Menon and Bhasin; Parker, Sigley, and Ram, this volume).[2]

Global events in the Catholic world during the 1960s—the Second Vatican Council (1962–65), the encyclical "On the Development of Peoples" by Pope Paul VI (1967), and the "Justice to the World" statement by the Synod of Catholic Bishops (1971) directed toward overcoming misery and justice—produced local effects. "Third World" churches, including those in the Philippines, declared their support for "the poor," and the right to national self-determination and development was proclaimed the new route to peace. Protestant world religions, represented especially by the World Council of Churches, increasingly became concerned about social justice and human dignity and organized the first world conference for women (Fabella 1993).

In the Philippines secular and clerical movements responded directly to global and national political and economic difficulties—foreign debt, the presence of U.S. bases, internal graft and corruption, and the ownership of resources by a minority elite. Protests became revolutionary in the late 1960s, when the communist New People's Army was formed. Poor rural farmers and workers took up arms against a government dominated by a rich and powerful elite, defended by the military and bolstered by a U.S. counterinsurgency program (Bello 1987, 1988).[3] Yet the communist NPA was not the only source of instability. The Moro [Muslim] National Liberation Front (MNLF) was fighting a nationalist and religious war against the state; military factions within the Armed Forces of the Philippines (AFP) in Manila staged several attempted coups, private armies of landowners (i.e., warlords) and companies threatened workers; and weaponry was in common use among the citizenry. The Philippines became known as a "gun culture."

Filipino citizens, particularly those who developed and expressed a critical consciousness, were threatened directly with violence; they were controlled (and punished) through military force or its threat, including arrest, torture, imprisonment, salvaging,[4] bombing, and strafing. Women were doubly punished, since violence against them is also sexualized. Fanon (1970), interpreted by Bhabha (1990), argues that demand and desire in a postcolonial state is pervaded by inequities and manifest in aggression. Violence or dissidence are not acknowledged as constitutive conditions of civil authority but, rather, vilified as obstacles to progress, misrecognitions, or alien presences. Leftist movements in the Philippines emphasized that the very inequities of daily life constituted violence: some classes were submitted to hunger, homelessness, unemployment, lack of health care and education, and exclusion from political participation. In any case liberal democracies (on which the Philippines and other postcolonial governments are modeled)[5] require "only minimal levels of activity and interest.... Anything more threatens the smooth working of the political system" (Pateman 1989, 147). Pateman suggests that citizens who do not consent to be governed—the crucial part of citizenship—must be punished.[6]

A chief protagonist in the Communist Party of the Philippines–New People's Army (CPP-NPA) war, especially in rural areas, was the progressive Catholic Church. As indicated earlier, it shares affinities with the church in Latin America, also heavily influenced by Spanish colonization. The theological effort of Catholic sisters in both places was significant (Gebara 1988), and the discourses and practices of feminist liberation theology were comparable. Nuns' positioning within both the hierarchy of the Catholic Church and among the citizenry yielded many connections, linking church and state. The relation between religious, political, and sexual spheres is examined in this chapter by focusing on politically active nuns in Mindanao during the 1980s.

Though rich in natural resources, Mindanao constitutes an outlying region where comparatively low levels of services and investment have been forthcoming from a government centralized in Manila and plagued by graft and corruption. Of all outlying areas of the Philippines, Mindanao is perhaps the most impoverished, as it is the location of both Communist and Islamic insurgencies, which reached their peak in the 1970s and 1980s. Nuns occupied pivotal roles in churches and communities beset by military violence. In Mindanao in 1986 this constituted at least 12 percent of nuns—170 sisters from twenty-four of sixty different congregations, the Daughters of Mary of the Assumption, and the Maryknoll Sisters (Sister Daniel Mitchell, interview 1988). They often led national and regional human rights organizations, thus challenging the traditional roles of women as protected, passive, and nonpolitical. Their reinterpretation and de/reconstruction of traditional forms of theology informed their practice in church, human rights, community, and women's organizations. Nuns shared similarities with other woman citizens involved in radical political organizations with whom they often lived and worked. The existence of both groups contradicts pervasive definitions of women as female citizens excluded from the public domain. But nuns, as celibate,[7] childless women, contest the notion of a maternal body as the perennial basis for imagining nations and female citizenship (Elshtain 1992; McClintock 1993; Parker et al. 1992). Rather, they represent a group of women relegated through biblical tradition to an asexualized, if celebrated, sacred category. For example, nuns in Mindanao are perceived to have advantages over laywomen: "People look up to sisters as people who are free from dishonesty, lies, graft and corruption for they represent the church" (Sisters Association in Mindanao [SAMIN] 1989, 25).

I arrived in the Philippines at the height of these struggles and undertook fieldwork in several rural and urban nontribal areas of Mindanao in the southern Philippines in 1988. I was studying the position of Christian Cebuano-speaking women in the intensely militarized but undeclared civil war between the communist New People's Army and the government's armed forces. Because of the close links between Gabriela, the key militant women's network with whom I worked, and SAMIN (one of several religious member organizations of Gabriela), I met several nuns engaged in nationalist struggles. I conducted interviews and participant observation in convents in militarized areas, where I stayed for safety, and in *barrios* (villages) where the sisters worked. I also interviewed several nuns who headed national church networks in Manila. Data were also collected from secondary sources, including parish records (1983–88), congressional proceedings (1985–89), and church newsletters (1988–91).

Theology and Citizenship

Liberation theologians have focused on justice for the poor and oppressed in the Third World. But not all theologians living in the Philippines and other parts of the Third World are liberation theologians—nor are all Third World theologies liberationist. Theologies of liberation aim to enhance citizenship among the poor. "Religiosity and poverty, each in its liberatory dimension, coalesced to forge a common front" (Pieris 1988, 88) that informed progressive church activities in the Philippines and other Asian societies.

Universal notions of theology have been challenged by Asian theologians (e.g., the Ecumenical Association of Third World Theologians [EATWOT], Fabella 1993). Asian Christian theologians need to take the experiences and aspirations of the "non-Christian" majority in Asia seriously (Pieris 1988). This has entailed a reexamination and reincorporation of both Asian and global religions including Christianity, Buddhism, Taoism, Hinduism, and Islam (Pieris 1988; Yeager 1988). The construction of a "utopia" of liberation theology in the Philippines, as in Latin America, is sensitive to place. Diverse liberation theologies reflect the different relations established between theological doctrine and pastoral practice in a plurality of historical and cultural situations (Scherer-Warren 1990). In the search for a relevant theology, tensions emerged among Third World church women about privileging class (being Third World) over race (being Asian) (Fabella 1993).

Moreover, although colonialism may have ended in 1946 as a formal historical relation, it is seen to persist in religious and other discursive practices. Thus, a critique of universal forms practiced in the Philippines as Eurocentric

158   Borders of Being

has led to a development of a liberation theology for Filipino and other Third World women, located between that attributed to Third World men and Western feminists. Asian women theologians—such as Virginia Fabella (1988, 1993), Mary John Mananzan (1987, 1988), Mercy Oduyoye (Oduyoye and Kanyoro 1992), and Marianne Sun Ai Lee Park (Lee Park 1989)—are anxious not to be classified as aping Western women, but their theology is perceived also as markedly different from that of men (Fabella 1993). They suggest, as do feminists of difference in the West, that claims of sexual and gender neutrality in religion are only possible to the extent that individuals are disembodied. They also proclaim that, if emerging theologies do not include women's views, then they cannot be considered relevant or liberating for church or society.

The Clerical Body as Citizen

But how does all this relate to how women were situated in earlier, indigenous connections between religion and politics? The literature suggests strong precolonial and early colonial links between church, state, and sexuality. Priestesses of the pre- and early-colonial Philippines,[8] namely *babaylan* (Bisayan) and *katalonan* (Tagalog), apparently "talked to the devil," interpreted wars, illnesses, and events in the community, determined village and individual activities, and even led insurrections against the Spanish (Guerrero 1992;[9] Veneracion 1992; and see Hilsdon 1995, for a more detailed discussion). The credibility and leadership of priestesses in the community seemed to be assured by their sexual and reproductive competence, but they were perceived as a threat to their colonial rivals, the Spanish priests, and many were accused and punished as witches (*brujas*) and goblins (*brujas y duendes*).[10] Eventually, indigenous priestesses and priests were discredited and converted to Catholicism, but religious and governmental control was never absolute (Aguilar 1988; Guerrero 1992; Veneracion 1992). The priestly profession reconstituted itself solely as a male domain by the end of the seventeenth century, and the rules on celibacy and virginity for women became more restrictive. Priestesses sought to join convents as *beatas* (nuns), headed by Spanish priests, but their positions were never comparable in scope with that of *babaylans* (Veneracion 1992).

Since the sixteenth century, female sexuality in the Philippines has been defined in the terms of Spanish Catholic Christianity. During Spanish colonization, male clergy instructed local women in virginity, chastity, and modesty. Seventeenth-century texts expound priests' manuals of instruction in this regard (Guerrero 1992). The *Lagda* and *Urbana at Felisa*, concerned with food, manners, and right conduct, were written in the nineteenth century, and, as in the catholicized West, the lives of various saints who died defending their virginity were told. Sexual intercourse and the corporeal pleasures of Adam and Eve were regarded as inherited sin, and their disobedience of God was referred to as the "original death," characterized by suffering, want, sin, mortality, and punishment forever in hell (Veneracion 1992). Salvation required the continual, conscious effort of preserving chastity. Through holiness one could atone for sins, thus making eventual death a renewal of life.[11]

Filipino women were, as in other states, identified as active transmitters and producers of national culture and as biological reproducers of the nation (cf. Yuval-Davis and Anthias 1989). But Pateman (1989) suggests that women have been incorporated into the civil order as subordinates, or "lesser men," and not as "men." Through giving birth, domestic service and child care, women represent the private—namely, all that is excluded from the public sphere—and their sexual embodiment prevents them from enjoying the same political standing as men (Pateman 1989, 4). Moreover, nuns in the Philippines as elsewhere were not, in general, allowed to participate in the religious sphere in the same way as men. Confined to the "private" sphere of convents and congregations presided over by a hierarchy of priests, nuns were expected to "decorate the church [and] be in charge of the choir" (SAMIN 1989, 25). They were excluded from official church functions, such as administration of the sacraments of forgiveness and healing and the celebration of holy mass, and prohibited from joining the priesthood (41). They were not able to participate in making church policy or decision making about the new direction of the church. "Sisters are not expected to say anything about hunger, malnutrition, poverty, exploitation, injustices and even killings. Such concerns are only for the [male] government officials or for civic organizations" (25).

Yet women, including nuns, were active participants in the nationalist struggle (Cass 1992;[12] Hilsdon 1995). But what was *their* relation to the dominant discourses of women as bearers of Filipino traditions as wives and mothers? As single women, without children, nuns were subjects who contradicted such hegemonic female images of nationalism, gender identity, and citizenship. How, then, are they implicated in "inventing" the Philippine nation?

Nuns as Clerics

Asian theologians (such as Fabella 1988; Jin 1988; Mananzan 1987; Mananzan and Park 1988; Tse 1988) advocate the primacy of praxis[13] to achieve ecumenical outcomes while working within present theological frameworks. For the church in the Philippines, Mananzan and Park (1988) identify a basis of unity that lies beyond "religious self-oriented interests of the churches" in solidarity, rather, with the struggle of the poor and oppressed, especially women. In Asian feminist theology

> the image of the human being transcends the dualistic body-and-soul relationship and has an optimistic view of the possibilities of personhood . . . body *and* soul are saved. (Mananzan and Park 1988, 81)

This conception is associated with the development of a separate Goddess theology, which Reuther (1983), a Western theologian, suggests is a correction to polarized masculinist beliefs and practices through an emphasis on worldly praxis and embodied belief.

Prior to the Second Vatican Council (1967), Filipino Catholic nuns were subjected to the same rigors of seclusion as nuns elsewhere—no newspapers, radios, contact with family, or participation in sacred ritual. But they were also culturally and linguistically isolated by serving in predominantly foreign orders (Barry 1992). After Vatican II, nuns shed their habits and were granted more active, if still secondary, roles within the church and in community work, but such roles seldom transcended the spheres of activity that "nature" and "God" assigned to women.

While the Catholic Church in the Philippines has assumed an extremely visible public and political role at local, regional, and national levels, its representatives have been predominantly male. Nuns have always been subject to the authority of male clerics. Priests were often responsible for adjudging nuns' suitability for sacramental ministry work, their form of dress, and organization of community life. As "brides of Christ,"[14] their mobility was restricted even if their marriage was construed as an asexual union of souls. As a "bride" a nun's experience of consent was different from that of a male religious: obedience to God was reinforced through obedience to the parish priest as God's earthly representative. Nuns did not help formulate basic church policy decisions but, rather, were restricted to the implementation of plans (Fabella 1988; Veneracion 1992).

Hence, clerical relationships with priests were often negotiated with difficulty because of gendered norms and expectations by male clerical authority about the gendered abilities of nuns. Some priests did not want nuns to work with them in the public sphere. As Sister Josie explained:

> We were told [by the Redemptorists] not to go to the "red" [communist-controlled] areas. They boycotted our meeting. I questioned. "It is not a matter of care and concern for [us], it's because you feel accountable," I

said to them, "I just want to concretize my vows. Teach people the rights of citizenship . . . to fight for the rights of citizenship . . . to become independent and organized."

Sister Annie told me about her relationship with Father Brian in Mindanao in 1988:

> He was okay for "dole out" (i.e., giving resources to the people); he was functional, but he did not have the feelings of the people. I am a threat to him because we are on equal footing in doing *kauban* (working together for the people). He wanted to be the authority. I told him, "If you expect respect you have also to respect us." After all, we do the work he writes about in his papers. We have a nice relationship now. You have to fight it out and sometimes he has the last say.

Several Asian feminist theologians critique the idea of woman as a nonperson and noncitizen. For example, Pui Lan argues:

> Women suffer from the millennia-old prejudices and discriminations of the male-dominated Eastern cultures, from rampant socio-political exploitations, and from their structured vulnerability. These big burdens join hand-in-hand to rob a woman of her personhood, to render her a nobody. (1986, 92)

Katoppo (1986), a feminist theologian, suggests that the theology for which women in Asia strive is a reconstructed familial relationship with a female deity: a maternal God comforting all the nonpersons (nonpersons because they are not rich, not male, not white) and assuring them that they are her beloved children. Asian feminist theologians begin from the premise that sexism against women is a universal sin (Fabella 1988; Jin 1988) that imposes an oppression additional to those of poverty, race, and class.[15]

Within contemporary theological frameworks, Catholic nuns in the Philippines deconstruct Scripture, dogma, and accounts of "traditional" religious practices as represented in biblical texts. Using inclusive language, they have reworked such texts in order to make new meanings of religious traditions (e.g., Mananzan 1988; Fabella 1988) and have uncovered women's hidden experiences in scriptural arguments, making justice and liberation the unifying message. Feminist theology has de-emphasized the masculinity of Christ and focuses instead on stories of his positive relationships with women and on his androgynous qualities of love and compassion. In this way they distinguish

Jesus from the other prophets, defining Christ as a symbol of human freedom and compassion while simultaneously rejecting, because of its demeaning view of humanity, the idea of supernatural salvation from human life. They emphasize the humanity of Christ and stories of his helpfulness to the poor and downtrodden, both in a material and spiritual sense.

For many religious women (e.g., Bacani 1988; Buhay 1988; Rose 1988) God was always female or androgynous, "a sweet, loving, caring and gentle mother" (Rose 1988, 155). Mananzan (1988) and Buhay (1988) are critical of a moral theology that focuses on "the sins of the flesh": where woman is represented as both "virgin-mother" (who it is impossible for women to emulate) and "Eve the temptress" (or whore, a pervasive trope in the Philippines as in other societies). "Mary," or the Mother of God, is deconstructed from an "up-there" image of grace, purity, power, fidelity, and physical virginity, the perfect embodiment of male control of women. She is remodeled (e.g., by Buhay 1988) as an image of unflinching faith, conscientized and committed in solidarity with the struggle of the poor and oppressed. This remodeling perforce reposes the question, What is the role of celibate or desexualized women?

The cooperation of priests and nuns in spiritual development was considered crucial by Filipino and other Asian feminist theologians (Fabella 1988). Priests appreciate women's capacity to enhance warm and loving human relationships and their ability to relate to a God who is personal (Mananzan and Park 1988). Yeager (1988), a Western theologian, also suggests that women, because of their marginalization, may be best able to understand the meaning of forgiveness and reconciliation. Yet the hierarchical church order is dually disadvantageous to women: they are vulnerable to the besetting consequences of the feminization of sin, and, even when they have managed to "break the hold of sin and reach toward reconciliation," their actions may be interpreted as "simply seeking hierarchical advantage . . . questioning of that order will *appear* to be self-serving" (Yeager 1988, 511).

Thus, a reconstruction of Catholicism in the Philippines has included a critique both of its masculinist and its Western forms, which are often associated. According to Fabella (1988), contemporary liberation theology recognizes that the rigid, cold, purely rationalist theology of the West needs spiritual flexibility and creativeness. For women in the church it offers

> more than a vertical relationship with God . . . [it is] an inner liberation, self knowledge, self acceptance [which] is equated with growing spirituality . . . nourished by their growing understanding of their self-image, which has been obscured by the roles that have been assigned to them by patriarchal society. (Mananzan and Park 1988, 83)

Yet the sexuality of nuns remains largely unexplored by contemporary Asian liberation theology. The first discussions of sexuality by nuns and priests reportedly took place only in 1993 (Fabella 1993). In Mindanao nuns' critiques of strict church laws on women's sexuality, such as those depriving them of their rights to birth control, divorce, and abortion, exclude the sexuality of women such as themselves (SAMIN 1989, 41). Are they celibate or desexualized? And do they engage in lesbian relationships? Their celibacy with respect to men was represented in magazine illustrations of solidarity in which they embraced *barrio* women and one another (SAMIN 1988, 56) but not men (SAMIN 1987, 10). The progressive Sisters Association in Mindanao actively advocated the development of closer relationships with one another (SAMIN 1989, 52), yet such relationships, as in other countries, are not openly sexual. Nuns seem to have become degendered and desexualized to accomplish their work leading poor and oppressed communities. Yet, like other Filipino women, they are perceived as the embodiment of "respect" and "protectiveness," imagery they use to advantage, like other political activists negotiating with the military. They can also actively desexualize themselves and their work. This is sometimes represented graphically, such as the reworking of St. Valentine's Day popularized images. In a congress on peace building, two large intertwining hearts inscribed with the words *peace* and *love* were depicted (SAMIN 1988, 55).

Nuns have acknowledged that their relationships in the community with male priests and members of the church hierarchy are stifled and they fear intimacy. Their awareness of and concern about community tensions about any reconstitution of their gender and sexual relations are revealed in their question: Do our congregations and communities love us enough to allow us to grow as we want to as persons? (SAMIN 1989, 25).

Merging Clerical and Political Bodies

As in Latin America (described by Molineaux 1983), the Catholic Church in the Philippines included: a traditionalist apostolic church comprising a conservative minority of bishops vaunting spiritual progress only; a modernizing majority church led by Cardinal Sin, based on a capital liberalist democracy aligned with ruling elites' interests; and a progressive church that sides with the poor in their struggle for a more equitable economic and political order.

Vatican II forged changes in values and experiences of daily life and facilitated religious activism (Barry 1992; Scherer-Warren 1990). Both liberation theology and socialism/communism express a utopianism founded in socioeconomic equality with political liberty a consequent result (Scherer-Warren 1990). Progressive clerics in the Philippines became aware of contradictions in the social system and the inadequacy of proposed political economic measures. They criticized the structures of power that created such forms of oppression, exploitation, and degradation (Rose 1988).[16] Bernales, who writes about Latin America, suggests that

> the Church, by means of new theological output and a new pastoral practice, helped in the process of awareness of the people. Here a new religious discourse appears, where the God of life is also a God of history and where history is made by a man [sic] fighting against the forces of death. (1983, 175)

Thus, being a nun in contemporary times meant being engaged in key social concerns and often being in the forefront of militant struggles (Mananzan 1988). Many were fully integrated into the National Democratic Movement[17] and, to a lesser extent, the National Democratic Front.[18] Nuns and priests ran several human rights organizations, such as Taskforce Detainees (TFD) and Concerned Citizens for Justice and Peace (CCJP). They worked closely with people whose citizenship had been compromised through the political power of rich over poor, government over citizens, capitalists over workers, elites over masses, colonialists over those colonized, and the power of men over women.[19]

The progressive church (Catholic and Protestant) resembled other new social movements in the Philippines. It was *for* national unity and sovereignty, including the reduction of foreign debt, removal of U.S. bases, and nationalization of industry, it was *for* the reduction or elimination of poverty, more equitable distribution of resources and collective rights in law and land, including women's rights. It was *against* militarization, imperialism, neocolonialism, and environmental destruction. To progressive church members religion was considered oppressive if it was limited to a personalized relationship with God, which "stagnated its followers to a stage of mediocrity by not challenging them to go beyond just receiving sacraments" (Ester 1988, 137–38). Clerical work resembled a stage of Paolo Friere's development of critical consciousness for liberation, that is, engagement in struggles for radical changes in the current social structure (Scherer-Warren 1990). Such practices were considered the "essence" of religion—not "mere God-talk" (Pieris 1988).

SAMIN stressed the participation of women religious in the church, the people's liberation struggle, and the women's movement. Members worked collectively or individually with the poor under the auspices of their specific religious denomination in basic Christian communities[20] or in cause-oriented organizations (see SAMIN 1989–91).

Filipino nuns, like their counterparts in Latin America (Gebara 1988), presented reconstructed Scripture and dogma highlighting representations of God as committed to the liberation of the poor, of Mary as an intimate interlocutor for women's problems, and of Jesus as less remote and more understandable—a Santo Niño (little Jesus), with whom Filipinos have a special affinity. Exceptionally strong religious faith, particularly in Mary and Santo Niño, was considered the basis from which rural peasants resisted poverty and injustice and nuns became their public and military spokeswomen.

Some nuns became involved in the people's movement through their work, teaching catechists and other lay church workers. Sister Annie, who became politically active after the late President Marcos's declaration of martial law (1972), told me in Davao City in 1988:

> I was a missionary, but there was something wrong. I wanted more of a challenge . . . so I asked Father Brian if I could work in a "red" [i.e., communist] area. . . . The families are so poor and depressed . . . sons are in the NPA and daughters work as medics. They want to change the system.

Nuns' work with the poor is perceived as connecting religion to survival by a spiritual and material indebtedness to those they "serve." Religious women, such as Sisters Annie and Josie, seek the "concretization of their vows" by working with the poor in the *barrios*. Sister Annie explained:

> The people live my vows, I do not; [and] I was shaken by that insight. In the hills you eat just salt. I think of the convent if I'm tired. I will go down to the city and relax and swim—so safe. The people teach me how to live. It is us who are evangelized by the poor, not the other way around. I've learned a lot.

Liberation theology has been adopted, however, only by a minority of bishops, nuns, and priests; most religious people did not work this way in the Philippines in 1988 (Cass 1992). Sister Josie told me in Surigao, Mindanao, in 1988:

> Not all of us can accept working in reality [i.e., with the people and the NPA]; some religious are for the people, but at a higher level. They don't go to the *barrios*. They don't get involved because they are afraid of communists.

Violence and Liberation

Throughout the 1980s, power mechanisms operating through the Roman Catholic and Protestant Churches influenced violent military control over civilians. The conservative Catholic Bishops Conference occasionally spoke out against militarization and especially human rights abuses (e.g., *Manila Chronicle*, 17 July 1988). But, as mentioned earlier, the progressive Catholic and Protestant Churches, especially in rural areas, became protagonists in the war between the CPP-NPA and the AFP. Appeals for human rights were used effectively by the church to curb militarization of civilians. Focusing primarily on attainment of basic needs and human rights for all, religious communities monitored the violations of notoriously abusive military commanding officers and their battalions as they were transferred from one area to another in rural Mindanao.

> Colonel Carmelius was terrible; with Colonel Guanco, there were isolated abuses, and abusive soldiers have been reprimanded and disappeared; he initiates dialogues with evacuees until their return to their farms; some [military personnel] build up cases [against civilians] to get even with charges of human rights abuses against them. (Cass 1992, 288)

Evacuated civilians usually preferred to be housed with the church, which was considered far less threatening than the military. This angered the AFP, which had plans for civic action and reform and attempted to control some evacuation programs (see my discussion of reform of civilians, Cass 1992, 290–31). "The military and clergy don't trust each other"—such was the claim of rural government officials, including Mayor Guasa of Bislig, Surigao Province. The military charged the clergy with supporting the NPA and speaking out about human rights violations by the military, whereas the clergy claimed that the political neutrality of evacuated civilians was not respected (Cass 1992).

Living and Dying like Christ

In their work Catholic nuns challenged boundaries of citizenship in ways other women did not. Bolstered by a spiritual power, borne of belief in God, they created new and powerful images of women. In so doing, they both dispelled and remodeled earlier images of chaste, passive women. They were involved, often directly as protagonists and victims, in militarized violence and its threat and have resisted militarization more effectively than other civilian women or men (Cass 1992). Like progressive Catholic priests, nuns had analyzed the influence of a colonial Catholic Church, which, they argued, had not only pacified the Filipino people but continues to contribute to the decline in the religion and way of life of cultural minorities in Mindanao. Nuns were more organized, active, and reportedly less fearful of the war than priests and bishops. Unlike them, nuns worked in highly militarized red *barrios* with Christians and cultural minorities. Like other politically active women, they critiqued patriarchal culture, which designated women's "inferior" position in war and peace. They actively adopted civic "masculine" roles, heading organizations, evacuating villages, sheltering communist suspects, confronting the military with their human rights violations, and leading protest rallies and demonstrations. This subsequently influenced their position both as nuns within all parts of the church hierarchy and as women citizens in the state.

Clerics who did not assume their rightful position in the state were punished. Entire Filipino congregations—for example, Redemptorist and Maryknoll groups—and individuals from particular congregations were spied upon, branded as communists, arrested, and sometimes killed. Consequently, as in El Salvador, this led to a "renewed interest in the efficacy of martyrdom . . . forced on the church because of the brutal destruction of life" (Grovijahn 1991, 20).[21] But Christian concepts about the martyrdom of women have been often focused on sexual assault and rape,[22] and new categories that bestowed other visibilities were required. Some nuns lived the actual experience of martyrdom daily—they knew its efficacy—and they modeled themselves on Christ. Sister Josie emphasized:

> If ever I work it is because I'm a Christian. Christ is my model. My religion is [modeled] on Christ's life. I will really die like Christ.

Nuns endangered their own lives to go to war fronts to defend life (Arellano 1988). They cared for evacuees including the sick and wounded, searched for "disappeared" community members, and witnessed the murder of loved ones. Sisters, like Annie and Josie, told me they were "with the people when they are risking their lives, to voice their needs, and to announce the bad deeds of the military." Women actually responded to whatever threatened or saved others—to them survival meant survival of the community. As in Latin America,

> [a] woman achieves fulfilment in the struggle by assuring a just life for all. . . . By constantly testifying to life, and choosing to act, to protect, and to defend life, women restore the power of choice and they also reveal an efficacy that goes beyond martyrdom as traditionally understood. Choosing is salvic. (Grovijahn 1991, 25–27)

Some nuns recalled when they first started to work in war zones in 1981 that priests invited Sister Lydia to work at the site of the first reported "hamlet-ing."[23] Now, when political activists are arrested, they call the sisters rather than priests to negotiate their release because "the military more or less respect us [as women]" (Sister Lydia, interview 1988). Nuns often worked in war zones. Sister Annie described the atmosphere in her red area (occupied by the NPA):

> Between three and five bombs were dropped each day and night, the earth shakes and the children are sick. The people asked for the bombing to stop; but instead they were pressured to become members of the Alsa Masa[24] to build a military detachment and to surrender as NPAs, after which they were trained as CAFGUs [Civilian Armed Forces Geographical Units]. Peace is for us to obey the AFP. We cannot do anything about it.

Bombing and encounters between AFP and NPA often resulted in evacuations (Cass 1992). Again, Sister Annie recalled:

> During an encounter in the village [where I was staying] there were two lines of military with guns trained on the bush—it was like a war. The people were packing to leave and they said [to me]: "You are baggage. Go back to the city." The military were coming and the people couldn't hide me. "You don't know where to run, and we are accountable [responsible] for you."

Sisters' work experiences in war zones were likened to biblical events, and they reinforced the alignment of the people's struggle with God. For example, Sister Josie compared her almost nightly evacuations to the exodus of Moses and the chosen people. Sister Josie told me that "they [the people] totally surrender to the Lord."

Conditions in evacuation centers were stressful because of the effects of militarily induced violence, hunger, malnutrition, ill health, and the threat of epidemics. Often personal quarrels erupted, and the sisters intervened. Sister Josie recalled:

> People want to fight with *bolos* [sugarcane knives]: they lose patience over the head of a dried fish; couples quarrel because opportunities for [sexual] intimacy are reduced; and children are often the recipients of their parents' aggression . . . my role was multipurpose . . . mother, guard, counselor, doctor. Sometimes I would just laugh at myself.

Awareness and change of values among the Philippine poor were stimulated "on the basis of group discussion and renewed interpretations of the Bible, mainly the Gospels and relating them to everyday life" (Scherer-Warren 1990, 18). Families met and shared problems through the inspiration of Gospels.

By working in war zones nuns crossed the given borders of female citizenship; they were suspected as communists, detained and tortured, their actions surveilled, and their lives threatened. Sister Lydia emphasizes nuns' social action despite the consequences:

> When people come to us, we do something. It is a risk for people to tell us. We write and publish the details of the [military] abuse they have suffered. When we do, the military get angry. We organize and talk to the government; we assist people to make their documents [of abuse] presentable to city councilors. Because of this we become targets.

AFP soldiers attended and taped Sister Annie's liturgy meetings and Sister Josie was monitored on public transport. Sister Annie recalled when the AFP raided her convent:

> At first I would not open the door. Then the soldiers did not believe that I and my companions were sisters, until I showed them the chapel. I was so angry I refused to help them, criticizing instead their lack of respect. I had to restrain myself from [physically] hurting the officer in charge of the raid and requested their names so that I could report them.

After the raid Sister Annie went to the cardinal, to the general of the Philippine constabulary, and to another military camp:

> If they cannot settle this, I said, I would bring it to a higher court. I was surveilled after that on public transport. I'm always being monitored. It is not good to let them know you're afraid. I always face them.

In defending the people against AFP intelligence operatives during evacuations, nuns like Sister Josie had her survival skills sharpened:

> The people would warn me if there were military of intelligence [operatives around] during evacuation. My role is one of throwing the questions back at them. I knew when they were lying; and we found ways of refusing to let them in.

Once, in 1988, heavily armed Alsa Masa and military men forced their way into a school on Human Rights Day, when a rally of unarmed marchers pursued by their gunfire sought refuge there. Armed troops surrounded the school and, amid accusations of concealing armed men, nuns were ordered to evacuate in two minutes the two thousand students already scared by the gunshots. The nuns bargained for a longer evacuation time, and, while their students were searched at gunpoint, they continued to dissuade the troops from shooting and to persuade them to enter into a dialogue with the marchers. Finally, religious and government leaders arrived to disperse the armed troops. The sisters denounced the aggression of military and paramilitary personnel and demanded that they be identified and prosecuted (SAMIN 1986–87).

A nun's residence (the convent), place of work (school), and her dress (the habit) became symbols of resistance, and the convent and school were suspected as places of concealment of enemies of the state. Similarly, in civil wars elsewhere (as in colonial Algeria and El Salvador) every veiled woman and every woman laden with a basket became suspected of concealing an arsenal (Cathcart 1991; Fanon 1967). Many nuns stopped wearing their habits on public transport and putting *sister* on their identification cards, so that they could revert to the status of a "protected" female citizen, relegated to the private sphere, perceived of as little threat in the public zone.

Some nuns "transgress" the borders of female citizenship more than others. Sister Mary affiliated with the government to work with the cultural (Lumad) minorities in the mountains of northern Mindanao, the heart of the logging industry. Lumad peoples are regarded as citizens only during elections; during the government census their area is considered uninhabited. As she worked, Sister Mary transgressed ideas of woman, citizen, and cleric:

> It was difficult at first to get the confidence of the male tribals. I had difficulties with the male chieftains. The *datu* [indigenous leaders] are men, not women. I have to deal with the men. Women are there, but do not talk. I went out with the chief to get timber. They accepted that it is possible that women [like me] could work [like them]. No one took the trouble to explain to them the history of the Philippines. I told them there were other groups struggling like them for self-determination.

Like other nuns, Mary John risked being identified as a communist:

> My knees would tremble with hunger and fatigue. We would confront the military who regularly bombed their homes. Once I borrowed an outboard, bought some gasoline to go to evacuate a father and his two children from a "red" area, because one child had a high fever. It was dangerous; the

barrio people thought I was crazy. We could have met the military. I thought it was worth dying for.

Nuns were implicated fully in the "red scare" in which citizens were considered to be either communists or government supporters. Influenced by AFP "black propaganda," villagers accused nuns of being NPAs. As Sister Lydia put it, "Because we expose data we are targeted. Graffiti on the wall says 'Assumption sisters—agents of Satan!'" (pers. comm. 1988). Hurt by such accusations, they acknowledged the inevitability of betrayal by people they assisted. Even within the church nuns were suspected of being NPAs and could be betrayed by priests. To quote again from Sister Annie:

> Father Brian thought that I was an NPA and was elated when I said that I wasn't. I kept telling him about the experiences of the people I work with, and the struggle between rich and poor. Now he has dropped the "being-used bit" and is no longer suspicious. Jun Palor, an Alsa Masa vigilante group member, issued death threats against Sister Lydia and other Assumption nuns on a radio program at the station he owns. She said she was afraid at first, because "it's harder to accept when he singles out my name, but I know he does not know [who I am]."

Clerical and political aims merged with military ones, however, when some nuns decided to work for CPP-NAP. Sister Josie assisted Communist Party officers in Mindanao: the NPA passed on its patients to her convent for treatment; she escorted their leaders to participate in secret dialogues with the bishop, government officials, and military leaders at AFP camps; and during the cease-fire (1987) she fed and housed NPAs. Several nuns and priests joined the communist New People's Army, but Sister Josie said she would take up arms only as a "last resort." Sister Annie concluded:

> I am not an NPA. I respect their role in the struggle, [but] I cannot really live with "one day, one eat." I cannot walk a "one day" walk. We [sisters] support those civilians out there without the guns, not the people with them.

Conclusion

Secular discourses of liberation in the Philippines associate citizenship almost exclusively with class and capitalism rather than gender and sexuality. Hunger and homelessness, lack of health care and education, and exclusion from politics are attributed totally to control by a rich, capitalist, elite-dominated government. But the clerical view of reforming the state is not only for the increased power of the poor as citizens but also for their human and spiritual dignity. As in Latin America, liberation theology in the Philippines aims to

> bring together people who suffer the same oppression with the aim of developing their group identity; promote the rediscovering of their dignity through this contact; increase their confidence in changing themselves and their society. (Scherer-Warren 1990, 17)

Christian feminist orientations such as those discussed here led to a critique of obdurate historico-cultural traditions that have given women a distorted image of their bodies, their abilities, their roles, their responsibilities, their dignity, and their destiny. Religion came to be considered a vehicle through which all women resist their oppression (Augustin 1987). In contrast with the extreme individualism and inflexibility they perceived in Western societies, Asian women were called on to restore inclusiveness, equality, and harmony in all human relationships (Fabella 1988; Tse 1988). Feminist theology and feminism were considered to "promote the equality of all human beings, and the ideology is derived from the experiences of women giving birth, and caring, and nurturing their children and family. . . . Here self and community are one" (Mananzan and Park 1988, 82). Thus, liberation theology may be best explained as a multiplicity of emancipations: inclusive of person and collective liberation, sexual and racial, as well as political freedom (Dussel 1978, 41). Nuns in Mindanao were able to discern their ministry according to needs of local people, not dictates of priests and bishops or a Westernized church; they developed a nuns' network in Mindanao and formed closer relationships with one another and with people in the *barrios;* they confronted governments and militaries to advocate for the citizenship rights of poor and oppressed communities. In so doing, they transgressed the boundaries of given female citizenship.

Although to some extent nuns have become the embodiment of "male" and "female" dimensions of the person, their sexual subjectivity, unlike that of the early priestesses, remains unacknowledged. In precolonial cultures the spiritual and civil status of priestesses in the Philippines was increased through sexual prowess and giving birth, which had important political implications for the Filipino state newly established by the colonizing Spanish (see my discussion, Hilsdon 1995). In contemporary times nuns occupy the same legal category as other women in the Philippines. Yet their lives, in the "private" sphere, are different from those of other women. They are advocates for the sexual concerns of other Filipino women citizens, while their own remain invisible. Intimate relations with priests and bishops remain problematic and, despite their professed convictions of being on an equal footing with priests as "companions," they can end up feeling like second-class church members with their talents repressed. As indicated earlier, nuns have resisted militarization effectively. Unlike other female political activists whose transgressive social action is punished by rape, nuns in this study were demonized rather than sexually abused. They had transgressed the sanctity of their sacred citizenship. Yet their assumed embodiment of "traditional" womanhood is evident too. Like other female political activists, it facilitated their political work, and they were physically abused less often than their male (priest) counterparts (Hilsdon 1995).

Nuns' political leadership is strengthened by a consciously developed community, yet their relationships within it are not yet overtly sexualized. Some, like Sister Josie, suggested that women are "stronger than men and have more stamina for suffering. Unlike men, they keep confronting government officials." Working alone and unaccompanied, nuns emphasized that their relationship was with God, their companion. Nuns identified sexually with the androgynous, celibate subjectivity of Jesus Christ and developed an asexual intimacy with God.

Barry (1992) suggests that in the Philippines the relationship of nuns with Christ was the ideal to which other citizens should aspire in the afterlife. Byrne (1990), a British theologian, contends that in Western Christianity the religious renunciation of sex resulted in the clerical state being regarded as more sublime than the lay. Such elevation of the religious life in the Philippines has facilitated the political leadership of nuns and their ability to resist and survive militarization.

NOTES

1. Liberation theology had its origins in Latin America:

The starting point is the liberation of the human person, the rediscovering of his/her dignity, the redefinition of his/her status of citizenship, the immediate freedom from several forms of oppression [economic, political, legal, racial, sexual, foreign exploitation]. (Scherer-Warren 1990, 17–18)

2. McClintock (1993, 61) suggests that, in shaping such nationalism, systems of cultural representation that "limit and legitimize people's access to the resources of the nation-state" are contested.

3. Profiles of congressional members and records of government members' links with, and ownership of, companies ranked according to wealth reinforce this claim. As a group, the elite profited from colonization, which enabled the development of a comprador strategy.

174   Borders of Being

4. Summary execution.

5. Philippines politics and government was shaped not only by Spain but, integrally, by the United States, which colonized it from 1898 until Independence in 1946.

6. Citizenship as a concept is used deliberately by Pateman (1989) instead of equality/inequality and equity, around which many debates about women and the state have clustered.

7. They were represented in the community as celibate, but it is possible they were involved in same-sex relations.

8. The Spanish colonized the Philippines from the sixteenth to the nineteenth centuries.

9. The outdoor (i.e., Guerrero) used missionary accounts in Spanish as sources.

10. Guerrero cites numerous examples of priestesses leading insurrections and being subjected to brutal military punishment and eventually being "converted."

11. Filipino government programs conducted to rehabilitate "surrendered communists" as government loyalists in the 1980s emphasized roles for men and women that closely aligned with these Christian ideals of chastity (see Hilsdon 1995).

12. In 1993 I changed my name from Cass to Hilsdon.

13. Primacy of praxis over theory is emphasized also by national liberation movements in the Philippines and in similar movements throughout Asia (Pieris 1988).

14. During their professing ceremony, nuns prostrate themselves on the floor at the church altar; renounce their names; take vows of poverty, chastity, and obedience; and wear a wedding ring as a symbol of Christ, their spouse (Sandra Close, pers. comm. 1992).

15. The discourse of sexism as sin contradicts the feminization of sin in biblical texts and church dogma now heavily critiqued in the Philippines (Veneracion 1992) and in the West (Yeager 1988; among others).

16. As other women and men in nationalist movements in the Philippines have done (Cass 1992, 314–63).

17. Militant left nationalist movement in the Philippines.

18. Underground leftist movement.

19. The latter, however, is not acknowledged by contemporary political theory (e.g., Pateman 1989).

20. A unit of organizational practice of liberation theology in the Philippines.

21. Such interest is not strictly clerical. See discussion of the martyrdom of political activists (Cass 1992, 338–39); for Latin America, see Sobrino 1985.

22. This was transmitted in the Philippines, for example, through teachings about the lives of saints, such as Agnes and Maria Goretti, both of whom chose death instead of being raped (and see my discussion of martyrdom and women in Hilsdon 1995).

23. A counterinsurgency strategy also used during the Vietnam War in which, in an effort to locate and disable guerrilla insurgents, the military carefully monitors the mobility and food supplies of civilians in a specific geographical area (hamlet).

24. A notorious rightist vigilante group.

REFERENCES

Aguilar, D. D. 1988. The low of high status. *Solidaridad II* 12 (1): 30–37.

Anderson, B. 1991. *Imagined communities: Reflections on the origin and spread of nationalism.* London: Verso.
Arellano, L. B. 1988. Women's experience of God in emerging spirituality. In *With passion and compassion: Third World women doing theology,* ed. V. Fabella and M. A. Oduyoye, 135–50. Maryknoll, N.Y.: Orbis Books.
Augustin, P. C. 1987. Women and politics in the Philippines. *Journal of Feminist Studies in Religion* 3 (2): 115–20.
Bacani, M. K. 1988. Autobiography—oppression and liberation. In *Woman and religion: A collection of essays, personal histories and contextualized liturgies,* ed. M. Mananzan, 113–18. Manila: Institute of Women's Studies, St. Scholastica's College.
Barry, C. 1992. Filipino Catholic nuns and the Rorschach test. Paper presented at the Australian Philippine Studies Conference, Australian National University, July.
Bello, W. 1987. *Creating the third force: US-sponsored low intensity conflict in the Philippines.* San Francisco: Institute for Food and Development Policy.
———. 1988. Counterinsurgency's proving ground: Low-intensity warfare in the Philippines. In *Low-intensity warfare: Counterinsurgency, proinsurgency, and antiterrorism in the eighties,* ed. M. T. Klare and P. Kornbluh, 158–82. New York: Pantheon Books.
Bernales, A. P. 1983. Les conditions sociales du surgissement d'une église populaire. *Social Compass* 30 (2–3): 175–209.
Bhabha, H. K., ed. 1990. *Nation and narration.* London and New York: Routledge.
Buhay, H. 1988. Who is Mary? In *Woman and religion: A collection of essays, personal histories and contextualized liturgies,* ed. M. Mananzan, 59–63. Manila: Institute of Women's Studies, St. Scholastica's College.
Byrne, L. 1990. Apart from or a part of: The place of celibacy. In *Through the devil's gateway: Women, religion and taboo,* ed. A. Joseph, 97–106. London: SPCK in association with Channel Four Television Company Ltd.
Cass, A. 1992. Sex and the military: Gender and violence in the Philippines. Ph.D. diss., University of Queensland, Brisbane.
Cathcart, S. 1991. *Walking on sticks.* A play written and performed by Sarah Cathcart. Produced by Performing Lines (Sydney) at La Boite Theatre, Brisbane.
Dussel, E. 1978. Barbarian theology. In *The scope of political theology,* ed. A. Kee, 37–43. London: SCM Press.
Elshtain, J. B. 1992. *Women and war.* New York: Basic Books.
Ester, Sr. (pseud.). 1988. Autobiography—oppression and liberation. In *Woman and religion: A collection of essays, personal histories and contextualized liturgies,* ed. M. Mananzan, 131–38. Manila: Institute of Women's Studies, St. Scholastica's College.
Fabella, V. 1988. A common methodology for diverse Christologies? In *With passion and compassion: Third World women doing theology,* ed. V. Fabella and M. A. Oduyoye, 108–17. Maryknoll, N.Y.: Orbis Books.
———. 1993. *Beyond bonding: A Third World woman's theological journey.* Manila: Ecumenical Association of Third World Theologians and the Institute of Women's Studies.
Fanon, F. 1967. *A dying colonialism,* trans. H. Chevalier. New York: Grove Press.
———. 1970. *Black skin, white masks,* trans. C. L. Markman. St. Albans, Herts.: Paladin.
Gebara, I. 1988. Women doing theology in Latin America. In *With passion and compas-*

sion: Third World women doing theology, ed. V. Fabella and M. A. Oduyoye, 125–34. Maryknoll, N.Y.: Orbis Books.

Grovijahn, J. M. 1991. Grabbing life away from death: Women and martyrdom in El Salvador. *Journal of Feminist Studies in Religion* 7 (2): 19–28.

Guerrero, M. C. 1992. Sources on women's role in Philippine history, 1590–1898: Texts and countertexts. Paper presented at the Fourth International Philippines Studies Conference, Australian National University, Canberra, 1–3 July.

Hilsdon, A. 1995. *Madonnas and martyrs: Militarism and violence in the Philippines.* St. Leonards, N.S.W.: Allen and Unwin.

Jin, Y. T. 1988. New ways of being church. II: A Protestant perspective. In *With passion and compassion: Third World women doing theology,* ed. V. Fabella and M. A. Oduyoye, 100–107. Maryknoll, N.Y.: Orbis Books.

Katoppo, M. 1986. Women that make Asia alive. In *New eyes for reading: Biblical and theological reflections by women from the Third World,* ed. J. S. Pobee and B. von Wartenberg-Potter, 96–100. Quezon City: Claretian Publications.

Lee Park, S. A. 1989. Envisioning a future church as an Asian woman. *Voices from the Third World* 12 (June): 64–94.

Mananzan, M. J. 1987. The Filipino woman: Before and after the Spanish conquest of the Philippines. In *Essays on women,* ed. M. J. Mananzan, 7–36. Manila: Women's Studies Program, St. Scholastica's College.

———. 1988. Woman and religion. In *Woman and religion: A collection of essays, personal histories and contextualized liturgies,* ed. M. J. Mananzan, 1–13. Manila: Institute of Women's Studies, St. Scholastica's College.

Mananzan, M. J., and S. A. Park. 1988. Emerging spirituality of Asian women. In *With passion and compassion: Third World women doing theology,* ed. V. Fabella and M. A. Oduyoye, 77–88. Maryknoll, N.Y.: Orbis Books.

Manila Chronicle, 17 July 1988.

McClintock, A. 1993. Family feuds: Gender, nationalism and the family. *Feminist Review* 44 (Summer): 61–80.

Molineaux, D. J. 1983. Latin America's three churches: Traditionalists, modernisers and prophets. *Latin America Press,* 1 September, 5–6.

Oduyoye, M. A., and M. R. A. Kanyoro, eds. 1992. *The will to arise: Women, tradition, and the church in Africa.* Maryknoll, N.Y.: Orbis Books.

Parker, A., et al. 1992. *Nationalisms and sexualities.* New York: Routledge.

Pateman, C. 1989. *The disorder of women: Democracy, feminism and political theory.* Cambridge: Polity Press.

Pieris, S. J. 1988. *An Asian theology of liberation.* Maryknoll, N.Y.: Orbis Books.

Pui Lan, K. 1986. God weeps with our pain. In *New eyes for reading: Biblical and theological reflections by women from the Third World,* ed. J. S. Pobee and B. von Wartenberg-Potter, 90–95. Quezon City: Claretian Publication.

Reuther, R. R. 1983. *Sexism and God-talk: Towards a feminist theology.* Boston: Beacon Press.

Rose, Sr. (pseud.). 1988. Autobiography—oppression and liberation. In *Woman and religion: A collection of essays, personal histories and contextualized liturgies,* ed. M. J. Mananzan, 154–58. Manila: Institute of Women's Studies, St. Scholastica's College.

SAMIN [Sisters Association in Mindanao] 1986–87. *SAMIN News,* issue 10 (December–February).

———. 1987. Proceedings of SAMIN Congress, Butuan City, 21–25 January.

———. 1988. Proceedings of SAMIN Congress, Cagayan de Oro City, 11–15 February.
———. 1989. Proceedings of SAMIN Congress, Davao City, 26 February–2 March.
———. 1989–91. *SAMIN News*.
Scherer-Warren, I. 1990. "Rediscovering our dignity"—an appraisal of the utopia of liberation in Latin America. *International Sociology* 5 (1): 11–25.
Sobrino, J. 1985. *The true church and the poor*, trans. M. J. O'Connell. London: SCM Press.
Tse, C. 1988. New ways of being church. I: A Catholic perspective. In *With passion and compassion: Third World women doing theology*, ed. V. Fabella and M. A. Oduyoye, 89–99. Maryknoll, N.Y.: Orbis Books.
Veneracion, J. B. 1992. From Babaylan to Beata: A study on the religiosity of Filipino women. Paper presented at the Fourth International Philippine Studies Conference, Australian National University, Canberra, 1–3 July.
Yeager, D. M. 1988. The web of relationship: Feminists and Christians. *Soundings* 71 (4): 485–513.
Yuval-Davis, N., and F. Anthias, eds. 1989. *Woman—nation—state*. Basingstoke: Macmillan.

CHAPTER 6

Fecundity and the Fertility Decline in Bali

Lynette Parker

The total fertility rate (TFR) in Bali dropped from 5.96 in the period 1967–70 to 2.28 in the period 1986–89 (Hill 1994, 135). The Indonesian National Family Planning Board (Badan Koordinasi Keluarga Berencana Nasional [BKKBN]) estimated that it would drop to 2.0 in the period 1990–95 (1992, 8). By any measure, this is an extraordinarily rapid decline in fertility. It seems likely that Balinese parents will not even be replacing themselves in the next century. Indonesia has experienced a nationwide fertility decline of over 40 percent in the period 1960–87 (i.e., the TFR declined from 5.61 to 3.33). Bali stands as the model province in this movement, followed by North Sulawesi (Hill 1994, 135–36). Writers such as Astawa, Soegeng Waloeyo, and Laing (1975); Freedman and Berelson (1976); Harrison (1978); McNicoll (1980); and Meier (1979) have attributed Bali's dramatic decline in fertility to the government family planning program, which took a distinctive form in Bali, the so-called *sistem banjar*. Under the *sistem banjar* the government supplied subsidized contraceptives and contraceptive services to the population via the *banjar*, the indigenous units of local government and social organization. Other writers—including Edmondson (1992); Hull (1978); Poffenberger (1983); and Streatfield (1986)—have taken broader approaches, explaining the fertility decline in terms of the potency and pace of social change, changing socioeconomic conditions, and interactions between preexisting features of the society and the family planning program.

This chapter explores some important but heretofore neglected causes and implications of the fertility decline in Bali. My perspective is that of a female anthropologist who has conducted fieldwork intermittently in Bali since 1980, studying the processes of rapid social change occurring there.[1] I lived and worked in "Brassika," a pseudonym for a village in east Bali, for one year initially and for shorter periods in 1989, 1992, 1994, and 1997. Data was mainly collected using participant observation. Two detailed village-wide surveys were conducted in 1982 and 1992. I have been struck by two aspects of the literature on the recent demography of Bali. The first is a large lacuna: the absence of the women who bear, or rather do not bear, the children who constitute the statistics. We have good statistical data about fertility rates, but we know very little about sex, sexuality, reproduction, and notions of fertility in Bali. It seems unlikely that they are unconnected. We are largely ignorant about women's motives for adopting contraception. The second feature of the literature is the dominance of the outsider (male) demographer's view of the family planning program. We know very little about the process by which married women were motivated to turn up at clinics to have intrauterine devices (IUDs) fitted. For these reasons I have focused on the experience of Balinese women. My research "frame" is everyday life rather than formal programs and institutions.

I will begin by outlining the nexus between female sexuality and fecundity and notions of the "good woman" in Balinese society.[2] Following that, the main body of the chapter falls into two sections. In the first I will examine the relation between the value placed upon fecundity and the transformation from a familial, peasant mode of production to a wage-labor mode of production. In the second section I will analyze decision making about fertility control in the context of the political incorporation of Balinese villages into the nation-state of Indonesia. I will argue that in Bali notions of female sexuality and reproduction have traditionally been fused. Within the context of male control, a number of historical changes have come together. There are economic pressures on women to work outside the subsistence household unit. Coincidentally, women have realized that babies are no longer likely to die, since there has been a decline in infant mortality rates. The government is simultaneously urging households to adopt the ideal of the small family, with family planning programs motivating women to use contraception. In the process, traditional notions of womanhood and motherhood have been radically redefined.

Fecundity, Sexuality, and Notions of the Good Woman

It is a puzzle for me that demographers have not expressed wonder at the volte-face of the Balinese in regards to fecundity, the reproductive worth of women, and the value of children to parents. Covarrubias, probably the most widely read authority on Balinese society, wrote, "A Balinese feels that his [sic] most important duty is to marry as soon as he comes of age and to raise a family to perpetuate his line" (1972 [1937], 122).

The artistic, anthropological, and archaeological literature on Bali is saturated with images of fertility, of male:female pairs, of pregnancy, of metaphors that associate the fertility of humans and rice crops, of offerings to ensure fertility, and of punishments for infertility (Bernet Kempers 1991, 58ff.; Brinkgreve 1987; Hunter 1988; Parker forthcoming; Pucci 1985). Women are considered responsible for successful reproduction. Given this overwhelming imperative for Balinese women to reproduce, one should ponder how it is that Balinese women have come to be persuaded to limit their fertility. The decline in fertility is not just a "demographic shift": it is also a significant transformation in ideas, motivations, strategies, and practices.

The Balinese have traditionally been preoccupied with fecundity rather than sexuality: women value and are valued for their reproductive capacity, which is seen as a source of unique power (Belo 1949; Lovric 1987; Parker forthcoming). Women are generally subordinate to men, and men seek to control their wives' fertility. The ideal woman was primarily a mother of sons and secondarily a faithful wife and hard worker at home, in the fields, and in the performance of ritual offerings (Covarrubias 1972 [1937], 120–59).

The basic social unit is the father-mother united in marriage, a subset of the patrilineal descent or ancestor group (Geertz and Geertz 1975). Traditionally, marriages were arranged or conducted by elopement, a method that allowed young people to elude parental and/or community disapproval and also allowed persistent young men to prevail over unwilling brides-to-be (on marriage and families, see Belo 1970 [1936]; Boon 1977, 119–44). Nowadays most marriages are not arranged. Elopement remains fairly common, yet parental approval is still considered desirable.

Endogamy is preferred within a variety of groups, including patrilineages, caste/status groups, and *banjar*. Among high castes, hypogamy was forbidden and direly punished; it remains an issue of great heat and significance. Women's endogamy maintains a group's identity by defining its borders and advertising its character as strong, vital, and pure. Notions and rules of purity and pollution regulate choice of marriage partner and many other aspects of women's sexual/reproductive life, such as menstruation and childbirth (Miller and Branson 1989).

Women's average age at marriage was very high by Indonesian standards in the 1960s and is probably rising (Hill 1994, 137; Streatfield 1986, 21). In 1964 women's average age at marriage in Bali was 21.7 years; by 1985 it was 22.3 years (Hill 1994, 137). Among high castes, female virginity at marriage is highly desirable. Among lower castes, premarital sex is not so much immoral as awkward. Upon pregnancy girls should be quickly married to the father of the unborn child. There is the feeling that, if unmarried, paternity can be difficult to establish and unwise marriages forced.

My hostess—the high-caste wife of the high-caste village head—and I were discussing Brassika's apparently model family of *brahman* man, Ida Bagus,

Fecundity and the Fertility Decline in Bali   181

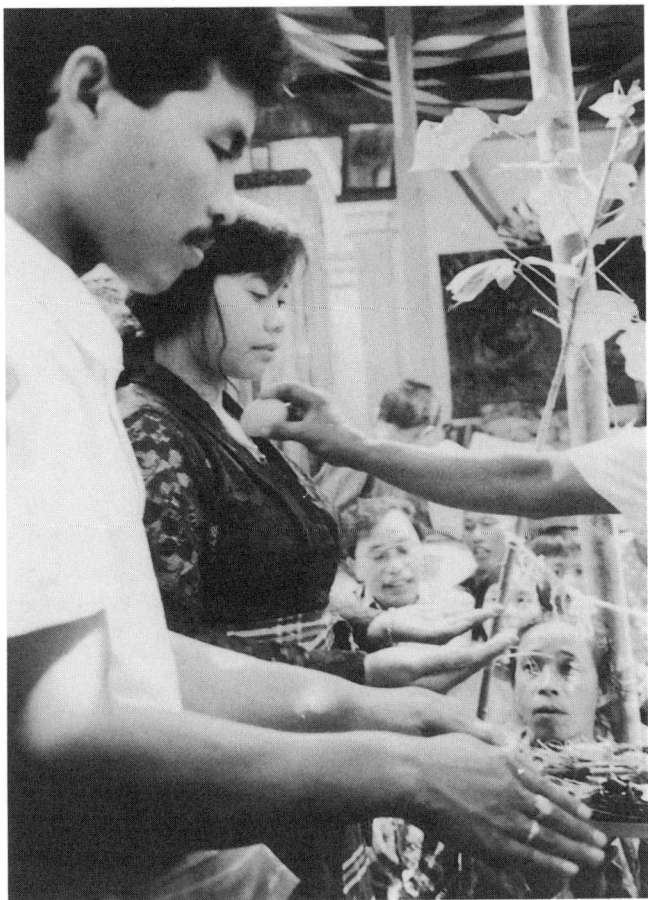

Fig. 4. Many stages of the Balinese wedding ceremony, such as the Egg Rite, express the wish that the bridal couple be fertile.

satria wife, Cokorda Isteri, and four children. Their "happy" marriage was contrasted with her own unhappy marriage. She said that, when Cokorda Isteri was still at school, "Ida Bagus and Cokorda Isteri were studying alone together one night, and the village head noticed that the light had gone out and that Ida Bagus had not come out [of the room]. It was assumed that they had had sex. The village head ordered them to be married (*dikawinkan*)" (field notes, 20 August 1992).

When a well-dressed newborn baby was left abandoned in the doorway of a nearby orphanage, most people thought it the product of an illicit union between a wealthy employer in the city and his village servant girl. It was assumed that she could not get him to marry her and was not brave enough to go home. It couldn't be like that in a village situation, they said, because everyone would know she was pregnant and force a marriage (field notes, 21 August 1992).

According to the small number of women with whom I could talk on such topics, sex is ideally initiated and controlled by men. The ideal wife is properly neither seductive nor lustful. In the early stages of a relationship or marriage, desire for sex and the creation of children are not separate.

Newly married women move into their husbands' house compound, co-residing with parents-in-law and brothers-in-law and their families. Until they produce a baby, especially a son, brides are in a weak and comparatively powerless position. The new wife is expected by her mother-in-law to take over the greater part of the housework, cooking, shopping, and laundry, and women have primary responsibility for child care. Mothers-in-law often perform much of the ritual work of the house compound, especially the making of offerings (on women's work, see Branson and Miller 1988; Connor 1983).

Divorce is traumatic and difficult for women, mainly because they must surrender their children to their husbands' patrilineage and also because they have no rights of access to family wealth and property. Women bitterly contrast their position with that of men, for whom divorce is easy, and usually explain that it is best "to accept, to receive" (*menerima*) and to stay in unhappy marriages in order to remain with their children. One village woman said, with regard to divorce:

> It's a shame, especially for the woman, because she usually has to leave the children when they are growing up. Usually if they are still young she can look after them and then they are given the choice to choose, and often they choose to go with the father because of the pressure of the inheritance and having a place. So the women lose their investment. (Field notes, 21 August 1992)

One son of the Palace had married a Javanese woman; they had had a daughter and were living and working in Java. When they were divorcing, the mother refused to give up her seven-year-old daughter, as it is customary in Java for divorced women to keep custody of their children. In a dramatic expression of outrage the grandfather rushed off to Java and, without the mother's permission, brought the girl back to Brassika, where she lived sequestered in the palace.

Polygyny is officially discouraged by the national government (e.g., through legislation and civil service penalties for promotion) but is nevertheless practiced, particularly by high-caste men. A sexual double standard operates by which sexual promiscuity is valorized for men, making them appear strong, potent, and attractive in the eyes of both men and women, but it is not condoned for women.

This is the cultural environment in which women's sexuality and fecundity are expressed. Women's fecund powers are valued (but also feared), and men seek to control women's reproductivity and sexuality. Past notions of women primarily as reproducers, however, have been transformed. Why and how has this come about?

Economic Transformations

The Balinese have long been aware that the area of agricultural land is finite, that the population is growing, and that access to a plot of rice land that will support a family is increasingly unlikely. Economic life has shifted from subsistence agriculture to commercial agriculture and wage-labor employment. Within the period of the dramatic decline in fertility, from the late 1960s to the late 1980s, there has been an efflorescence of wage-labor employment opportunities in Bali and a rapid expansion in parental investment in children's education. There has been a shift in women's labor away from family work (both reciprocable and unpaid) to wage labor, a great increase in the economic cost of children, and a decline in the economic contribution of children to family fields. Consequently, since the mid- to late 1970s there have been powerful economic incentives for married women to limit family size drastically.

These economic motives for adopting contraception are those most often mentioned by Balinese women, in combination with their stated perceptions that any children born are now likely to survive to adulthood. In the past, they say, it was a sensible strategy to bear more children than necessary because of the likelihood that some would die. Their perceptions are borne out by the macro-level statistics, which show a dramatic decline in infant mortality rates in Bali, from 121 deaths of infants under one year of age per 1,000 live births in the late 1960s to 49 in the late 1980s (Hill 1994, 141).

Women's work and control of household finances have usually been hailed by observers as signifying that Balinese women have an extraordinary degree of economic autonomy. My argument is the opposite: that in the past most women traded and kept pigs for sale, and, more recently, they labor on the open market and perform other marginal and lowly work because they have heavy financial responsibilities within the family, are expected to work hard, and cannot inherit the main traditional means of production: *sawah* (irrigated rice fields). Even high-caste women, who are sequestered behind high walls, have a tradition of earning money by weaving, keeping pigs, or setting up stalls suspended from the walls of their house compounds.

Agriculture is still the main source of income for village men. *Sawah* is owned by men, not by women. Land is inherited through the patriline and nowadays can be bought and sold, pawned, and sharecropped. In the Klungkung area the few women who control *sawah* are widows, and the only women to head households are widows. In 1981, in Brassika, the village where I lived, only 15 out of 439 *sawah* owners were women, all widows.[3] Women frequently expressed outrage to me that they could not inherit land. This sense of injustice is probably informed by recently acquired knowledge about national laws that require equal inheritance rights for sons and daughters and about traditional inheritance laws in other parts of Indonesia. The clash of local and national laws on this topic is not (yet) a subject for public discourse as an issue or problem, but in a seminar paper Desak Putu Parmiti stated that

> it can be said that Hindu religion views women and men as having the same position in matters of faith and deed, as well as in occupation, except in the division of inheritance, which follows the patrilineal kinship system, recognizing only the *purusha* (male) line of descent. (1992, 103; my trans.)

She then went on to outline the ways in which the patrilineal system elevated the position of men over women. The participants at the seminar did not debate the issue.

Before the Green Revolution of the 1970s to 1980s, women were valued as unpaid family workers in the *sawah,* particularly in the harvesting and pounding stages. As recently as 1981, they were very active in voluntary harvest groups and exchanged their labor directly for rice. Now virtually all harvesting is done on a commercial basis by small, efficient harvest teams, while rice-hulling machines have made hand pounding obsolete. The labor inputs from wives (and children) for each rice crop are much reduced. Both men and women are searching for new sources of income. The diversification of villagers' occupations and sources of incomes is a striking feature of the transformation of the village from peasant subsistence economy to wage-labor market economy. While this type of transformation is not uncommon in Indonesia, the pace and magnitude of the shift away from the agricultural sector and the expansion of the workforce in the industrial and service sectors in Bali is extraordinary (Bendesa and Sukarsa 1980, 32; Oey-Gardiner 1993, 211; Team Pengembangan 1984). Likewise, the level of participation of women in the workforce, always high in Bali compared with other areas of Indonesia, is growing rapidly (Abdurochim

1986, 49–50; Hugo et al. 1987, 244–49; Oey-Gardiner 1993, 210; Team Pengembangan 1984, 19). The fast pace of industrialization and internationalization of the economy is mainly a result of the tourism industry in Bali. The burgeoning industrial and service sectors, which are largely financed by national (Jakarta) and international capital, have piggy-backed on the international marketing networks, advertising linkages, and political power of the tourism industry (Aditjondro 1995, 19–20).

Balinese women now commonly work alongside men as laborers for government departments and for private companies that are contracted for public works projects, especially roads, and on building sites. Laboring is a lowly occupation, and positions are usually offered for a particular construction job or project, not as a permanent attachment to an employer. There is usually no job security and no protection against time off for injury, pregnancy, or sickness. People who have no land, no education, no skills, no money, and no contacts are forced into laboring. The work is hard and hot, hours are long, and laborers bundle themselves against the burning sun. Higher-caste people will not labor in Bali but have been known to do so in Java and overseas.

Laborers are usually paid daily wages; laboring women receive two-thirds to three-quarters the male rate. Some women, usually the younger unmarried women, attach themselves to a large company, live in Denpasar, or other towns, and follow the company to the site of a contract. Women work in gangs, sometimes with men, carrying head loads of sand or gravel or rocks, shoveling materials on to or out of trucks, breaking rocks, tending the fires to heat drums of tar, spreading blue metal, sometimes supplying male bricklayers with mortar and bricks. Usually, the more skilled and better-paid jobs in construction, such as setting up form work or string lines off plans, are male jobs, as are foremen positions. Tradespeople—stonemasons, electricians, mechanics—are men.

More recently, it is the expanding industrial sector, especially the textile, garment, and handcraft industries, that has especially attracted female workers. In these industries there is great variation in work arrangements: labor-intensive manufacture of finished items performed in the home, including items such as cut-work clothes (*bordir*), carving and painting wooden statues and trinkets, and sewing sequined or embroidered clothes and shoes; small, backyard factories equipped, for instance, with sewing machines or soldering irons and bellows, employing a small number of male and/or female workers, who frequently live on site or in rented rooms; and full-scale weaving or jewelry-making factories employing hundreds of workers. The first two arrangements are frequently practiced in villages that are distant from towns such as Denpasar. The last two types of factories are mostly in urban or peri-urban areas. In these factories one finds many nonlocal workers, including many from outside Bali. The pace of much of this work is driven by the timing of the orders received from middlemen or, less commonly, middlewomen. It is rare for women sewing at home to work steadily for several months, but they may work frantically for a couple of weeks to fill an order. Likewise, wages are usually not steady and are paid on completion of an order and according to productivity: the speed and skill, and thus output, of the worker determines the wages.

By 1981 poorly educated young women from villages were frequently leaving home at the age of fifteen to eighteen to go to Denpasar, Sanur, Kuta, and other towns and tourist centers in search of work. Many had no jobs lined up, and some had no accommodation organized. Parents were usually aware of the open-ended nature of these trips. Sometimes daughters came back home after a couple of days; some trips ended more profitably; and some ended with the daughter back home and pregnant some months later.

Better-educated, high-caste, and better-placed women have taken up new posts in the tertiary sector, for instance, in teaching, medicine, the civil service, the hospitality industry, in insurance, and banking. Still, in general, they do not occupy the apical positions in occupational pyramids.

It is well-known that women control and operate the markets in Bali and that trading has traditionally been the main independent source of income for women. Markets for food and everyday goods are still dominated by women, but it appears that larger-scale trading, for instance, in rice, cars, and cattle, has been largely taken over by men. Some commentators have presented women's independently acquired cash as "money for a rainy day" and as the property of the woman (e.g., Covarubbias 1972 [1937], 155–56), but in my experience women's income now contributes to the household purse in order to meet everyday needs. Women often control this purse for daily expenditures, such as food, clothing, medical costs, treats, and school fees, but many claims on it are beyond their control—for instance, amounts to be contributed for community rituals and public works are determined by men, as are contributions for major family rituals, such as cremations. Young unmarried women working and living away from home are apparently very conscientious about sending wages home.[4]

Balinese women appear to be strong and are usually thought to be careful and clever economic managers. Yet they cannot be said to enjoy economic autonomy. Women in Bali are supposed to be hard workers and to contribute productively to the household economy. These norms are held by both men and women. Women take considerable pride in their material wealth and strength, particularly with regard to their children's appearance, health, well-being, progress in school, and so on, for which they often claim major responsibility and credit. Although Balinese women have no ownership rights to the major traditional means of production, land, the implementation of these strong norms enhances their feelings of self-worth and provides them with considerable incentive to find sources of income and a degree of economic independence.

Balinese women have traditionally been very much tied to the house yards into which they are born and later marry. Yet dramatic changes in virtually all aspects of living—public transport, marketing, rice distribution, water supply, education, supply of trees—are transforming women's work at home: women can easily buy and sell produce, every day if necessary, because motorized transport has penetrated most villages; many offerings and foods formerly produced or processed at home can be bought ready-made, for example, rice is now bought husked and ready-to-cook; most villages have piped water, either to public taps or into houses; kerosene stoves are replacing wood fires; and schools have proliferated such that almost all children aged seven to twelve are enrolled at primary school.

Thus, in the last twenty years women's work at home has been considerably reduced in terms of time and energy required; simultaneously, the adoption of Green Revolution technology has caused the decline of much women's work associated with the rice crop; nonagricultural employment opportunities have increased; the pressure and economic incentives to send children to school have risen; and families' needs for disposable cash incomes have risen sharply.

Balinese women are now much more physically mobile for school and work than they were twenty years ago. Young, unmarried village women usually leave home to go to high school or university and to compete in the labor market; if they find somewhere to live and work, they are physically, though not morally, largely outside the control of their families. With marriage, however, they are once again controlled and tied. Some married women can afford servants in town to help with child care; some with children return to the village for help with child care; and some send their children to their grandparents in the village in order that they can keep working in the towns. This is becoming so common that it seems likely that pressure will mount for the development of day care centers in urban areas.

Most women said to me that it was the opportunity to work that motivated them to limit family size. A keyword, and one frequently employed by village women, was *bebas* (free): that using contraception after they had had two or three children allowed them to be free to move around to search for work and to be able to work.

Incorporation of Villagers into the Nation-State

After the Suharto government came to power in 1966–67 it lost no time in instituting a national family planning program as part of its economic development program. By 1970 the National Family Planning Board was operational and concentrating its contraceptive campaigns in Java and Bali. By 1974 two features of the Indonesian family planning program that are unique to Bali and important in explaining its success were being implemented: the *sistem banjar* and the advocacy and use of the IUD as the method of contraception.

The IUD has often been used as the preferred first, or pioneer, contraceptive in family planning programs in the Third World. The IUD is an invasive but once-only device—unlike the pill, once accepted its use is out of the woman's control until such time as it is extracted. It is effective without the user understanding how it is effective; it requires no knowledge of anatomy, no memory of menstrual cycles, and no memory or foresight to use it (unlike the pill and diaphragm) on the part of the user.

The pill is the most common contraceptive in all Indonesia, followed by the IUD—14.8 percent of married Indonesian women took the pill in 1991, and 13.3 percent used an IUD; 31.1 percent of new acceptors of contraceptives in 1990–91 took the pill, and 20.2 percent used the IUD—but the general trend is toward a diversification of contraceptive methods, with injections, Norplant arm implants, and sterilizations becoming more common (BKKBN 1992, 3; Hill 1994, 142). In Bali the IUD was adopted as the preferred contraceptive by the provincial branch of BKKBN from the beginning: 49.3 percent of new contraceptive acceptors adopted IUDs in 1975–76 and by February 1990 the figure had risen to 69.96 percent (Kantor Statistik 1988[?], 24; Kantor Statistik 1990[?], 23).

Although convenient and effective as a contraceptive, the IUD often causes significant health problems, such as bleeding, pain, and infections, which are not adequately attended to by village medical staff. In other societies the IUD has been seen as potentially unpopular because of the embarrassment or shame of women at the time of insertion. In Bali, however, this is rarely expressed as a problem, partly because women are often attended by female clinic staff and partly because Bali is unusual in having a tradition of male traditional birth attendants. Village women who knew that there were other methods of contraception usually stated their preference for the IUD in terms of not having to remember to take it, unlike the pill. Yet real knowledge and experience of oral contraceptives are abysmally absent: in 1994, for instance, the local "experts," the clinic staff, asked me for information about how to take the pill. The head of BKKBN in Bali noted this selective knowledge and stated:

Field workers are trained to devote special attention to the IUD in providing information about the program. Clinic personnel are instructed to recommend the IUD above other methods, to encourage continuation among IUD users who are considering having the IUD removed or changing methods, and to encourage users of other methods to shift to the IUD. (Astawa, Soegeng Waloeyo, and Laing 1975, 95)

This method has been so successful that the term *IUD* is used in rural Bali to mean "contraception," and most women do not use a word that generally signifies contraception.

I explain the comparative frequency of IUD use in Bali mainly as the result of the government's totalitarian methods of disseminating information about contraception and of delivering contraceptive services and supplies. Knowledge about female anatomy, reproductive processes, and contraceptive choice is inadequate even among those medical and paramedical staff who have been "trained." Further, the IUD is the "easiest" method of contraception (second to sterilization) in terms of cost and distribution of supplies, education, motivation, and permanency of "contraceptive status" (i.e., adopting women cannot easily renege on their decisions). On this last point, Astawa, the head of BKKBN in Bali, stated that the "high continuation rates" of IUD acceptors was the principal reason that his organization promoted the use of the IUD (Astawa, Soegeng Waloeyo, and Laing 1975, 95). One village official of BKKBN stated in a conversation with me about the prevalence of the IUD that it was suitable (*cocok*) because it didn't require much desire (*keinginan*) on the part of the woman (field notes, 19 June 1994). Within the context of Balinese male control of women's sexuality and fertility, it is not surprising that a form of contraception that, once inserted, is largely beyond the control of its female users is the only form made available.

The second aspect of the family planning program unique to Bali is the so-called *sistem banjar*. The term *banjar* can be glossed as "hamlet" and "local council." A *banjar* is usually, but not always, a discrete geographic area; it is a cohesive moral and religious community commonly consisting of 50 to 150 households. It is an organization of married men that meets once a month to decide matters of local government, community ritual, public works, and sometimes problems of marriage or inheritance. It is formally equipped with corporate rules, fines for infringements, and elected leaders with specific duties. Increasingly through the 1970s and 1980s, the *banjar* has become a channel through which government policy on development matters, such as health and hygiene, school attendance, and family planning has been implemented (Parker 1989, 326–29, 443–48; Warren 1986,

1990, 1993). Its status as an autonomous, democratic local government has thus been seriously corrupted.

Under the *sistem banjar* of the national family planning program, elected *banjar* heads are responsible for reaching targets of contraceptive acceptors—for example, one target that was mentioned to me in 1980 was that 90 percent of "eligible couples" (ElCos) (married couples of childbearing age) were to become acceptors of contraceptives. Unmarried women are not able to receive contraception through the government program and are thus not included in such registers. Heads of *banjar* are now paid a small salary; candidates for the position are vetted by government officials; and most spend considerable amounts of time compiling paperwork, implementing government development programs and attending government meetings and training courses. Although they are not civil servants, they can now be seen as administrators and for the most part as an extension of the government bureaucracy.

The *banjar* head must make a household map and register of all ElCos in his hamlet. The register for each ElCo includes name and age of woman, husband's name, date on which she accepted family planning, numbers of dead and alive children, as well as current details of contraceptive status. The *banjar* heads work in bureaucratic tandem with village clinic staff and BKKBN fieldworkers, who are public servants. Clinic staff and fieldworkers have medical training, though villagers are often unaware of their differing levels of training and professional status. They distribute supplies of contraceptives, such as pills, but only the more senior clinic staff can fit IUDs.

The "contraceptive status" of any married woman and eligible couple—most usually whether a woman of childbearing age is using an IUD—is part of the personal knowledge of *banjar* heads.[5] It is also common knowledge in any *banjar* and, if unacceptable, is acted upon by the *banjar*. Normally, if an eligible couple is procrastinating about using contraception after the birth of a child, the matter is raised casually by friends and neighbors as well as by clinic staff in postnatal checks and immunization visits. Truly recalcitrant couples may find themselves the topic for discussion at the monthly *banjar* meetings and/or visited by *banjar* heads as well as by government medical and administrative staff.

Balinese women are excluded from the major local decision-making organization, the *banjar*, but they are bound by its decisions and expected to implement them. The local Balinese model of women's exclusion from decision making and of their subordination by and dependency on men for political action is present at all higher levels of the Indonesian nation-state. Coupled with this political exclusion is the expectation that women will accept (*menerima*) orders and act on them.

Although a national family planning program, its local deployment highlights the "Balineseness" of the campaign (Streatfield 1986, 55). The Parisada Hindu Dharma, the quasi-government Hindu umbrella organization, published assurances in book form that "The Hindu Religion Does Not Forbid Family Planning"; in television advertisements women in traditional dress extol the economic advantages of having small families; some posters employ the local, rather than the national, language; and the whole campaign has a local flavor because of the *banjar* implementation system.

Further, the target-driven nature of the campaign, which has probably also contributed to the promotion of the IUD as the contraceptive par excellence, has cashed in on a distinctive characteristic of Balinese institutions: their competitiveness. Clinic staff, fieldworkers, *banjar* heads, and the institutions they represent are assigned performance credit points according to the number of acceptors they can muster, winners get prizes, including trips to Jakarta, losers may find their villages designated *desa tertinggal* ("left-behind villages"). This competitiveness operates at all levels of BKKBN and health services administration such that even village-level personnel often told me proudly that Bali was the first (or third, depending on the period) province for family planning success in Indonesia.[6]

The family planning program has been accompanied by a comprehensive public health program aimed principally at women of childbearing age in order that they take partial responsibility for the modern health care of the next generation. The program includes vaccinations, weighings, and nutritional supplements for children under five, antenatal and postnatal checks for women—including checks on their "contraceptive status"—and a birthing program that has moved parturient women from homes to clinics and hospitals.

Infant mortality rates have dropped substantially in the period of fertility decline. The infant mortality rate in the late 1960s for Bali was 121 and by the late 1980s had dropped to 49 (Hull in Hill 1994, 141). (The rates for Indonesia as a whole were 132 and 69.) Female informants perceived that nowadays babies are more likely to live to adulthood than they did when they were young and frequently mentioned this as one reason they would restrict the number of births.

This bombardment of state policy and government programs is present in most of Indonesia and is not unique to Bali. Balinese "enthusiasm" for contraception cannot, therefore, be solely attributed to government health programs and propaganda. As BKKBN realized in the early 1970s, however, Bali is a small, densely settled island, with a socially cohesive and, until recently, relatively homogeneous society that enjoys a good supply of clinics and medical and paramedical staff, easily articulated with its indigenous *banjar*. In Bali the net of government health and contraceptive services has been densely interwoven

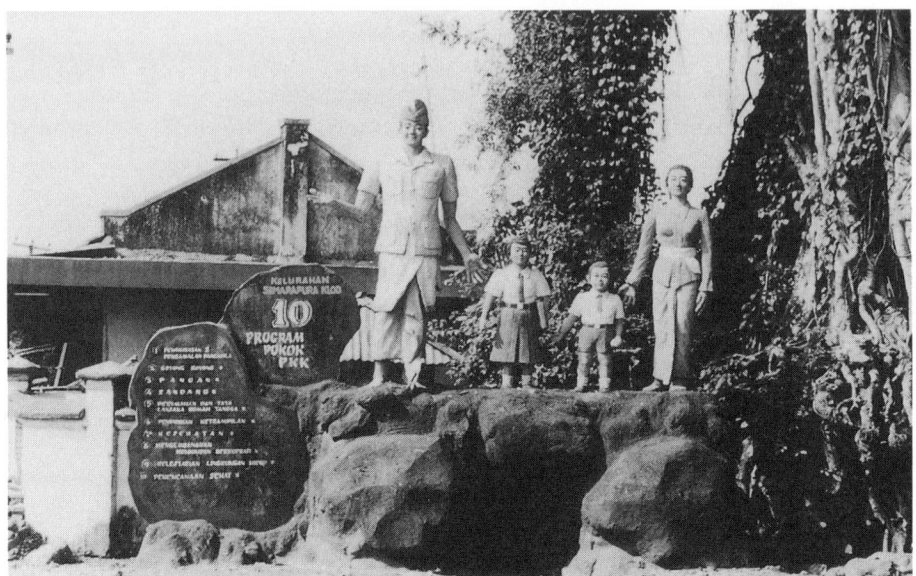

Fig. 5. Statue at a crossroads in Klungkung, East Bali, advertising the Ten-Point Program at the PKK and the "Small Family Norm" of the Family Planning Program

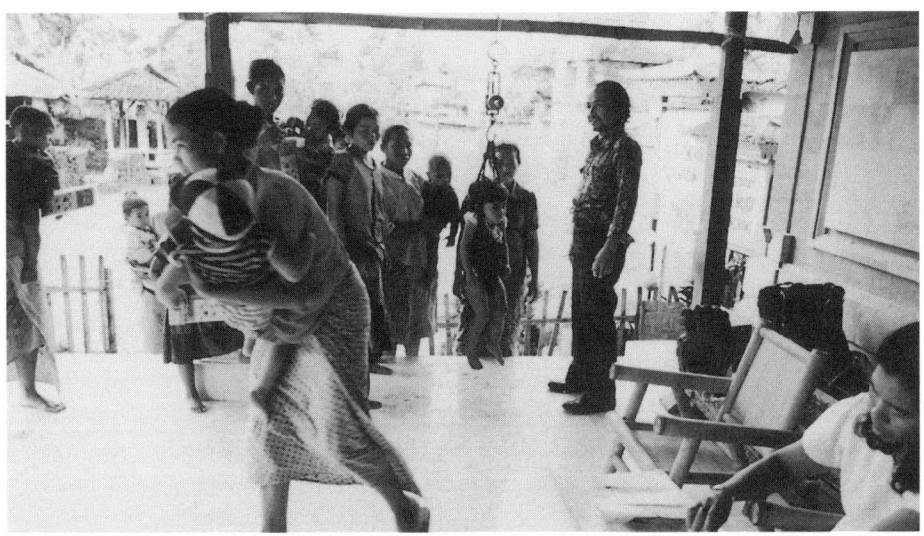

Fig. 6. Monthly weighing of babies is now institutionalized, *banjar* "Anjingan," East Bali

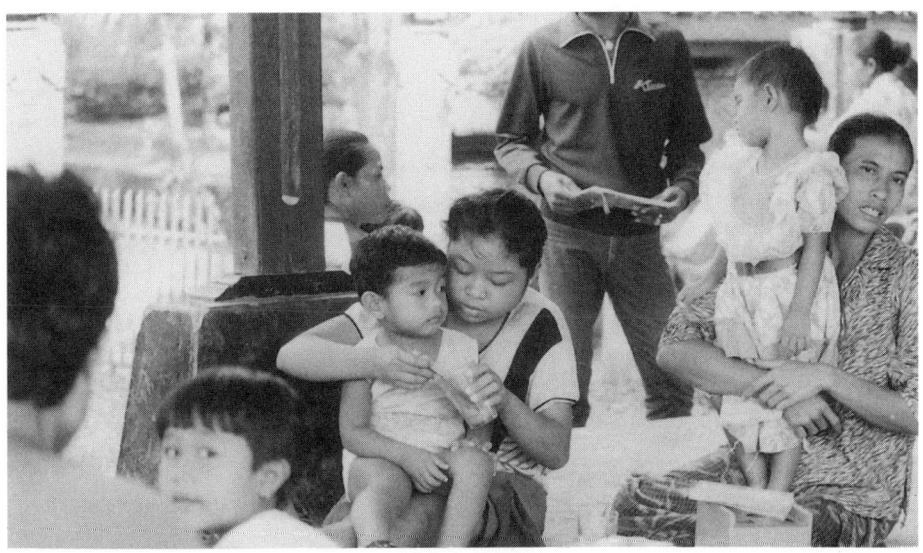

Fig. 7. The introduction of toys to the "under-fives" (*anak balita*) at the monthly weighing meeting, *banjar* "Tirtawangi," East Bali

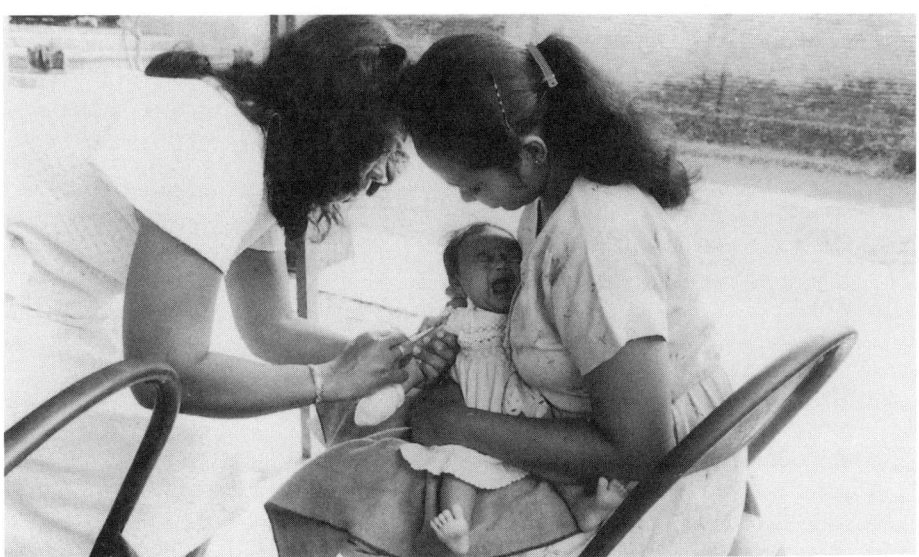

Fig. 8. Immunizations of babies are now routine in Bali

with the decision making of local government forums (*banjar* meetings and leaders) and the moral force and identity of local communities (*banjar*).

The incorporation of Balinese villagers into the Indonesian state via contraception not only occurs within the health care and local government systems. Formal teaching about the need for contraception begins in the first year of school and continues in all subjects and all grades of school.[7] For instance, in a fifth-grade Indonesian language lesson in a village primary school I witnessed a lesson on the value of small families. The main point was that the purpose of family planning is to achieve happy and prosperous families. The textbook stressed the happy side: in small families the parents could shower more love and attention on the children, but in large families the parents would always be cross with the children and always fighting.[8] It was the teacher's extemporizing words on the economic advantages of family planning that rang true for Hindu Bali:

> If I have a kilogram of rice to divide among four people, there's enough, but if I have to divide it among seven people, there will not be enough and I will have to go looking for more money again. (Field notes, 10 February 1992)

At all levels of society, including the *banjar,* the basic political unit in Bali, the government has set up a PKK (Family Welfare Organization) to mobilize women's participation in development. Each PKK is headed by the (unpaid) wife of the government official of that stratum or group, such as the wife of the *banjar* head.[9]

The PKK signs posted in villages throughout Indonesia proclaim the duties of a woman as

1. producer of the nation's future generations
2. wife and faithful companion to her husband
3. mother and educator of her children
4. manager of the household
5. citizen.

(Hull 1982, 122)

This government emphasis on women as caregivers, supporters, and nurturers neglects the important contribution that women make as producers and providers, as workers in the labor force (see Sullivan 1991 on the rhetoric and implementation of this ideology at all levels of society). Control over women's reproduction has accompanied a move in women's labor away from family work to wage-labor; women are moving away from the home, but they do not have a proper place to go. According to its own ideology, the Indonesian state has no place for women as breadwinners, community leaders, or engineers. The message is that the men of power, the men of action, produce, manage, decide, and control, while the women serve, accept (*menerima*), maintain, and reproduce—the latter in moderation!

The ideal woman, the "good woman," of the Indonesian state is a shrunken figure compared to the real-life Balinese woman. According to the state stereotype, women are only home-bound, dependent wives and mothers. In the quotidian experience of Balinese women, however, extradomestic practices and relations are often sources of personal satisfaction, social and self-worth, freedom and enablement. They often involve women in personal moral conflicts— the risk of incurring gossip if a young woman leaves home to try to find work in a town, the anguish over whether or not to work away from home for wages but leave children in the care of others. The working woman has satisfaction but also overwork and many stresses as a result of what is commonly known as *peranan ganda,* her double/multiple roles. Many women see their work in terms of a tripartite division: home, work, and ritual, the latter being an extraordinarily heavy obligation in Bali. This phrase and the overload of work and pressure of time that it connotes are now the usual topics of discussion whenever women's issues are raised in public. *Peranan ganda* is an accepted part of public discourse in a way that unequal inheritance rights or custody rights are not—as yet.

Balinese gender norms, at least those of female and lower-class culture, provide women with a positive valuation if they choose the path of wage labor. For Balinese women, using family planning is a means by which they can help to reconcile the often conflicting roles of mother and worker.

The IUDs in the statistics on fertility decline are not used by government officials or even by men sitting in *banjar* meetings. They are inserted in the bodies of married women who do not attend meetings but who must be sufficiently well-motivated to turn up to clinics to be fitted. Not unexpectedly, most women with whom I have discussed such matters have said that they decided to become family planning acceptors after discussing the matter with their husbands.[10] Nevertheless, in Klungkung, Karangasem, and Gianyar, at least, there appear to be significant differences in contraceptive acceptance rates according to *banjar* (Poffenberger 1983, 54–55; Streatfield 1986, 147–52; Warren 1993, 219–24). These differences could reflect the decisions made or not made by the councils, variations in the moral cohesiveness and homogeneity of communities, and also the enthusiasm and industry of *banjar* leaders. Women's comments and the statistically significant differences between *banjar* acceptance rates point to two crucial intersections of social, religious, and government life in Bali: the importance of the structural inequality between the sexes in Bali, such that men are thought to have the right to control the sexual and reproductive life of their wives and female fellow citizens, and the public nature of decisions about fertility control.

Women informants do not generally perceive, however, that their acceptance of contraception has been forced upon them: one high-caste woman removed her own IUD and had a tubal ligation without her husband's knowledge, and another well-educated woman, the mother of eight, refused to comply with her husband's and *banjar*'s demands that she use contraception, because she had not yet produced a son. Most women see the adoption of contraception after the birth of two or three children as a means of liberation. Contraception enables women to seek employment and income, which will enable them to provide a more healthy and comfortable standard of living for their small families. But my own assessment is that this recent contraceptive freedom occurs in a context of un-freedom, that deep historical and cultural forces structure new strategies and decisions. The mother of eight girls acts "freely" in order to comply with a societal norm that makes sons more desirable than daughters. The woman who secretly went off to have her tubes tied did so after her husband had assured her that he had had a vasectomy but then made her pregnant.

Fertility Decline and Its Implications

I contend that the success of the family planning program in Bali has occurred in a complex cultural context of male domination and control of female sexuality and reproductivity combined with economic and political transformations that have had considerable potency in persuading women to use contraception. The last twenty years of demographic change in Bali imply some profound shifts in sociocultural values and beliefs.[11] The positive productive value of children to subsistence families and households has reversed and become a negative value: instead of being a valuable labor resource and source of economic security and prosperity on the family farm, children have become an absolute economic cost, a burden and a responsibility, unless or until they can be successfully accommodated in modern, secure employment (cf. Caldwell 1982).

A concomitant of the fertility decline seems to be a qualitative shift in the care and valuation of children in a family. There is now a comparative concentration of parental (and, often even more pronounced, grandparental) attention to the quality of upbringing, talents, special qualities of each child, an individualization of the few children in a family. This is a new feature of Balinese family life: each child is more coddled, paid more attention, offered more opportunities, and lives longer than children of former generations. Fewer children are more precious children.

Currently, the government family planning program in Balinese villages only offers services to married women and men with children. The demands, however, of ever-longer periods of schooling, of employment in urban centers, and of boarding away from home are causing young people to delay marriage and yet live in comparatively free environments. In such circumstances reports of an unprecedented number of abandoned babies and of premarital pregnancies are not surprising. It is likely that there will be increasing demand for sex education, contraceptive advice, and services for young, unmarried, and childless women. At the moment women who want to terminate a pregnancy are limited in their choices. If they are wealthy and "in the know," they can see a doctor privately and clandestinely and get an illegal abortion. Less advantaged women might risk a dangerous backyard abortion. Unmarried women who want to avoid a pregnancy can, if they have the means and nous, consult a private doctor and get advice about and buy appropriate contraceptives. Others can buy oral contraceptives over the counter from a chemist—other types of contraceptives require examination by medical personnel. Most, however, risk pregnancy. There is not a lot of pressure on men to take responsibility for contraception. During the 1990s the Suharto government encouraged the privatization of contraceptive services. The growth of the urban population and of the education level and (tenuous) wealth of this population (the new middle class of Bali) means that medical services in urban areas are increasing. There is growing realization that HIV/AIDS exists in Bali and that it will not be restricted to "immoral" people, such as prostitutes.[12] Among other effects of the AIDS epidemic, it seems likely that sexuality will become a topic for public discussion; as a result, subjects such as the sexual double standard for men and women might also be aired.

Balinese notions of fecundity and sexuality, once fused, are becoming separated. The possibilities for new ways of living—of sex before and outside marriage, of not being married, of not having children—are increasing. On the other hand, government ideology has taught strict adherence to an assumed "Indonesian" pattern of living based on a nuclear family, headed until recently by the Father of All, Bapak Suharto. It remains to be seen if this rigid and hierarchical family model will prevail.

How have notions of the good woman and of femininity in Bali changed as a result of the dramatic decline in fertility? Health workers and public servants at monthly health checks at *banjar* halls, school textbooks and teachers, public health and family planning advertisements on television, and glossy women's magazines teach that family health and well-being are women's responsibility.[13] The producer of the nation's future generations is responsible for family nutrition, cleanliness, politeness and public presentation, family planning, medical treatment, child care, child socialization, and moral education. The dominant image of femininity displayed by the mass and government media is that of the beautiful, responsible, and consuming housewife: buying deodorant, a washing machine, contraception, sending children to university, getting her aging mother's eyes checked for glaucoma.

I showed some village women an article in the *Bali Post*, which put forward the view of an eminent Balinese female professional that the "rights and emancipation" (*hak dan emansipasi*) of Balinese women were "already quite good" (*sudah cukup baik*). My hostess was quite bitter and vehement in her opposition to this: "Yes, rights and emancipation can be talked about, but what about if there's already a set situation like the husband here? You can't do anything and it's better just to put up with it and shut up than to argue" (field notes, 13 August 1992).

Balinese women are now employed in wage work and incorporated into the global capitalist economic order. They have adopted contraception in a cultural context of male control of female sexuality and fertility and in a political context of male policy making and program implementation. Balinese women are no longer merely sexual partners and reproducers for their husbands' lineages; they now have separate identities based on their new productive, reproductive, sexual, and consuming duties. What is not clear, however, is that these new identities will translate into new rights and emancipation.

NOTES

1. Fieldwork was sponsored by Lembaga Ilmu Pengetahuan Indonesia and Universitas Udayana, and financed by the Australian National University and the Spencer Foundation, Chicago.

2. A detailed account of the Balinese identification of sexuality and fecundity can be found in Parker forthcoming.

3. Twelve of these widows had "inherited" their husbands' land, and three had been given land by their fathers—in all cases these were young widows with children, and the transfer of land was seen as temporary. The widows could not sell, pawn, or give away this land without permission of their children or the dead husbands' families.

In areas further west, especially in Tabanan, it appears that sonless families commonly adopt other, usually agnatically related, males (*sentana*) as heirs or adopt daughters as legal males. A daughter with jural male status inherits her father's land and responsibilities, and her husband may not inherit from his father. Sons of such marriages inherit from their mother.

4. Caldwell (1982) has posited the theory that the breakdown of the traditional

economic obligation of children to support parents accompanies the modernization process and is the motivation for parents to create smaller families. This theory has been provisionally tested for Bali by Edmondson. She concluded that

> there is no evidence that children are forgoing these obligations due to the inculcation of western values of parent-child relations, or any other aspects of modernization. . . . New wealth flows from educated children to parents are continuing . . . [and] have provided a major vehicle for upward mobility during the past decade. (1992, 2)

5. It was assumed at all levels of government that pre- and extramarital sex was rare and that only married couples need to be targeted. These assumptions were to have important ramifications for policy development for dealing with the HIV/AIDS epidemic.

6. Nevertheless, I have recently heard some opposition to Bali's wholehearted adoption of family planning on the grounds of potential loss of ethnic identity: some urban, educated Balinese are beginning to feel threatened by the numbers of Javanese and other islanders walking their streets and fear the continuing diminution of the Balinese population.

7. Examples of school lessons that focus on family planning can be found in Parker (1992a, 108–10; and 1992b, 63–65).

8. The textbook reading passage was titled "My Younger Sibling Is One." It celebrated the happy family life enjoyed by the narrator and his or her younger sibling with their parents and concluded: "The slogan 'The Small Family Norm Is Happy and Prosperous' (Norma Keluarga Kecil Berbahagia dan Sejahtera, NKKBS) is indeed correct" (Muslich 1988, 2).

9. The health and vitality of the various PKK organizations fluctuate, and in many *banjar* at any time PKK exist on paper only. See Sullivan 1991.

10. Likewise, in a comprehensive survey of village women in rural Klungkung, Streatfield asked women to identify who, apart from themselves, had been involved in their decision to accept family planning. He found that 68.8 percent of 712 respondents said that their husband was the only other person involved in the decision; only 7.4 percent of women said it was their decision alone; 8.3 percent nominated the BKKBN fieldworker as instrumental in their decision (Streatfield 1986, 118).

11. This is not the place to explore those shifts that do not relate directly to women. Here I will only mention a possible cosmogonic concomitant of recent changes to notions of fecundity. In Balinese cosmology there is a crucial interaction between the forces that animate and make fruitful humans and rice plants. The ritual metaphors that express these—for example, the offerings that mark the pregnancy (*beling*) and the performance of the marriage (*masakapan*) of the rice plants—are based on a positive valuation of fecundity, a belief in the possibility of the efficacy of human intervention, and a holistic belief that events and actions in one sphere (*buana*) have effects in other spheres. I am as yet unable to determine the cosmological significance of human intervention in human fertility; one hopes that there is not a directly proportional effect on rice fertility!

12. The usual term for prostitutes is (*Wanita Tuna Susila* WTS; lit. women without morals).

13. Many major road intersections and village government offices in Bali are fes-

tooned with government messages and slogans, such as a concrete statue or emblem advertising the ten brightly painted basic points of the PKK program:

1. Vitalization and supervision of *Pancasila*
2. Helping each other
3. Food
4. Basic necessities (clothing)
5. Housing and household management
6. Education and skills
7. Health
8. Developing a cooperative existence
9. Sustainable environment
10. Healthy planning.

REFERENCES

Abdurochim. 1986. *Profil kependudukan Indonesia*. Jakarta: Kantor Menteri Negara Kependudukan dan Lingkungan Hidup dan Lembaga Demografi, Fakultas Ekonomi, Universitas Indonesia.

Aditjondro, G. 1995. Who owns Bali? *Inside Indonesia* 44 (September): 19–20.

Astawa, I. B., Soegeng Waloeyo, and J. E. Laing. 1975. Family planning in Bali. *Studies in Family Planning* 6 (4): 86–101.

Belo, J. 1949. *Bali: Rangda and Barong*. American Ethnological Society, Monograph no. 16. Seattle: University of Washington Press.

———. 1970 [1936]. A study of a Balinese family. In *Traditional Balinese culture: Essays*, ed. J. Belo, 350–70. New York: Columbia University Press.

Bendesa, I. K. G., and I. M. Sukarsa. 1980. An economic survey of Bali. *Bulletin of Indonesian Economic Studies* 16 (2): 31–53.

Bernet Kempers, A. J. 1991. *Monumental Bali: Introduction to Balinese archaeology and guide to the monuments*. Berkeley: Periplus Editions.

BKKBN [Badan Koordinasi Keluarga Berencana Nasional]. 1992. *Kumpulan data: Kependudukan dan keluarga berencana Indonesia*. Jakarta: Badan Koordinasi Keluarga Berencana Nasional.

Boon, J. A. 1977. *The anthropological romance of Bali, 1597–1972: Dynamic perspectives in marriage and caste, politics and religion*. Cambridge: Cambridge University Press.

Branson, J., and D. B. Miller. 1988. The changing fortunes of Balinese market women. In *Development and displacement: Women in Southeast Asia*, ed. G. Chandler, N. Sullivan, and J. Branson, 1–16. Clayton, Vic.: Centre of Southeast Asian Studies, Monash University.

Brinkgreve, F. 1987. The *cili* and other female images in Bali. In *Indonesian women in focus: Past and present notions*, ed. E. Locher-Scholten and A. Niehof, 135–51. Dordrecht: Foris Publications.

Caldwell, J. C. 1982. *Theory of fertility decline*. New York: Academic Press.

Connor, L. 1983. Healing as women's work in Bali. In *Women's work and women's roles: Economics and everyday life in Indonesia, Malaysia and Singapore*, ed. L. Manderson, 53–72. Canberra: Development Studies Centre, Australian National University.

Covarrubias, M. 1972 [1937]. *Island of Bali*. Oxford: Oxford University Press.
Edmondson, J. C. 1992. Bali revisited: Rural economy, intergenerational exchanges, and the transition to smaller family sizes, 1977–90. MS. Denpasar: Pusat Kajian Budaya, Universitas Udayana.
Freedman, R., and B. Berelson. 1976. The record of family planning programs. *Studies in Family Planning* 7 (1): 1–40.
Geertz, H., and C. Geertz. 1975. *Kinship in Bali*. Chicago: University of Chicago Press.
Harrison, P. 1978. And in Bali . . . *banjars* show the way. *People* 5 (1): 14–17.
Hill, H., ed. 1994. *Indonesia's new order: The dynamics of socio-economic transformation*. St. Leonards, N.S.W.: Allen and Unwin.
Hugo, G., et al. 1987. *The demographic dimension in Indonesian development*. Singapore: Oxford University Press.
Hull, T. 1978. Where credit is due: Policy implications of the recent rapid fertility decline in Bali. Paper presented at Population Association of America Meeting, Mexico City, 14 April.
Hull, V. 1982. Women in Java's rural middle class: Progress or regress? In *Women of Southeast Asia*, ed. P. van Esterik, 100–123. DeKalb: Center for Southeast Asian Studies, Northern Illinois University.
Hunter, T. M. 1988. Crime and punishment in Bali: Paintings from a Balinese hall of justice. *Review of Indonesian and Malaysian Affairs* 22 (2): 62–113.
Kantor Statistik Provinsi Bali. 1988[?]. *Statistical pocketbook of Bali 1987*. Denpasar: Kantor Statistik Provinsi Bali.
———. 1990[?]. *Statistical pocketbook of Bali 1989*. Denpasar: Kantor Statistik Provinsi Bali.
Lovric, B. J. A. 1987. Rhetoric and reality: The hidden nightmare. Myth and magic as representations and reverberations of morbid realities. Ph.D. diss., University of Sydney.
McNicoll, G. 1980. Technology and the social regulation of fertility. Working Paper no. 46, Center for Population Studies, Population Council, New York.
Meier, G. 1979. Family planning in the *banjars* of Bali. *International Family Planning Perspectives* 5 (2): 63–66.
Miller, D. B., and J. Branson. 1989. Pollution in paradise: Hinduism and the subordination of women in Bali. In *Creating Indonesian cultures*, ed. P. Alexander, 91–112. Sydney: Oceania Publications.
Muslich, M. 1988. *Bahasa Indonesia SC, Untuk Kelas 5, Catur Wulan 3, Sekolah Dasar*, 2d ed. Klaten: Intan Pariwara.
Oey-Gardiner, M. 1993. A gender perspective in Indonesia's labour market transformation. In *Indonesia assessment 1993. Labour: Sharing in the benefits of growth?* ed. C. Manning and J. Hardjono, 203–13. Proceedings of Indonesia Update Conference, August 1993. Political and Social Change Monograph 20. Canberra: Department of Political and Social Change, Research School of Pacific Studies, Australian National University.
Parker, L. 1989. Village and state in "new order" Bali. Ph.D. diss., Australian National University, Canberra.
———. 1992a. The quality of schooling in a Balinese village. *Indonesia* 54 (October): 95–116.
———. 1992b. The creation of Indonesian citizens in Balinese primary schools. *Review of Indonesian and Malaysian Affairs* 26 (1): 42–70.

———. Forthcoming. Flowers and witches in Bali: Representations and everyday life of Balinese women. In *ReOrienting the body: Embodiments of women in Asian cultural forms*, ed. V. Mackie and F. Freiberg. Wild Peony Press.

Parmiti, D. P. 1992. Konseptualisasi diri wanita Hindu di Bali (The self-conceptualization of Hindu women in Bali). Paper presented at the Annual Meeting of the Society for Balinese Studies, Denpasar, August.

Poffenberger, M. 1983. Toward a new understanding of population change in Bali. *Population Studies* 37 (1): 44–64.

Pucci, I. 1985. *The epic of life: The Balinese journey of the soul.* New York: Harper and Row.

Streatfield, K. 1986. *Fertility decline in a traditional society: The case of Bali.* Indonesian Population Monograph Series, no. 4. Canberra: Department of Demography, Australian National University.

Sullivan, N. 1991. Gender and politics in Indonesia. In *Why gender matters in Southeast Asian politics*, ed. M. Stivens, 61–86. Clayton, Vic.: Centre of Southeast Asian Studies, Monash University.

Team Pengembangan, Pengolahan dan Penyajian Data Statistik Pembangunan Daerah Bali. 1984. *Kesempatan kerja dan angkatan kerja di propinsi daerah tingkat I Bali.* Denpasar: Bappeda Tingkat I Bali, Fakultas Ekonomi Unud and Kantor Statistik Propinsi Bali.

Warren, C. 1986. Indonesian development policy and community organization in Bali. *Journal of Contemporary Southeast Asia* 8 (3): 213–30.

———. 1990. The bureaucratisation of local government in Indonesia. Working Paper no. 66. Clayton, Vic.: Centre of Southeast Asian Studies, Monash University.

———. 1993. *Adat and Dinas: Balinese communities in the Indonesian state.* Kuala Lumpur: Oxford University Press.

CHAPTER 7

Empowerment or Control? Northeast Thai Women and Family Planning

Andrea Whittaker

Thailand is considered a model of a successful "reproductive revolution," as it has achieved a rapid fertility decline during a period in which the majority of the population has remained rurally based (Knodel, Chamratrithirong, and Debavalya 1987, 6–7; Krannich and Krannich 1983). In northeast Thailand the family planning program has been associated with a decline in total fertility rates from 7.63 births per woman in 1969 to 1.98 births per woman in 1997 and a contraceptive prevalence rate of 72.2 percent (IPSR 1997; Knodel, Chamratrithirong, and Debavalya 1987, 56). In this chapter I explore the effects of the family planning program in northeast Thailand on a number of levels. First, I describe the application of family planning to a specific population so as to suggest the relations of power and ethnicity implicit in the targeting of the northeast. Next, I describe the ramifications for women in the small rural community of Baan Srisaket, exploring the traditional construction of gender within the village and the ways in which reproduction is viewed and managed. There has been a shift from reproduction as a process that was managed by women and the community to one that is located in the realm of the state.

At one level the objectives of state policy and that of village women coincide, since they relate to women's desire to have control over their own fertility and their views of themselves as having primary responsibility over reproduction. Yet, for all the positive benefits, the administration of family planning and the side effects of the contraceptives used create a gulf between women's subjective well-being and state objectives. This tension is most acute with regard to abortion.

Paradoxically, while family planning choice is understood in international development circles to be a cornerstone of women's empowerment and contraception provides the opportunity for Isaan women to gain control over their own bodies, the acceptance of family planning also makes women subject to regulation by the state. In their dealings with health authorities, who are middle-class bureaucrats, often of Sino-Thai or Central Thai background, northeastern women negotiate their inferior class and ethnic position and are made targets of reform, carrying the burden of state policies. Yet this relationship cannot be characterized simply as the extension of patriarchal control over women, for it is a process in which many women are enthusiastic volunteers. At the same time, women are sensitive to the relations of power inherent in family planning programs, revealed in their experiences of encounters with government staff and the restrictions placed on their autonomous control of reproduction.

This chapter is based upon eighteen months of ethnographic research in northeast Thailand in 1992–93. Ten months was spent in the remote ethnic Lao community of Baan Srisaket,[1] Roi Et Province, which has 740 households and a population of 3,926 people. Participant observation, focus group discussions, semistructured and informal interviews, and two household surveys were employed in the study, supplemented by hospital and clinic observations concentrating on gynecological, obstetric, and family planning services (Whittaker 1995).

Thailand and the Thai Nation-State

The region in which this chapter is based is known colloquially as "Isaan," a Pali Sanskrit term meaning northeast. This term reflects the marginal orientation of the region in relation to the social and economic center of Thailand: the central plains and Bangkok. The majority of the population is ethnically distinct: Lao-speaking people who express a collective identity based upon domestic language, cultural practices, and regional history distinct from central Thai people. At various moments in history this distinct identity has intensified various separatist movements, such as the communist insurgency of the 1960s and 1970s (Keyes 1967, 1989).

The integration of Isaan within the Thai state since 1893 has largely resulted in its subordination both economically and socially. The sense of physical isolation far removed from the center is reinforced by socioeconomic differences. The northeast is the least developed and poorest region of Thailand, with the highest incidence of poverty, calculated at 36.3 percent of the population in 1988 (Krongkaew 1993, 412–13). Rice farming is the principal productive activity. The average income per capita officially reported for households in the northeast in 1989 was 11,981 baht (US$480), about one-seventh the per capita income of Bangkok (Sheehan 1993, 32). Historically, the northeast has been a problematic region of the Thai state. In the 1950s, against the backdrop of the growing anticolonial movements in Vietnam and Laos, there was an increasing fear of communist insurgency in the northeast. Under the military rule of General Sarit and throughout the Vietnam War, and revolution in Laos, the northeast was seen as a security problem and raids on "communist separatists" became common (Keyes 1966, 1967; Tandrup 1982). The "development" of the northeast was seen as a counterinsurgency measure to alleviate the poverty, which the government feared made the northeast vulnerable to the communist cause (Demaine 1986, 98; Keyes 1989, 158; Phongpaichit 1980).

"Rural development" policies sought both to improve infrastructure—the expansion of roads, communication, transport, and trading networks—and to increase living standards to reduce support for communist subversion. Brown states that "the emergence of a concern for rural development in the peripheral regions was based not so much on welfare considerations as such but rather on the economic, political and security needs of the Bangkok-centred state" (1994, 174). The Community Development Program was initiated in 1960. Advised by the United States Operations Mission, the Thai government developed Mobile Development Units (MDUs) targeting villages in "pink zones" where the communist movement had local support. The MDUs aimed to legitimize the extension of social control to these areas through medical treatment, economic development, and village security volunteer programs with anticommunist education (De Beer 1978; London 1977, 61–66; Prizzia 1985). It was in this period that health services were first made available to villagers as counterinsurgency measures. The decline of communism in the northeast led to a consolidation of state penetration into the region (Brown 1994, 200).

The process of political and economic incorporation of the northeast region into the Thai state has been accompanied by ideological and cultural integration. As Reynolds states:

> As the power of the centre grew and expanded, the Thai state encountered regional and minority cultures different from its own. These encounters engendered reflection on what the dominant, national culture should be, and by the 1930s the government was undertaking strenuous efforts to codify and promote a national culture. (1991, 5)

Central Thai culture is regarded as the "elite" culture of Thailand, both for Central Thai and Isaan people. The discourses of national identity and national culture serve to legitimate the authority of the state and function to "exclude and subordinate other ethnic groups" (Reynolds 1991, 18). Dominant discourses in government and mainstream media portray the northeast in imagery of marginality and cultural inferiority (Brown 1994, 203). Modern, urban, educated, wealthy, and progressive Central Thais are commonly contrasted with traditional, rural, ignorant, poor, and backward Lao/Isaan villagers (Whittaker 1995, 36–37). Through such representations, the moral authority of change and modernity mediates ethnicity and class position, aligning inequalities, exploitation, and underdevelopment with Lao-ness and a failure of peasants to adapt to modern times.

The discourses that constitute ethnicity are important, as they are the basis by which the nation-state assigns resources and they determine the ways in which people are categorized and treated by members of the dominant group. Essentially, they reflect and shape the relations of power between a group of people and the nation-state. Through them, Isaan villagers are constituted as ignorant subjects in need of development and education (Hobart 1993, 6; see also Ram, this volume).

Within health services such public definitions of Isaan culture affect health providers' perception of their clients and community practices. The practices and policies operating in health care settings often revolve around assumptions of ignorance, mediating the subordinate economic and ethnic status of villagers. The mediation of Isaan/Lao ethnicity and class thus runs as a subtext throughout this chapter.

State Population Policies and Thai National Development

Population control through family planning has been an important strategy of Thai national development since 1970. Until 1959 the official Thai government policy was strongly pronatalist, influenced by successive military leaders who viewed the expansion of the population as a necessary defense against Chinese expansion (Keyes 1989, 13). In 1959 the World Bank economic mission recommended that the government consider the adverse economic impact of high population growth and advised the dissemination of birth control information (Sittitrai 1988, 139–40). By 1968 a Population Unit was established in the National Economic and Social Development Board (NESDB). With the public support of the king of Thailand, by 1970 a formal population policy was announced supporting the use of family planning as a measure to reduce population growth.

A National Family Planning Program was incorporated into the Third National Economic and Social Development Plan (1972–76). Prior to this national program, birth control pills and condoms were already available in Bangkok and some provincial centers, and sterilizations were being practiced in some urban centers (Cunningham, Yoddumnurn, and Ratanasupa 1970; Prasartkul and Sethaput 1982). In 1976 the contraceptive pill, the intrauterine device (IUD), and sterilization were offered free of charge at all government health stations, and there was a rapid increase in contraceptive acceptors. Sittitrai states that by 1971 there were 408,000 new acceptors, with an average of 450,000 new acceptors in each succeeding year (1988, 342). In 1995 there were 529,816 new acceptors across Thailand (Thailand, National Statistical Office 1995, 257). In addition to government programs, nongovernment organizations also have been involved in the promotion of family planning, notably the Population and Community Development Association, which has been conducting community-based family planning projects since 1974 (Soonthorndhada, Buravisit, and Vong-Ek 1991).[2] The family planning program has been accompanied by an extensive maternal and child health program.

As Demaine (1986) notes, the key concept of the Third National Economic and Social Development Plan was "human resource development," and it marked the first time that the word *social* was used in the title of the national development planning document. This emphasis on "the social" indicated a change in development discourse by the Thai government. Previous emphasis had been on infrastructure and economic planning. In the Third Plan the problem of development was conceived as the inability of the population to take advantage of available opportunities because of their poor living standards and lack of education:

> Human resources play a leading role in the effort to increase the national productive capacity . . . The increase in efficiency of the rural labour force is very closely related to raising incomes and living standards of rural people. (NESDB 1972, qtd. in Demaine 1986, 100)

The Sixth Plan (1987–91) formulated a strategy of community participation in family planning programs and promoted the use of village health volunteers and village health communicators to encourage villagers to use family planning (see Soonthorndhada, Buravisit, and Vong-Ek 1991, 30–36). In this plan, development was explicitly linked to population control as a means of improving quality of life and as a precondition for raising rural incomes and producing an educated, productive, and healthy work force.

The Seventh National Economic and Social Development Plan (1992–96) directly links the control of population growth to the "international competitiveness of the economy" (Thailand, NESDB 1992, 149) and identifies specific populations as "remaining problems" in need of intervention. The targets set are to

> reduce population growth rates to 1.2 per cent by the end of the Seventh Plan period . . . with special focus on the target groups in the northeast, and

the south, and the special target groups such as hill tribe peoples, Thai nationals of distinctive cultures in the south, slum dwellers and industrial workers. (Thailand, NESDB 1992, 149)

This "special focus" upon subordinate classes and ethnic groups reveals an agenda apart from the improvement in health status. The implementation of these programs extends the incorporation and regulation of these marginalized ethnic and class groups within state structures. Within the historical context noted earlier, the targeting of the northeast for family planning can be seen as not only a reflection of the poverty and high birthrates of the region, but an extension of state concern over a population that has emerged in the national imagination as a potential threat to state solidarity. The population of the northeast is also problematic to the Thai state because of increasing rural-urban migration. Each year large numbers of northeasteners migrate to Bangkok in search of work, cramming into the slums of Bangkok. Despite the economic benefits that a large supply of surplus labor has for the economy of the Central Plains, in Bangkok the effects of overpopulation are made most evident to policy makers.

Family planning programs provide an opportunity and a rationale for numerous points of intervention into specific populations and individual bodies. They require the mobilization of female bodies, the allocation of resources, and the justification of practices of surveillance and regulation. Foucault has termed this the practice of "bio-power": "the insertion of bodies into the machinery of production and the adjustment of the phenomena of population to economic processes" (1984, 141). In the case of the northeast, the adjustment of the population by the Thai state is motivated not purely by concerns for the quality of life of the citizens but also by economic and political objectives.

Traditional Forms of Contraception

> In the past we got married and we were so young. After we got married we had children right away. But now we have got family planning.
> —Aunt Som

Before the availability of modern contraceptives, women of Baan Srisaket practiced a number of techniques to control their fertility. Fertility control was personally managed with resources within the community (Whittaker 1996, 212). Although a number of authors claim there were no "traditional contraceptives" other than abortion, herbal and magical means were also used for the control of fertility (Hanks 1963, 16–17; Mougne 1978, 82; Riley and Sermsri 1974, 13; cf.

Poulsen 1983). Grandmother Sow, a traditional midwife, demonstrated the grinding of two types of bark into a powder that she said "makes the uterus *hiaw* [dry],[3] so your menstruation will come, but you will not get pregnant." The powder is mixed with water and drunk every day. Grandmother Sow also said that eating white clay was a contraceptive, "but now we have *yaa khum* [contraceptive medicine] and women don't have to eat clay."[4] "Drying out the womb," through the postpartum practice of staying by the fire, is still practiced to delay the next pregnancy:

> If you stay by the fire you will have children slowly, in one to five years, you don't have to take any contraceptives.
> —Grandmother Sim

Other traditional means of contraception include herbal concoctions made efficacious through sacred spells. These continue to be drunk through the postpartum period to delay the next pregnancy (Poulsen 1983, 224). Periods of abstinence were not mentioned as a means of delaying or avoiding pregnancies, nor is withdrawal a widely used technique (Knodel, Chamratrithirong, and Debavalya 1987, 108). Avoiding certain foods was also used in the past to help prevent pregnancy. The foods avoided were metaphorically linked either to sexual desire or fertility. One grandmother recalled being told not to eat *plaa kheng* (cramming perch), which is said to increase desire for sex, which will lead to more children. All of these forms of contraception were used in the past and, to a limited extent, continue to be used in the present, although women recognize the greater efficacy of modern contraceptives. It is common for grandmothers in the village to state that they had "two children in three years," which implies that prolonged breastfeeding and subsequent postpartum amenorrhea may also have had a limited effect in spacing births.

Reproduction and Constructions of Gender

Popular Buddhism reinforces and celebrates an image of women as nurturers of men and religion (Keyes 1984, 1986; Kirsch 1985). Men must "reject" their potent nature/sexuality for the discipline of monkhood in order to obtain Buddhist merit, whereas a woman is required to "realize her 'nature' as a mother" in order to obtain merit through the ordination of her sons and nurturance of the religion (Keyes 1986, 86–87). Whereas village men confirm their adult status through ordination into the monkhood, for a woman it is through enduring the suffering of pregnancy and the pains of childbirth and postpartum that her status as a full adult is confirmed. In the past, the successful rearing of a large number of children conferred prestige and merit upon a woman. Muecke writes that childlessness was considered legal grounds for divorce: "While women could live without husbands, they could not live without children" (1984, 462).

The importance of the reproductive role of women in Isaan society is reinforced by traditional bride-price, postmarital residence, and inheritance patterns, all of which locate women as the key household members through which household resources are obtained and regulated (Keyes 1975, 295; also Podhisita 1984). To marry, the groom must pay bride-price to the bride's parents to compensate for his access to the matrilineal land that she will inherit. After marriage the groom resides with the bride's family. Ritual symbolism reinforces the domestic authority of women, as they are the custodians of each household's domestic ancestral spirits.

Context of Change

The economy of northeastern villages has shifted from one based on subsistence rice production to one dependent on cash crops and labor migration. This extension of capitalist relations of production into daily village life has eroded many of the former bases of women's status in village communities, separated the reproductive sphere from the productive sphere, disrupted links to land and matrilineal kin through labor migration, and exposed villagers to new, "modern" values, practices and representations of women. Simultaneously, new status markers and meanings are evolving for women, yet often these are beyond the access of village women with little formal education and few economic resources.

Education and wealth have become new sources of prestige for men and women (Muecke 1984) and have become synonymous with modernization and the development of the Thai state. Within Baan Srisaket traditional discourses of constrained sexuality, motherhood, and nurturance still operate but are competing with persuasive messages of what it is to be a modern Thai woman. In Baan Srisaket, although increased numbers of young people are studying to high school level, raising their expectations above rice farming in their own and the community's eyes, few have the opportunity to work in anything but low-status, poorly paid positions. In northern Thailand, as Muecke (1984) describes, the prospects for most women from lower socioeconomic backgrounds to achieve social mobility through education and the accumulation of wealth depend upon the removal of gender-specific barriers, such as lack of access to legal abortion, lack of equal pay, and lack of time due to heavy domestic responsibilities. Muecke suggests women are making rational choices to "make money, not babies" through the practices of urban migration, prostitution, and abortion (1984).

The introduction of modern contraception has released Baan Srisaket women from constant childbearing and freed them to work in the cities but simultaneously deprives them of a traditional source of status as mothers of many children. Traditional values are being renegotiated, but the experience for many women is one of ambivalence. The sections that follow will explore the ways in which modern contraception is welcomed by women and the ways in which it also deprives them of a degree of autonomy with regard to reproduction. The involvement of the state in the implementation of family planning programs adds a further ethnic and class-specific character to the relationship.

Birth and Contraception as Women's Responsibility

From the outset the state family planning program has been gender specific, targeted at women. Stated objectives of the Third National Plan were "to inform and motivate eligible *women,* particularly those living in rural and remote areas" and placed family planning in the context of maternal and child health services (NESDB, qtd. in Sittitrai 1988, 341; my emph.). The emphasis placed on female use of contraception continues to the present and is reflected in the low number of condoms being distributed by village health stations and the low numbers of men having vasectomies (see also Prasartkul and Sethaput 1982; Sukdis, Taendum, and Na Pattalung 1982).[5] Records of the local district hospital nearest Baan Srisaket show only two men were admitted for vasectomies in 1992, whereas, according to hospital records, eighty-three tubal ligations were performed. Female sterilization remains the most used method of contraception in Thailand (Archavanitkul and Pramualratana 1990, 38; Chintana 1986). For example, 1996 data for Khon Kaen province shows 43.14 percent of women who are married and living with their husbands are sterilized, while only 0.58 percent of their husbands have had vasectomies (Khon Kaen Public Health Office 1997).

The low participation of men in contraceptive use reflects cultural attitudes concerning masculinity and fertility. Men are ideally characterized as the economic mainstays of families and as the ones most responsible for productive labor in the fields and elsewhere. Their potency is understood as linked to their strength. Vasectomies are unpopular with men and women, as it is feared that they deplete a man's strength and virility, weakening and making him incapable of the heavy, hard work necessary in the fields. Female sterilization is also understood to make the woman weak, but villagers say "women only have to sit at home and look after children, but men have to do heavy work," despite the fact that, in practice, women share much of the heavy labor in the fields with men. Contraception is considered a woman's responsibility; it allows women to retain control over their fertility and is seen as an extension of their domestic and procreative responsibilities. People also consider it more important for men to retain their fertility in the case of remarriage:

> Men have to work the fields and do heavy work. If they have a vasectomy they can't do heavy work. I know a man who had a vasectomy and then his first wife died and he married another woman and now she wants to have children, but he can't.
> —Aunt Wii

Women's Views of Modern Contraceptives

Official village records report that 87 percent of couples between the ages of fifteen and forty-four use some form of contraception in Baan Srisaket (Thailand, Department of Rural Development 1989, 1990).[6] Local health station data state that 152 people in a total of 667 visits used the family planning services in 1992. Sixty-seven percent of clients used the contraceptive pill, 30 percent injectable contraceptives, and 3 percent received condoms.[7] Health station staff stated they only give contraceptives to married women. Unmarried women have to buy their supplies from drugstores in the district town.

Family planning is being used to space children after the birth of the first child and to prevent further pregnancy rather than to delay childbearing (see also Knodel and Chayovan 1989). The average number of children of clients was 1.8 children. Only 0.3 percent of users had no children. Use of contraception before the fertility of a couple has been confirmed by the birth of a first child is believed by some to make the body weak and possibly jeopardize fertility. Uncle Wan warned me, "If you take the pill, contraceptives, for a long time before you have a baby, the womb is no good and the baby won't have good health, won't be strong."

New contraceptive technologies have freed women from "balancing the water buckets on a pole over one shoulder, having a baby in a sling at your breast and another child on the hip" (Grandmother Sian). As the figures presented above imply, women of Baan Srisaket have embraced family planning. A consistent theme from older women was the lack of control over their fertility in the past. "In the past we didn't have contraceptive medicines. If you had children you had them, ten, twelve children. We only had the local doctors and the midwives. Some died in childbirth." Grandmother Seen, who is now fifty-five, says she was the first woman in Baan Srisaket to take the pill. She had "two children in the first three years" of her marriage. After six children and one miscarriage she simply "didn't want to have any more children." She heard that medicine that stopped you from having more children was available from the health station and took the pill for ten years.

Village women speak positively of the changes in reproductive attitudes and behavior. The desire of women to control their fertility coincides with state population policy. A trend toward smaller family sizes is acknowledged by young and old. Younger women consistently stated that "two children are enough" as an ideal family size. They said that after two children they would have a tubal ligation. The financial burdens of feeding many children and sending them to school are the factors most frequently stated for smaller family sizes.[8] Several women also indicated that having only two children allows them to continue working and remain economically productive, which would not be possible if they had more children. Sittitrai et al. write that small families are viewed by villagers as better able "to adapt to new opportunities afforded by modernisation" (1991, 32; see also Havanon, Knodel, and Sittitrai 1990). Similarly, Muecke found that childbearing had become so expensive for women in Chiang Mai that "the best survival strategy for both economic and moral ends was to have fewer children than their parents had" (1984, 467; see also Mougne 1978, 93). The advantages of small families have been reinforced by family planning promotions that stress in posters and jingles the better quality of life for parents and children in one or two-child families. The "two children and a ligation" ideal is promoted in most antenatal clinics. A poster in one antenatal clinic shows a picture of two children, a girl and a boy, declaring: "Our mother loves us. She has had a tubal ligation already!"

Disjunctures between Women and State Policies

The objectives of the state and of women coincide at various points but vary at others, making the adoption and administration of family planning difficult to characterize as purely the product of patriarchy, as women clearly desire to control their fertility. Whereas modern contraceptives are viewed positively by village women as a means of controlling their fertility, such an advantage comes at a cost. Contraceptives are understood as the source of a range of unwanted side effects that affect women's well-being. The administration of family planning also involves a series of encounters with government representatives in which women are subject to monitoring and subtle reinforcements of their subordinate status. Finally, the disjuncture between the desires and autonomy of women and the state is most acute in matters concerning abortion. The following section describes these disjunctures and the ambivalent relation of women to the state that results.

Unwanted Side Effects

Many of the contraceptive side effects described by women are culturally specific and refer to humoral concepts of wetness and dryness, heat and cold, and the perceived linkage between fertility, regular menstruation and vitality. Stories of side effects and changing contraceptives in an attempt to find one suitable to their body and lifestyle are commonly discussed among women. The side effects described for modern contraceptives usually highlight the effect of the contraceptive on the humoral balance of the body.

The human body is understood to consist of four (elements), derived from Ayurvedic traditions, namely *din* (earth), *fai* (fire), *naam* (water), and *lom* (wind). Disequilibrium in one of these, due to eating wrong foods, fluctuations in climate, or behaviors that jeopardize the balance of these elements, increases one's vulnerability to ill health (Manderson 1981, 1986). Modern methods of contraception are understood to disrupt the bodily balance leading to a range of complaints, the most common of which is a loss of vitality and an inability to work hard.

> In the past we didn't have the pill and so I had seven children and then, after that, I went and used an IUD. It was painful and I got a lot of *maat khaaw* [discharge] and I smelled so strongly that I couldn't get close to other people. I got the doctor to take it out and I had another child right after it was taken out. After that child I took the pill and I got a dry throat and I didn't feel well, so I stopped and then I had another child, and after that child I made the decision to have a tubal ligation. That was three years ago. After the tubal ligation I get really tired and can't sleep and have vision problems.
>
> —Aunt Uay

> After I had the injections [Depo Provera] I never menstruated, I was thin and cold and I had to take warm water baths, whereas in the past I could always use only cold water.
>
> —Aunt Naam

Women's reproductive health is invested with complex meanings. Their strength and vitality is intimately linked to the positive values of their fertility, motherhood, and sexuality. The cycles of menstruation, pregnancy, and parturition also leave women vulnerable and weak, however, and exposed to dangerous fluctuations in the humoral balance of their bodies (Irvine 1982, 258–84). A heavy regular menstrual flow of red blood is indicative of a healthy body. This ensures that the "bad" blood that builds up in a woman's body has been expelled. Irregular menstruation, or blood that is "thin" or "black, bruised and congealed," or any discharges (*maat khaaw*), are signs of ill health and bodily imbalance. The retention of bad blood within a woman's body may cause varied bodily and emotional states: weakness, bad moods, irritability, insanity, skin rashes, headache, dizziness, ulcers, and paleness (Chirawatkul 1996). The presence of leucorrhea and other discharges signifies a "dirty" womb and is associated with an inflamed or infected uterus requiring cleansing and drying out through the restriction of "hot foods." Any contraceptives that disrupt menstruation or increase discharges are thus understood to jeopardize a woman's physical and mental well-being. Table 3 lists the most common side effects mentioned by village women in interviews and focus groups.

While women may experience side effects that are not considered serious medical conditions, the effects attributed to contraceptives are understood to be consequences of the interference with the normal reproductive processes balancing the female body. Despite the controversy surrounding the use of Depo Provera in some countries,[9] women in Baan Srisaket appreciate the convenience of the injectable contraceptives, as there "is no need to remember to take a pill every day." In addition, injections are valued highly in the local culture (Reeler 1990). Yet injectable contraceptives are frequently associated with

TABLE 3. Common Side Effects Attributed to Contraceptives by Isaan Women

Contraception	Common Complaints
Pill[a]	dry throat, tiredness, lack of appetite, skin problems, thinness, dizziness, obesity, abdominal pain, lower back pain
IUD	abdominal pain, heavy discharge, inability to work hard
Injectable (Depo Provera)	headaches, thinness, weakness, amenorrhea, dizziness and confusion, coldness, obesity, eye problems, blotchy skin
Tubal ligation	lower abdominal pain, weakness, discharge, forgetfulness, waist and back pain, leg pain, change in consistency of menstruation, amenorrhea
Vasectomy	weakness, inability to work hard
Condom	reduces sensitivity
Norplant	weak, tired arms, inability to work hard, implant moves through body

[a] *Yaa met khum gamnoet* is the term used by women to describe all forms of the contraceptive pill. Only in a few cases are women able to identify the brand of pill used; hence it is not possible to identify which form of contraceptive pills may be associated with particular problems. Rather, the categories used in this chart reflect women's categories of different contraceptives, which are referred to by the mode of administration.

side effects, such as tired arms, amenorrhea, thinness, weakness, and chills, as the bad blood that is normally expelled through menstruation accumulates in the body causing a cold state. The contraceptive pill is associated with dizziness, blotchy skin, weight gain, and tiredness. IUDs are known to cause bad-smelling discharges and pain.

Likewise, a newly introduced contraceptive method, Norplant, is associated with similar effects on the body. Norplant consists of five small tubes containing laevonorgestrel that are inserted beneath the skin of the upper arm and offer contraceptive protection for five years (Sivin et al. 1980). As part of the local campaign to introduce Norplant by one local district hospital, 488 women had Norplant inserted en masse in April 1992. When I visited the district hospital, many of the women were having the rods removed, complaining of sore, tired arms, tiredness, weakness and dizziness, amenorrhea, irregular bleeding, and a fear that the rods could move through the body. Staff of the district hospital did not acknowledge the cultural understandings of the clients nor try to address their fears (see also Charoenchai and Thongkrajai 1985, 89–90; Stayapan, Kanchanasinith, and Varakamin 1983).

Tubal ligations are the most common form of permanent sterilization and have become the norm for women of Baan Srisaket. Women encourage each other to have ligations, and, although women complain of chronic tiredness and weakness, an inability to sleep, vision disturbances, and abdominal pain after a tubal ligation, they say that the benefits and relief of knowing that they will not fall pregnant again outweighs the ill effects. Having two children and then a tubal ligation has become conventional behavior for women within Baan Srisaket. Tubal ligations are free and usually performed directly after birth.[10]

Women's discourses relating to modern contraceptives reveal a perceived disruption of the traditional ordering and balancing of the female body caused by the new technologies. While women acknowledge the benefits of the control over their fertility, this is perceived to be achieved at the price of their vitality and strength, to the extent of interfering with their productive capabilities. Many women say that women who have tubal ligations have more problems with their health and are not capable of as much hard work, because *bor dai yuu fai lang het man* (they did not stay on the fire after they had a tubal ligation). In this statement the disruption of traditional feminine sources of social and physical strength and status, exemplified in the traditional postpartum ritual, is blamed upon modern contraception.

Delivery of Services: Embodying Ethnic and Class Status

Government hospitals and clinics remain the most important source of supply of contraceptives and clinic procedures (Chayovan, Kamnuansilpa, and

Knodel 1988). Whereas women of Baan Srisaket regard contraception as a means of control over their bodies, their experiences of family planning services within government clinics are encounters that are far from empowering. Once within the clinic space, women become "contraceptive acceptors," with the doctor or nurse as the superior knowing agent and the woman as ignorant passive recipient of this knowledge. Observations of government clinics reveal a range of micro-relations of power enacted in clinic procedures and counseling. Staff in these clinics are often of elite Central Thai or Chinese Thai backgrounds with middle-class aspirations, who look down upon Lao-speaking village women who come wearing cotton *phaasin* skirts, clearly marking their class and ethnicity (Cohen 1989, 164–65; Maxwell 1975, 484–85). Little detailed counseling is given to clients, and they have few opportunities for questions.

The spatial organization and service provided at the district hospital family planning clinic near Baan Srisaket subordinates the needs of clients to the priorities of staff members. The family planning unit is in a room positioned between a secretarial administration room and the outer hall, and, consequently, staff are constantly passing through the room down the passageway between the benches of the patients and the desks of the staff. Clients to the clinic are forced to stand in order to speak to nurses sitting behind their desks, as no chairs are provided. No private space exists for consultation or counseling except for the brief period when a woman is positioned in a vulnerable posture on the examination bed to be injected in the buttocks or examined for an IUD. While clients are consulting, any number of nonmedical staff pass through the room and overhear conversations. As may be expected, the behavior of most clients I observed was passive, with little conversation or questions asked of the nurses:

> One young woman came at 9.30 A.M. into the family planning room filled with clerks and other staff reading magazines. She handed her card to the first staff member, whose greeting was *"chiit yaa* [injection]." She was pointed in the direction of the examination table and had to negotiate her way between the staff standing talking between the desks. There was much interest in the raffle tickets the police were selling to the nurses at 20 baht each. Eventually the curtain was pulled around the bed and she was given her injection and told the date to come back.

Within the village health station, the experience of women seeking contraceptives is similarly a perfunctory consultation with few questions asked about difficulties women may be experiencing with their contraceptives. Women in Baan Srisaket are aware of the subtle discrimination operating with many officials and criticize staff for neglecting their needs, "speaking rudely," and failing to give information to them.

Attitudes of professional health providers are informed by discourses that represent Isaan villagers as dirty, ignorant, and naive. Within a provincial hospital jokes circulate among staff of the "real stories" of Isaan women clients seeing gynecologists:

> An Isaan village woman was told that she should wash herself before coming to see a gynecologist, so the next time she did . . . she washed her hands.

> An Isaan village woman was told by a nurse to go to the bathroom and clean up before seeing the doctor. One hour later they realized that she hadn't returned. So they went to the toilets, and there she was, cleaning the toilets.

When discussing gynecological problems of village women at a provincial hospital, I was told by one group of interns that "the reason they [village women] get problems is because they are not clean and their hygiene is poor. This is because they have low education."

Such stories of the dirtiness and ignorance of villagers are frequently repeated by the urban middle class and in official discourses about village health (Cohen 1989, 165). Descriptions of Isaan villagers as dirty articulate their marginal status in the eyes of the elite. It forms a part of the common discursive contrasts, described earlier, between Lao villagers as ignorant, uneducated, poor, traditional, and dirty, and the Central Thai elite as educated, wealthy, modern, and clean. Attributions of dirtiness also carry with them assertions of pollution, immorality, and impurity. Health and disease thus become coupled with class and ethnic-specific discourses. Isaan village women's bodies mediate these discourses in their interactions with health staff and institutions.

Even posters of babies in clinics and hospital environments reinforce these subtle messages concerning class and ethnicity. Clinics are replete with glamorous images of beautiful pale-skinned mothers in Western clothes and clean modern urban surroundings, lovingly rubbing baby powder over the soft white skin of their chubby (usually male) babies. At the same time that such imagery glorifies motherhood, these images are used in family planning posters to stress the need for poor rural Isaan women to reduce their fertility. Ethnic and class difference is subtly reinforced in these images, where regulated motherhood is modern, clean, pale skinned, apparently wealthy, and not Isaan. The discursive oppositions captured in these images address poor rural "traditional" dark-skinned Isaan women as objects of reform, not only for their own advancement but also for the development of the Thai state.

Abortion: Women's Autonomy versus State Prohibition

The question of abortion in Thailand lies at the core of state control of women's bodies and reproduction, and the cultural and social meanings of gender and reproduction. Abortion is illegal in Thailand, unless performed by a medical practitioner for the sake of a woman's health or if the pregnancy is the result of rape, incest or unlawful sexual contact (Population Council 1981, 101–2). The state prohibition of abortion is derived from Buddhist beliefs, as it is considered a sin to kill a sentient being.[11] For women with appropriate knowledge and resources, however, abortions are readily available by sympathetic registered physicians. Yet the majority of village women are unaware of the actual availability of abortion options, and many women attempt to induce abortions or consult untrained abortionists. Field and hospital-based studies suggest that, despite the illegalities, induced abortions are common, with between 200,000 and 300,000 performed each year by a variety of methods, with a high number performed inadequately, resulting in complications including injury, infection, infertility, and maternal death (Chaturachinda et al. 1981; Ladipo 1989; Narkavonnakit 1979, 227; Population Council 1981; Thailand, Ministry of Public Health 1990).[12] As Germain writes, the question of access to safe abortion services is important to women's health status throughout the world:

> An estimated 200,000 or more Third World women die needlessly every year due to botched abortions. Additional uncounted thousands suffer severe morbidity, including infertility and chronic health problems due to unsafe clandestine abortions. (1989, 1)

The most common method of fertility control in the past appears to have been abortion. Older women say that in the past, despite the Buddhist demerit involved, traditional birth attendants and massage doctors were skilled at massaging and "squeezing" a fetus out. The present massage doctor claims she does not perform abortions, as it is *baap*, a Buddhist sin. Stories of women who had abortions in the past are still surrounded by secrecy. In a conversation with Grandmother Mai and a group of her friends, I was told: "No, no one we know ever did an abortion." Yet a later conversation with the daughter of Grandmother Mai revealed that Grandmother Mai did know of one case, involving her husband's younger sister:[13]

> I remember that my Aunt died from an abortion. When I was a girl I was shown the slivers of wood that were inserted into her vagina to cause the

abortion. I think that maybe they were poisonous. I don't know how old she was. She had had five pregnancies before that. Other women have the baby pushed and massaged out. Grandmother Wan has done two or three that I know of. She is a *mor tam yae* [midwife] and a *mor sen* [massage doctor]. And you know Grandmother Pau, she has to go to a clinic to get injections, as she has a *mot luuk buam* [swollen uterus] from her many abortions.

The Population Council reports that the most common methods used by women in Thailand to induce abortions are massage, uterine injections, or a combination of methods (1981, 8). It reports an abortion incidence of thirty-seven per thousand among rural women aged fifteen to forty-four (1981, 13). A survey of abortionists by Narkavonnakit (1979) found an average annual caseload of 356 procedures per practitioner, ranging from only a few each year to over ten each day. Fees for abortions are based on a charge related to the month of pregnancy, due to the increased risks of complications with late gestational cases, a practice confirmed by some of my informants (Narkavonnakit 1979, 225). In my interviews and focus groups women reported induced abortions by the use of saline injections by *mor tahan* (army-trained medics who sell their services), massage, the insertion of vaginal abortifacients, and the consumption of traditional emmenagogues:

> I was pregnant and so I bought herbs from a traveling doctor, some herbs which I put inside me. This worked and I aborted, but afterwards I had *maat khaaw* [discharge], for twenty-one days, very heavy. I still haven't healed. I bought some medicine at the shop, *yaa satrii "phenpaa"* [a brand of "women's medicine"], and I had *yaa tom* [a medicine from boiled herbs], but I still haven't healed.
>
> —Aunt Thii

In addition, drugs such as Kano (500 mg tetracycline) or the contraceptive pill, which specifically state that they should not be taken by women who are pregnant, are sometimes taken in the hope that they will produce an abortion:

> I had four children but one died. My third pregnancy I gave myself an abortion. I bought a tablet at the store for 15 baht when I was one month pregnant and then I aborted at three months. I had very bad pain for four hours, much worse than giving birth, and that was that.
>
> —Aunt Bunlaai

> I had an IUD for six months and then I bled for eight days. I went to see the doctor and he performed an abortion for me. It and the IUD came out. The

second time after I knew I was three months' pregnant I took the pill. I tried lots of medicines for taking out the baby, so I don't know what worked. I took them until nine months and when it [the baby] came out it was dead already.

—Aunt Yii

Many women consume large quantities of "hot" medicines in attempts to induce late menstruation. This use of dietary manipulation, herbal medicines, and hard work to bring back their menses is not viewed as abortion but, rather, a form of menstrual regulation. Such a view is supported by traditional medicinal texts such as the *Khamphee prathom chindaa* (Thai Book of Genesis), which describes the early stage of pregnancy as little more than a lump of blood (see also the description in Hanks 1963, 34–35):

At the time of conception they say that [the embryo] is the finest particle, so fine . . . having been conceived in the mother's womb it can become liquefied more than seven times a day, it is so difficult to retain. After seven days, first a cell is formed from the blood. . . . When the pregnancy has lasted seven days without miscarriage the blood becomes thicker, like water which has been used to wash meat. After another seven days it becomes flesh. (Mulholland 1989, 17)

At this early stage intervention to induce menstruation is considered to expel the blood and reverse the process through which it gradually becomes flesh (see also Nichter and Nichter 1987, 24). In such a way women evade the normative definitions of abortion and thereby avoid the legal and social implications of their action. Apart from the consumption of hot medicines, a variety of contraceptive pills are available by the sheet in drugstores and can be purchased and taken by a woman to "bring down" late menstruation. Herbalists sell packets of herbal "tablets" for late menstruation.

When my menstruation didn't come normally I didn't go to the doctor but brought a packet of *yaa dong lau* [pickled medicine] and put it in the alcohol and drank it. After I drank the whole lot my menstruation came.

—Aunt Kaew

There is an unmet need for access to safe legal abortions for Isaan women. The local district hospital near Baan Srisaket reported only one thirty-six-year-old woman presenting with an "incomplete criminal abortion" in 1992.[14] Yet records also show another 13 cases of "incomplete/inevitable abortions," of which some would have been induced. Four abortions were performed at the district hospital. The provincial hospital in Roi Et reported 111 abortions in 1992, and across Roi Et Province there were 1,129 admissions of women in 1992 with complications from unspecified abortions (91.46 per 100,000 population) (Roi Et Provincial Health Office, pers. comm. 1992).[15] The district doctor said that he sees many women seeking abortions and makes his decisions on a case-by-case basis: "Some I help, others I send away. I always wonder if they will go to a quack and come back here with a septic abortion."

In inducing abortions, women are actively resisting state regulation and asserting control over their reproductive bodies. Yet, in seeking late abortions through untrained practitioners or by consuming drugs, they are forced to place their lives at risk. The difficulty in obtaining an abortion through government hospitals was described by Aunt Uay, whose story highlights the linkages between class and wealth and access to a safe abortion:

> I wanted to have the abortion because my husband wasn't here and I didn't think that I could look after the baby. I had it when I was four months' pregnant. I had an injection from the *mor phu'n baan* [local doctor]. I was very sick and thin and couldn't eat any food. After it was out it was very painful from 3 P.M. to 8 P.M. . . . I did the abortion at home, because at the hospital they ask lots of questions and you have got to have enough reasons not to keep your baby. If you're in the city, [having the baby] will cause lots of problems for you and the doctor might do it [an abortion] for you, but for people in the village they try to force you to keep the baby even though you don't have lots of money. The pain was worse than when you give birth, not the same at all.

Thorbek similarly documents the plight of poor women in Bangkok seeking abortions, for whom money makes the difference between painful and dangerous abortions by untrained practitioners and safe, quick, and less painful abortions in a clinic (1987, 100–102).

The pressure placed upon women not to have abortions became evident in an abortion counseling session I witnessed at a major teaching hospital in Khon Kaen.[16]

> I enter the room where the intern counselor, a nurses' aide, and a patient are sitting. On the wall of the room, which doubles at other times as an examination room, are several posters. One depicts a man and woman in a pink heart promoting a two-child family. There are several baby posters showing cute, chubby, fair-skinned babies, and one photograph, placed strategically at eye level next to where the patient sits, showing a woman on

a stretcher with an intravenous drip with the caption "This is a woman who self-aborted at four months. It is very dangerous and leads to shock and death."

A young woman in her second year of high school sits facing the doctor with her head lowered. Her mother sits behind her. She is two months pregnant after attending a birthday party with a girlfriend and five young men. She says she drank five or six drinks and can't remember with whom she had sex. She says it was her first time. The counselor speaks accusingly, asking for all details of the night: "You went to this party? With how many girls? How many boys? And drinking?" Tears well in the girl's eyes.

The intern asks, "And what will you do about contraception? Or this will happen again, won't it? If you take the pill you will just forget to take it, you should have an IUD or maybe the new drug that goes into your arm that works for five years."
  She asks the girl if she has slept with this boy before.
  "No, I never have," the young woman replies.
  The intern doesn't believe her and keeps questioning her. The intern suggests that the mother should find out who the father is and they should ask him about the baby's fate. The doctor goes to consult with another doctor. The nurses' aide says to the mother, "We see cases like this all the time of young girls who go out riding on the back of their boyfriends' motorbike." The intern comes back and says, "There are no indications for an abortion."

Another woman comes and explains that she had been having Depo Provera injections and has fallen pregnant. When she did not menstruate she saw a doctor, who told her she was not pregnant, and was given another injection of Depo Provera. Now she is four months' pregnant and wants an abortion. The doctor replies that it is unfortunate that her contraceptive failed, but that there are no indications for an abortion and as she is four months' pregnant it is too dangerous. The nurses' aide goes to call in the woman's husband, who explains that he doesn't want the child as they have three children already.
  "How are your other children?" the counselor asks.
  "We have two girls and a boy," he replies.
  "Why don't you want another child just as lovely? The doctor said that you should think of the two lives [the baby and the mother]." The couple remain silent.

> "In another five months you will have another baby! It's just too dangerous to abort."
>
> The husband expresses the fear that the child might be deformed because of the Depo Provera injection: "It might have six fingers or something."
>
> "That's nothing, we'll just cut it off!" the counselor replied jokingly.
>
> Finally, the intern says to the nurses' aide, "Go and show the couple the pictures of a four-month-old fetus. You'll see what you have inside you; it's a little baby already. Go and get the model."

Despite the first case being a possible rape and the second late gestational case apparently caused by contraceptive failure, neither woman was granted an abortion. Another woman who attended was mute and intellectually disabled and four months' pregnant to an unknown father. Through a village friend who accompanied her, she indicated that she did not want the child. The doctor showed her the photograph of the woman who had died from a late abortion and told the interpreter to tell her that if she died that way she would become a terrible *phii* (spirit).[17] The friend signed to her that if she did anything to herself she would die or else the police would take her away. In the end the doctor suggested that when she saw the baby her natural maternal desire would make her accept it.

Through a heavy use of moralistic discourse on motherhood and Buddhist values of not taking a life, the counseling I witnessed offered few choices to the women. It did not empower women to make a decision nor support them if they were over four months' pregnant and could not have an abortion. "Responsible" control over one's fertility through contraception was contrasted with "irresponsible" desire to control fertility through abortion, even when contraception had failed. The sanctity of motherhood and maternal desire and the authority of the husband/father, supported by appeals to religious and social tradition, were placed in discursive opposition to imagery of sexually wanton young women and evil female spirits. Medical students and nurses said that when women are granted an abortion at the hospital some doctors perform the procedure with no anesthetic or pain relief.

The numbers of women seeking abortions indicate that state morality as codified in Thai law is inconsistent with the realities women face in controlling their fertility. As long as the Thai government fails to acknowledge publicly the need for safe therapeutic pregnancy terminations on demand, women will continue to utilize unsafe abortifacients and untrained abortionists.

Thailand has an extensive and successful family planning program that has institutionalized the motto Two Children Are Enough in the minds of its citizens and has been responsible for a large reduction in the average birthrate in the last two decades. A range of contraceptive technologies are widely available through village health centers and through social marketing. Family planning programs have enabled women to control their fertility and release them from the pattern of high parity and high maternal mortality that their mothers describe. In this respect the objectives of the state programs coincide with the desires of women to control their fertility. Yet, at the same time, access to legal abortion is denied. In inducing abortions, women are actively resisting state regulation and asserting control over their reproductive bodies but in that same act they also risk their lives.

Traditionally, fertility regulation, pregnancy, and childbirth were conditions to be managed within the community, often with the services of the village midwife. Modern contraceptive techniques, while appreciated for their effectiveness, have shifted control of fertility from the intimate realm of the personal into the public realm of the state. Thus, the wombs of women are being managed and disciplined as the locus of interventions and new technologies in family planning, birthing, breastfeeding, and child care. These technologies have effects that become explained and experienced through local understandings of the body and health. New contraceptive technologies are understood to dry out the womb, and tubal ligations negate the need to stay by the fire but lead to longer-term weakness and ill health. Women are strongly encouraged by health workers to be sterilized immediately after the birth of their second child, an act that both frees them from further strains of pregnancy and birthing but which they believe will weaken them and leave them unable to work as hard as they did in the past.

In their interactions with service providers women are made participants in a process of medicalization specific to female bodies. In this process women also carry markers of their subordinate ethnicity. They are addressed as targets of reform whose high fertility and, by extension, their poverty and lack of education may be reversed through a pill, IUD, or tubal ligation so as to become part of the modern, developed Thai state.

NOTES

    1. All names of villages, districts, and informants in this chapter are pseudonyms.

    2. Other nongovernment organizations involved in family planning include the Planned Parenthood Association of Thailand, the Association for Strengthening Information in the National Family Planning Programme, and the Thailand Association for Voluntary Sterilization (Soonthorndhada, Buravisit, and Vong-Ek 1991).

    3. The transcription of Thai and Lao words in this chapter is based upon the Thai Royal Transcription system, with some modifications (see Whittaker 1995). It is used

throughout this chapter except when referring to the title of works that may have used a different transcription system. Tones are not represented in this system. Double letters indicate long vowels.

4. According to Grandmother Sow, eating clay, also termed *pica* or *geophagy*, is another common practice for pregnant women in Isaan. Biscuits made from dried clay are still sold in some shops in the northeast for pregnant women to eat grilled.

5. The low number of people (only 3 percent) being supplied condoms included some of the village health volunteers, who were given up to thirty at a time to distribute, and so actual usage of condoms may be slightly higher than the percentage of users indicates. Condoms continue to carry an association with commercial sex and so are considered by many villagers to be inappropriate for long-term contraceptive use, despite the advent of HIV/AIDS. Approximately 560 condoms were distributed by the health station at Baan Srisaket in 1992, according to its figures. This number remains low given the population and may be due to the fact that condoms are easily purchased elsewhere, which people may prefer given their association with commercial sex.

6. The accuracy of local government statistics is uncertain, as there is no indication how they are derived. A more accurate picture of local patterns of contraceptive use by women in Baan Srisaket is presented in this chapter. It is derived from the family planning data I collected from the village health station for 1992 for the entire *tambon* (subdistrict), consisting of twelve *muubaan* (administrative villages). As this data refers to people who used the local health station for their family planning services, it may not represent all people using contraception in the twelve villages, as these services are also available elsewhere in district and regional centers. It also does not include any people who have been sterilized, since sterilizations are not performed locally and do not appear in local records.

7. This local picture differs from the overall pattern because it describes services available at the local health station level. Hence, it fails to give the percentages of couples using sterilization that is do ne at the district hospital level and so is not counted in this data. Recent 1996 data for Khon Kaen Province shows that 87.56 percent of women who are currently married and living with their spouses are using some form of contraception, with 13.6 percent using Depo Medroxyprogesterone Acetate (Depo Provera, or DMPA), 16.7 percent using the pill, 13 percent using IUDs, 0.84 percent using Norplant, 0.58 percent using male sterilization, and 43.14 percent using female sterilization (Khon Kaen Public Health Office 1997).

8. See also Knodel, Chamratrithirong, and Debavalya 1987, 123–37; and Knodel, Havanon, and Sittitrai 1990, for a discussion of factors contributing to a smaller family size.

9. The injectable contraceptive known as Depo Provera has not been approved by the Food and Drug Administration in the United States due to reports of higher incidence of breast cancer in beagles and evidence of congenital malformations among infants if accidentally exposed to the drug early in pregnancy (Stephen and Chamratrithirong n.d.). After a review, however, the United States Agency for International Development (USAID) recommended that Depo Provera should be made available to other countries that request it. The international controversy over the use of injectables has centered around the questions of long-term cancer risks of DMPA and the ethics of its use in developing countries. A review by Archer (1985) for Save the Children Fund concluded that any long-term cancer risks are outweighed by the hazards of uncon-

trolled fertility for women in developing countries and noted that such risks also exist for other hormonal methods that provided highly effective, simple-to-use, and undetectable contraception (1985, 17–18).

10. Humoral notions underlie local descriptions of tubal ligations, as either "wet" ligations or "dry" ligations. Wet ligations are those done very soon after birth and are said to be less painful, whereas dry ligations are those performed at times other than after birth.

11. For further detail regarding Buddhist understanding of abortion, see Hardacre 1997; and Keown 1998.

12. Statistics on the consequences of illegal abortion in Thailand state that 0.7 percent of thirty-seven hundred women who had illegal abortions died as a result (Koetsawang, cited in Thailand, Ministry of Public Health 1990, 79).

13. Bleek writes of similar "lying informants" in a study including questions about birth control and abortion in Ghana. He suggests lying "is a strategy for survival, a code to preserve one's own and other people's self-respect" (1987, 319). Although it seems that the secrets of women's abortions, domestic violence, and prostitution are widely known, they are an unspoken currency rarely articulated to the outsider/anthropologist who does not share the history of the community. In some ways my role of living in the community and talking with many families made it even more important for Grandmother Mai, with whom I lived, to keep her secrets, to preserve my respect for her and to negotiate her identity and history as she saw fit.

14. As English is the technical language used in medicine in Thailand, doctors often write their diagnoses in English in the hospital records. "Criminal abortion" refers to a case where there is evidence of the abortion having been induced, or the patient has admitted to seeing someone to induce the abortion. Due to the legal restrictions on abortion, most cases of induced abortion are therefore illegal. In my visits to several hospitals it is clear that the designation of such cases as criminal abortions varies from doctor to doctor. The hospital records indicate the name and address of each patient; such a designation clearly leaves the woman vulnerable to possible legal action.

15. Hospital admission records do not generally distinguish between admissions for incomplete natural abortions and incomplete induced abortions. Therefore, it is not possible to state that all of these cases are the result of induced abortion. It is also unlikely, however, that all clients developing complications of induced abortions are admitted to hospitals.

16. In contrast to the women attending the outpatients' antenatal clinic who wore pregnancy dresses even in the first trimester, women who were seeking abortions were all dressed in pants, even those who were already four months' pregnant. This clothing suggests a denial of their pregnant condition.

17. Women who die in childbirth or in unnatural circumstances are said to become *phii taai hoog* (fierce spirits).

REFERENCES

Archavanitkul, K., and A. Pramualratana. 1990. Factors affecting women's health in Thailand. MS.

Archer, E. 1985. *Injectable contraceptives: The role of long-acting progestagens in contraception in developing countries.* London: Save the Children Fund.

Bleek, W. 1987. Lying informants: A fieldwork experience from Ghana. *Population and Development Review* 13 (2): 314–21.

Brown, D. 1994. *The state and ethnic politics in Southeast Asia*. New York: Routledge.

Charoenchai, A., and E. Thongkrajai. 1985. *Reasons for family planning method switching in northeastern Thailand: An experimental study of a motivational strategy*. Khon Kaen: Khon Kaen University.

Chaturachinda, K., et al. 1981. Abortion: An epidemiologic study at Ramathibodi Hospital, Bangkok. *Studies in Family Planning* 12 (6–7): 257–62.

Chayovan, N., P. Kamnuansilpa, and J. Knodel. 1988. *Thailand demographic and health survey, 1987*. Bangkok: Institute of Population Studies, Chulalongkorn University.

Chintana, P. 1986. *Contraceptive method choice in Thailand*. Bangkok: National Statistic Office of the Prime Minister.

Chirawatkul, S. 1996. Beliefs of blood in a transitional culture of northeastern Thailand. In *Maternity and reproductive health in Asian societies*, ed. P. L. Rice and L. Manderson, 247–59. Amsterdam: Harwood Academic Publishers.

Cohen, P. T. 1989. The politics of primary health care in Thailand, with special reference to non-government organizations. In *The political economy of primary health care in Southeast Asia*, ed. P. T. Cohen and J. Purcal, 159–76. Canberra: ASEAN Training Centre for Primary Health Care Development.

Cunningham, C. E., B. Yoddumnurn, and W. Ratanasupa. 1970. Aspects of maternity and birth control in two Saraphi villages. In *Studies of health problems and health behaviour in Saraphi district, North Thailand*, ed. C. E. Cunningham, T. C. Doege, and H. N. Bangxang, 157–74. Chiang Mai: Faculty of Medicine, Chiang Mai University.

De Beer, P. 1978. History and policy of the Communist Party of Thailand. In *Thailand: Roots of conflict*, ed. A. Turton, J. Fast, and M. Caldwell, 143–57. Nottingham: Spokesman Books.

Demaine, H. 1986. Kanpatthana: Thai views of development. In *Context, meaning and power in Southeast Asia*, ed. M. Hobart and R. H. Taylor, 93–114. Ithaca, N.Y.: Southeast Asia Program, Cornell University.

Foucault, M. 1984. *The history of sexuality*, vol. 1: *An introduction*. London: Penguin.

Germain, A. 1989. The Christopher Tietze international symposium: An overview. *International Journal of Gynecology and Obstetrics* (supp.) 3:1–8.

Hanks, J. R. 1963. *Maternity and its rituals in Bang Chan*. Ithaca, N.Y.: Cornell Thailand Project, Cornell University.

Hardacre, H. 1997. *Marketing the menacing fetus in Japan*. Berkeley: University of California Press.

Havanon, N., J. Knodel, and W. Sittitrai. 1990. The impact of family size on wealth accumulation in rural Thailand. Report no. 3, May 1990. Project on socio-economic consequences of fertility decline for the Thai family. Bangkok: Institute of Population Studies, Chulalongkorn University.

Hobart, M. 1993. Introduction: The growth of ignorance? In *An anthropological critique of development: The growth of ignorance*, ed. M. Hobart, 1–30. London: Routledge.

IPSR [Institute for Population and Social Research]. 1997. Population statistics as of July 1, 1997. *Mahidol Population Gazette*, IPSR, Mahidol University, 6 July, no. 1, 1–2.

Irvine, W. 1982. The Thai-Yuan "madman" and the "modernising, developing Thai

nation" as bounded entities under threat: A study in the replication of a single image. Ph.D. diss., University of London.
Keown, D., ed. 1998. *Buddhism and abortion.* Basingstoke: Macmillan.
Keyes, C. F. 1966. Ethnic identity and loyalty of villagers in Northeast Thailand. *Asian Survey* 6 (9): 362–69.
———. 1967. *Isan: Regionalism in northeastern Thailand.* Ithaca, N.Y.: Southeast Asia Program, Cornell University.
———. 1975. Kin groups in a Thai-Lao community. In *Change and persistence in Thai society,* ed. G. W. Skinner and A. T. Kirsch, 274–97. Ithaca, N.Y.: Cornell University Press.
———. 1984. Mother or mistress but never a monk: Buddhist notions of female gender in rural Thailand. *American Ethnologist* 11 (2): 223–41.
———. 1986. Ambiguous gender: Male initiation in a northern Thai Buddhist society. In *Gender and religion: On the complexity of symbols,* ed. C. Walker Bynum, S. Harrell, and P. Richman, 66–96. Boston: Beacon Press.
———. 1989. *Thailand: Buddhist kingdom as modern nation-state.* Bangkok: Editions Duang Kamol.
Khon Kaen Public Health Office. 1997. *Komuun kan wang phaen khropkhru'a pii 2539 cangwat khon kaen* (Family planning statistics for Khon Kaen Province). Khon Kaen: Khon Kaen Public Health Office.
Kirsch, T. 1985. Text and context: Buddhist sex roles / culture of gender revisited. *American Ethnologist* 12 (1): 302–20.
Knodel, J., A. Chamratrithirong, and N. Debavalya. 1987. *Thailand's reproductive revolution: Rapid fertility decline in a Third World setting.* Madison: University of Wisconsin Press.
Knodel, J., and N. Chayovan. 1989. *Health and population studies based on the 1987 Thailand demographic and health survey.* Bangkok: Institute of Population Studies, Chulalongkorn University.
Knodel, J., N. Havanon, and W. Sittitrai. 1990. Family size and the education of children in the context of rapid fertility decline. Report no. 2, January 1990. Project on socio-economic consequences of fertility decline for the Thai family. Bangkok: Institute of Population Studies, Chulalongkorn University.
Krannich, L., and C. R. Krannich. 1983. *The politics of family planning policy: Thailand—A case of successful implementation.* Lanham, Md.: University Press of America.
Krongkaew, M. 1993. Poverty and income distribution. In *The Thai economy in transition,* ed. P. G. Warr, 401–37. Melbourne: Cambridge University Press.
Ladipo, O. A. 1989. Preventing and managing complications of induced abortion in Third World countries. *International Journal of Gynecology and Obstetrics* (supp.) 3:21–28.
London, B. 1977. Is the primate city parasitic? The regional implications of national decision making in Thailand. *Journal of Developing Areas* 12:49–67.
Manderson, L. 1981. Traditional food classifications and humoral medical theory in Peninsular Malaysia. *Ecology of Food and Nutrition* 11:81–93.
———. 1986. Food classification and restriction in Peninsular Malaysia: Nature, culture, hot and cold? In *Shared wealth and symbol: Food, culture, and society in Oceania and Southeast Asia,* ed. L. Manderson, 127–43. Cambridge: Cambridge University Press.

Maxwell, N. E. 1975. Modernization and mobility into the patrimonial medical elite in Thailand. *American Journal of Sociology* 81 (3): 465–90.

Mougne, C. 1978. An ethnography of reproduction: Changing patterns of fertility in a northern Thai village. In *Nature and man in South East Asia,* ed. P. A. Stott, 68–106. London: School of Oriental and Asian Studies, University of London.

Muecke, M. A. 1984. Make money not babies: Changing status markers of northern Thai women. *Anthropology Today* 26 (4): 459–70.

Mulholland, J. 1989. *Herbal medicine in paediatrics translation of a Thai Book of Genesis.* Canberra: Faculty of Asian Studies, Australian National University.

Narkavonnakit, T. 1979. Abortion in rural Thailand: A survey of practitioners. *Studies in Family Planning* 10 (8–9): 223–29.

Nichter, M., and M. Nichter. 1987. Cultural notions of fertility in South Asia and their impact on Sri Lankan family planning practices. *Human Organization* 46 (1): 18–28.

Phongpaichit, P. 1980. The open economy and its friends: The "development" of Thailand. *Pacific Affairs* 53 (3): 440–60.

Podhisita, C. 1984. Marriage in rural Northeast Thailand: A household perspective. In *Perspectives on the Thai marriage,* ed. A. Chamratrithirong, 71–109. Bangkok: Institute for Population and Social Research, Mahidol University.

Population Council. 1981. *Abortion in Thailand: A review of the literature.* Bangkok: Population Council.

Poulsen, A. 1983. *Pregnancy and childbirth: Its customs and rites in a north-eastern Thai village.* Copenhagen: Danish International Development Agency.

Prasartkul, P., and C. Sethaput. 1982. Women's role and status in family planning. In *Women in development: Implications for population dynamics in Thailand,* ed. S. Prasith-rathsint and S. Piampiti, 234–53. Bangkok: National Institute of Development Administration.

Prizzia, R. 1985. *Thailand in transition: The role of oppositional forces.* Honolulu: University of Hawaii Press.

Reeler, A. V. 1990. Injections: A fatal attraction. *Social Science and Medicine* 31 (10): 1119–25.

Reynolds, C. J. 1991. National identity and its defenders. In *National identity and its defenders: Thailand, 1939–1989,* ed. C. J. Reynolds, 1–41. Melbourne: Centre of Southeast Asian Studies, Monash University.

Riley, J. N., and S. Sermsri. 1974. The variegated Thai medical system as a context for birth control services. Working Paper 6. Bangkok: Institute for Population and Social Research, Mahidol University.

Sheehan, B. 1993. *Thailand—An introduction to Thailand, its people, trade and business activity.* Melbourne: Australia-Thailand Business Council.

Sittitrai, W. 1988. Rural transformation in northern Thailand. Ph.D. diss., University of Hawaii.

Sittitrai, W., et al. 1991. Family size and family well-being: The views of Thai villagers. Report no. 5, January 1991. Project on socio-economic consequences of fertility decline for the Thai family. Bangkok: Institute of Population Studies, Chulalongkorn University.

Sivin, I., et al. 1980. Norplant: Reversible implant contraception. *Studies in Family Planning* 11 (7–8): 227–35.

Soonthorndhada, A., O. Buravisit, and P. Vong-Ek. 1991. *Ascertaining the user perspec-*

tives on community participation in family planning programme in Thailand. Bangkok: Institute for Population and Social Research, Mahidol University.
Stayapan, S., K. Kanchanasinith, and S. Varakamin. 1983. Perceptions and acceptability of Norplant implants in Thailand. *Studies in Family Planning* 14 (6–7): 170–76.
Stephen, E. H., and A. Chamratrithirong. N.d. *Side effects of contraceptive methods in Thailand.* Bangkok: Institute for Population and Social Research, Mahidol University.
Sukdis, T., P. Taendum, and R. Na Pattalung. 1982. Role, status and problem of Thai women in family planning. In *Women in development: Implications for population dynamics in Thailand,* ed. S. Prasith-rathsint and S. Piampiti, 208–33. Bangkok: National Institute of Development Administration.
Tandrup, A. 1982. *Thailand: Internal colonialism and revolutionary war.* Copenhagen: University of Copenhagen.
Thailand, Department of Rural Development. 1989. *Baep sorpthaam khormuun phu'nthaan radap muubaan. Muubaan* 1, 5, 8, 9, 10, 11 (Village survey data Baan Srisaket. Village 1, 5, 8, 9, 10, 11) (in Thai).
——— . 1990. *Baep sorpthaam khormuun phu'nthaan radap muubaan. Muubaan* 1, 5, 8, 9, 10, 11 (Village survey data Baan Srisaket. Village 1, 5, 8, 9, 10, 11) (in Thai).
Thailand, Ministry of Public Health. 1990. *Statistics on women and health in Thailand.* Bangkok: Thai Population Information Centre, Ministry of Public Health (in Thai).
Thailand, National Statistical Office. 1995. *Statistical Yearbook Thailand,* no. 43. Bangkok: National Statistical Office, Office of the Prime Minister.
Thailand, NESDB [National Economic and Social Development Board]. 1992. *The Seventh National Economic and Social Development Plan (1992–1996).* Bangkok: NESDB, Office of the Prime Minister.
Thorbek, S. 1987. *Voices from the city.* London: Zed Books.
Whittaker, A. M. 1995. Isaan women: Ethnicity, gender and health in Northeast Thailand. Ph.D. diss., University of Queensland.
——— . 1996. White blood and falling wombs: Ethnogynaecology in northeast Thailand. In *Maternity and reproductive health in Asian societies,* ed. P. L. Rice and L. Manderson, 207–25. Amsterdam: Harwood Academic Publishers.

CHAPTER 8

Mutual Goals? Family Planning on Simbo, Western Solomon Islands

Christine M. Dureau

I had been on Simbo, in the western Solomon Islands, only a couple of weeks when Ani,[1] a young married woman, offered to take me to her garden to talk about women's business and I delightedly accepted. When we arrived there, we sat and rested before weeding her sweet potato garden. She wasted little time coming to the point. After a few pleasantries—asking me about my own family, how many children my siblings had, whether my parents were alive, how they felt about me coming to the Solomons, why my husband had allowed me to go so far without him, why my family had allowed me to bring my young daughter with me—she made a comment that I was to hear many times: "The life of a woman on Simbo is hard, Christina."

I looked at her garden, thought of the time it had taken us to climb up there, of the two netbags she had brought up to carry back the food for the next few days, and presumed she meant the physical work that all women do. I was partly right, but she went beyond the work to one of its causes. We European women were lucky, she pointed out. We were not poor, we "gardened in the store," our husbands were not "cross all the time," our children were well clothed. I agreed, with some qualifying remarks about economic inequality and domestic violence, which she clearly disbelieved. Then she abruptly asked what contraceptives we had in Australia. In the course of the afternoon, we did a little weeding, dug up a few sweet potatoes and talked at length about reproduction on Simbo.

Ani was in her mid-twenties. She had three small children, one of them an infant and, I learned some months later, had had a fourth child, who died of a bleeding disease at three months. How was it, she demanded, that I had only one child? How did I achieve that? She did not want, she said, to have more and more children. Look at those women with many children—

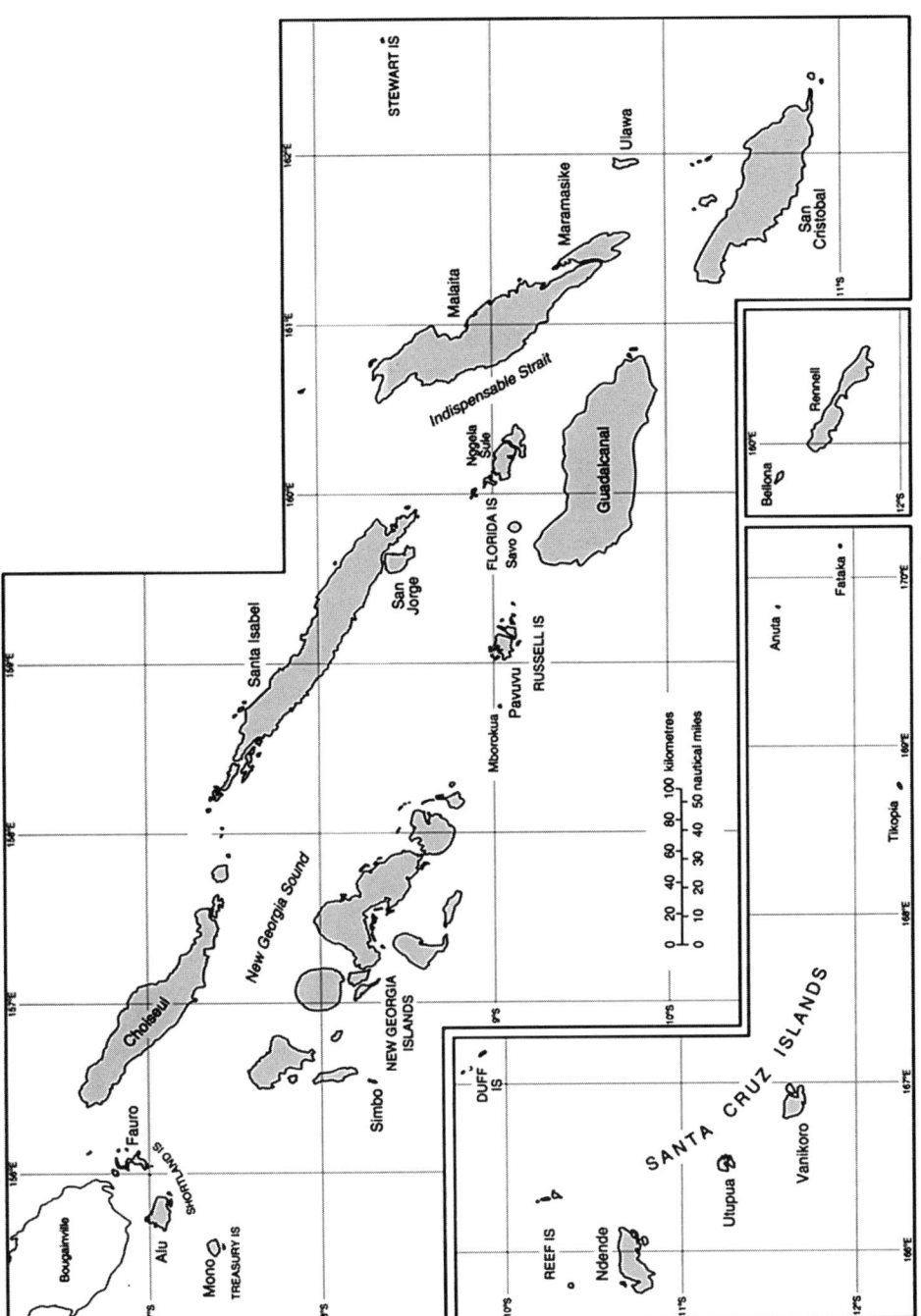

Map 2. The Solomon Islands, showing location of Simbo in the West

no money for clothes or school fees and permanently tired from the work of supporting them. We talked about the contraceptive methods available in Australia. She asked what else there was. I denied any further knowledge. She was too polite to disagree, but once again looked dissatisfied with my answer. Eventually I learned the reason from other women, who asked the same questions and made similar comments about their lives. They, like Ani, hoped that I had some secret European women's knowledge to share with them. Things in Australia were better than things in the Solomons. Why wouldn't we have better contraceptives, too? Throughout my time on Simbo, this was a recurrent theme in talk with women of childbearing age.

On Simbo, at first sight, the fertility goals of a number of actors apparently coincide. Local people are eager to address resource depletion; most married women seek greater control over their bodies; and the state wants to limit the growth of population. Each of these groups hold that women should bear fewer children and that the official state family planning programs should provide the means of achieving this. What might have been a family planning triumph, however, remains a field of contention. This, I will argue, is because each group's apparently mutual goals are in fact discordant, and there are three factors informing these differences.

First, the way in which all groups focus on female fertility obscures their distinctive interests. Thus, while they share local anxieties about declining land and marine resources, women are also motivated by concerns over their personal well-being. Young and middle-aged men publicly state their alarm at local population levels, but they are simultaneously concerned to constrain their wives' reproductive autonomy. And the state, preoccupied with the limited means it has available for providing services for the national population, has limited interest in the well-being of individuals and small local populations. Second, the means for addressing the perceived problem of female fecundity are generally rejected. The government proffers a range of biomedical contraceptive technologies through the local clinic, but neither men nor women find them appropriate. Men tend to regard them as threatening their domestic authority, whereas women find them physically and conceptually unsuitable. Finally, as the articulation of the problem as one of female fecundity suggests, women's bodies are sites of struggle for control—between themselves, their husbands and brothers, and the state.

This is also a clash between different levels of organization—the state, through its family planning service; men, who tend to be collectively concerned about controlling both women and resources, a double concern that sees them articulate contradictory policies of reducing reproduction and denying women access to contraception; and women, who struggle to have the question of their personal well-being considered in all the debates over their bodies. Women's bodies, then, are different entities to each of these groups. To the state, they are both the source of the problem and a means to its resolution: they bear too many children but, if they "accept" contraception, can potentially arrest the growth of population. To men, women embody contradictory potentials: the dangers of unrestrained female sexuality versus the possible birth of children, and the prospect of domestic strife or harmony. They find themselves caught in tensions between domestic sexual politics and local reproductive and ecological concerns. Contraception is linked with female sexual license but also enhances their wives' well-being. It reduces family size and thereby available labor but also reduces pressure on land and resources. For women, however, reproduction and contraception fundamentally impinge on their embodied personhood. Rather than seeing their bodies as sites of technological or conjugal or state control, they are, themselves, *in* their bodies (cf. Martin 1987). As such, contraceptive technologies are an ideal means to their own ends of corporeal and, thus, personal autonomy.

While men are torn by contradictory desires, those of the state and women need not conflict despite their different objectives. The state, after all, wants women to use contraceptives, and women want to do so. Yet the contraceptives offered by the local clinic and the Solomon Islands Planned Parenthood Association (SIPPA) are largely unacceptable to Simbo women. There are problems in fitting such medical treatments to women's bodies: the intersection of biomedical and local conceptions of how bodies work; and the politics of the state's urge to control as against women's quests for autonomy and health.

Overview

Simbo is a small island of less than four square miles, located on the far western side of the New Georgia Group of the western Solomon Islands (see Map 2). About one quarter of the island is rendered infertile by an active sulphuric volcano, although megapode eggs, laid on its lower slopes, provide a source of food and income to those with land rights. The remainder of the island, with soils ranging from rich volcanic loam to heavy clay, has long been fertile. With a growing population, however, fallow periods have been much reduced, and people across the island express concern about falling productivity.

Tinoni Simbo (People of Simbo) are subsistence horticulturalists, mainly raising sweet potato and cassava. Taro, a staple throughout much of the Solomons, seems never to have grown on Simbo (Hocart n.d.a). Fish provides most dietary protein, and pigs are usually reserved for weddings, when they are eaten in small quantities.² Local subsistence production is augmented by purchased rice, noodles, and tinned fish, which are consumed in sufficient quantities to regard them as staples.³ Indeed, with a population of some two thousand, I doubt that subsistence needs could be met without such supplements. Cash is usually obtained through copra and pandanus mat production on the island or via wage migration and remittances from close kin living in urban and development areas. Petty sums are raised through small surpluses of oranges, watermelons, megapode eggs, and, occasionally, sweet potato or other crops, which are sold at the provincial capital, Gizo.

Fertility Practices and Demographic Changes

The last census (1986) recorded 1,328 people on Simbo (S.I. [Solomon Islands] Census Office 1988, table A). By my reckoning, based on my own censuses between 1990 and 1992, approximately 400 to 500 Tinoni Simbo were not enumerated, because they were elsewhere on the night. At the national rates of increase reported by the census (3.5 percent per annum), the resident population would now be approximately 2,077 and the total number of Tinoni Simbo about 2,687. On an island of less than four square miles, this represents a population density of approximately 673 persons per square mile.⁴ Although Simbo is, in many respects, typical of the New Georgia Group, it is unique in this high population density.⁵ This lends an intensity to reproductive politics on Simbo. While women's sentiments echo those of women in other parts of the group, I do not think that resource management features as prominently in the debates about family size and reproductive autonomy on other islands. Elsewhere, then, the ways in which gender relations and reproduction are articulated are somewhat different because men, in particular, are less likely to be enmeshed in the kinds of contradictions that I describe later.

This population picture clearly represents a new situation. In 1908 Hocart conducted ethnographic research in the New Georgia Group and estimated the Simbo population at 400 (Hocart 1931). The resident population has thus increased remarkably within about ninety years and today's high fertility rates reflect that change. The Solomon Islands have one of the highest growth rates in the world, with a total fertility rate (TFR) of 6.4 births per woman (S.I. Census Office 1988). By comparison, my genealogies suggest that Simbo women have a lower TFR of about 5.5.⁶ This situation arises from radical transformations in local epidemiology and reproductive behavior since the end of headhunting and the successful establishment of the Christian churches.

These shifts are partly due to epidemiological changes. When Hocart and Rivers visited Simbo in 1908, the average number of children per woman was about two.[7] Rivers saw this as a manifestation of the "depopulation of Melanesia," which he attributed to the "extent [to which] the zest has gone out of their lives," following the forced abolition of cultural practices, such as head-hunting (1922, 102). Oral accounts, however, suggest the deliberate restriction of births—in a situation of endemic raiding, with women having no more children than could safely be carried into the bush to escape raiding parties. A woman with two children could carry the younger and flee, holding the older by the hand (see also McDowell 1988, 238; Ogan, Nash, and Mitchell 1976, 541). The actual birthrate would have been higher than this. Claims about running away with two children imply that women had only one or two *small* children at any given time. Until recently, people kept shallow genealogies and oral accounts tended to omit the names of those who did not live to adulthood. Death rates were high due to malaria, polio, and environmental hazards. Indeed, in a few cases, I collected data that show women with up to ten live births, of whom only one or two survived to adulthood. Whatever the precise birth and death rates, though, it is clear that women did not generally have more than one or two children who reached maturity during that time.

Contemporary claims that births were restricted by ritualized celibacy, contraceptives, abortifacients, and infanticide must be pondered in the context of the epidemiology of the time, then. Although I cannot give precise figures, many married women's fecundity was almost certainly made problematic by high infant mortality and low fertility. Rivers, for example, claims mortality rates of 31.1 percent and 14.8 percent for male and female children respectively in the first decade of this century (1922, 98). Bennett suggests even higher rates, estimating that some 40 percent of infants died of malaria alone in the Solomons prior to pacification (1987, 9; see also Scragg 1969, 1977).[8] To this must be added the spontaneous abortion levels associated with chronic malaria and yaws, and the possible infertility caused by gonorrhea introduced by passing traders in the nineteenth century (Bennett 1987, 9, 38, 98; Ogan, Nash, and Mitchell 1976, 538–39). Finally, epidemics of polio, influenza, and measles swept the area in the early twentieth century (Bennett 1987; Edge-Partington 1907; Jackson 1978; Rivers 1922, 86), killing young and old and leaving many disabled. Under such circumstances, even if the ideal number of children was, as contemporary women argue, a maximum of two at any one time, achieving this may have been difficult.

The issue of *who* practiced fertility control is debatable. Given the epidemiological conditions outlined here, it is unlikely that many married women were concerned about containing their fertility—some probably were. Yet adoption was frequent (Tinoni Simbo actively sought young children for adoption on their head-hunting raids), which would have further reduced the number of women needing to limit their fertility. Contraception, abortion, and infanticide probably involved negotiations between opposite-sex siblings rather than husbands and wives.

In the period prior to pacification, gender relations were structured by inequalities between opposite-sex classificatory siblings (*luluna*, reciprocal term). Marriage was characterized by the relative autonomy of men and women. Women oversaw most household matters as well as were influential in land distribution, domestic economy, and lineage affairs. Their dwelling houses were said to belong to them, irrespective of whether residence was virilocal or matrilocal. Men were also influential in lineage affairs and land distribution as well as occupied with warfare, ritual, or trade. While husbands were concerned with women's sexuality and adultery was regarded seriously by the couple's lineages, husbands had little explicit authority over their wives. In particular, violence was not considered a legitimate sanction within marriage.

To the extent that men did exert direct personal control over women, it was in their capacity as brothers or *luluna*, but their concern was more with containing the corporeality of married and unmarried sisters rather than with women's productive and parental activities. Female sexuality was always constrained by women's fear of their *luluna*. Revelation of any aspect of a woman's corporeality, but particularly any implicit or explicit disclosure of her sexuality, elicited violent reactions. While there was no norm of marital virginity (Hocart n.d.a, n.d.b), lovers had to be extremely careful, as they are now, to ensure that a significant number of men did not learn of their intrigues. Tinoni Simbo are unanimous in reporting the violence with which men responded to any knowledge of their *luluna*'s corporeality or sexuality (see Dureau 1998 for extended discussion).

This seems to be at odds with reports of both the sexual freedom of unmarried New Georgian women and their exploitation as prostitutes by their fathers (Bennett 1987, 70; Hocart 1931, 6).[9] Writing about nearby Roviana Lagoon, Hocart (n.d.a, n.d.b) is certain that girls used contraceptives and that children of unmarried women were uncommon and disapproved,[10] and a European trader living on Simbo in the early twentieth century also reported the use of effective contraceptives made from local plants (Cambridge University Library).[11] Premarital sexuality, then, was not associated with high rates of pregnancy. Under such conditions of liberal sexuality and rigid corporeal decorum, it is hardly surprising that there was a strong notion that reproduction was "women's business." Further, it seems likely that those who were most in need of fertility control methods were unmarried women facing death at the hands of their *luluna* if they became pregnant.

This is not to presuppose the effectiveness of local contraceptives and abortifacients.[12] It is possible that indigenous medications were not very successful or that girls remained unmarried for only a short period after menarche, and were anovulatory for much of that time. Irrespective of the physical need for or worth of contraceptives, though, this has long been a contracepting society. These practices have shifted radically, however, from a focus on primarily premarital female contraception and abortion to one of exclusively conjugal, female-focused contraception.

Cultural Historical Framework of Fertility Changes

The Australian (later New Zealand) Methodist Mission arrived on Simbo in 1903, shortly after the abrupt elimination of head-hunting by the British Administration (1896–1900) (Bennett 1987, 107). Mission and later government health initiatives, religious, economic and political forces were associated with phenomenal social and demographic changes.[13] The mission placed heavy emphasis on providing health services at a time when the protectorate's resources were reserved for Europeans and plantation laborers (Bennett 1987, 98, 113, 210, 216). Yaws, polio, leprosy, tuberculosis, and maternal and infant health were prime foci of missionary interventions. The first three have now been almost eradicated thanks to missionary, government and Rockefeller Foundation programs, and there have been concerted efforts at controlling tuberculosis and malaria, although the latter remains a serious problem. National infant mortality had plunged to 40 per 1,000 for males and 36 per 1,000 for females in 1986.

Such interventions may have demonstrably improved the general health of the population, but contraceptives were never included in mission or, until recently, government health programs. Missionaries regarded local medical treatments, which were accompanied by prayers to ancestral spirits, as a mixture of devil worship and native malpractice. They campaigned effectively against them, promoting their own cures and prayers in their place. They were particularly opposed to indigenous fertility control, on the additional grounds that it promoted female promiscuity or inappropriate female conjugal autonomy. The acceptance of Western medicine was regarded by both sides as proof of the acceptance of Christianity and rejection of ancestor veneration.

Under missionary influence, birth and infancy were progressively relocated from forest to clinic. Despite its undoubted health benefits, this was at the cost of subjecting women's reproduction to the surveillance of both husbands and medical personnel (see Dureau 1998). Women, then, lost reproductive autonomy at the time that much higher survival rates for infants and children were assured. Whatever the motivations behind medical interventions, then, such reforms have been of equivocal benefit to women who had to cope with an explosion in family size. From about 1930 the rate of reproduction began to climb precipitously.[14] In the generation following the suppression of head-hunting and the arrival of the Methodist Mission (1903), the average number of children per woman grew to about eight, according to oral accounts, a rate that has since declined to present levels.

The epidemiological revolution provided the biomedical environment for the population surge. Reproductive bodies are not biological constants, however, so much as outcomes of culturally generated actions, engagements, and practices (e.g., Ginsburg and Rapp 1991, 329–30; Rosaldo 1980, 393–401). So, how did a society in which contraception was commonplace come to be characterized by high birthrates that seemingly no one regards as desirable?

The most immediate effect of suppressing warfare was the decline of men's "communal houses" (*paile*), which had been maintained by powerful semi-hereditary leaders (*banara*) as part of the patron-client relationships of local politics. Prior to bonito or head-hunting expeditions, men remained celibate in these houses for extended periods, avoiding intimate contact with their wives and other female kin.[15] Pacification, which involved the systematic destruction of the houses and the canoes and enemy skulls kept in them, dislocated the connections between the sea, economy and political leadership. *Banara* abruptly lost much of their power and the capacity to build new *paile*. Male celibacy disappeared even before the last of the houses (see Nag 1980, 576–77, 579). If the end of head-hunting destroyed such intimate ties between polity, marriage, and sexuality, it was local engagements with Methodist missionaries that shaped later social practices. They were determined to replace indigenous marital and residential practices with a form of nuclear family that included transformed attitudes to conjugality and kinship and increased male control over their wives and their bodies.

There has been an almost continuous Methodist presence since 1903, with the entire population converted to Christianity by about 1930.[16] The missionaries, from Fiji, Tonga, and Samoa, lived in Simbo villages and took local children into their homes for education or employment as domestic helpers. They introduced sewing and new forms of weaving, literacy in the vernacular, floored housing, and new kinds of yams, among other innovations. As far as possible within their power, they replaced indigenous forms of medical treatment with their own remedies and strove to prevent women going to the forest to give birth without medical attendants. Old women alive today speak of the missionaries' significance in changing family practices. Thus, they say, they shortened the period of breastfeeding to twelve months because the missionaries told them it enfeebled women. While it is doubtful that changes in social practice initiated by missionaries were unproblematic or as immediate as people today perceive them to have been, the messages of these Pacific missionaries nonetheless had far-reaching effects on bodily and familial practices.[17]

The end of prolonged lactation and celibacy obviously enhanced conjugal fertility, but the new ideologies reinforced these effects, with patterns of authority and responsibility reconstructed. In particular, local interpretations of biblical passages enjoining wifely obedience buttress the novel view that women's bodies belong to their husbands. This is most clearly expressed in terms of women's sexuality and reproductivity and less often in terms of rights to labor and productivity. Today, a model of family relations derived from Saint Paul and other New Testament Gospels is consistently invoked in discourses about conjugality and family relations. The most cited or quoted biblical passage, in church services and out, was Ephesians 5, 22–25, in which wives are urged to be obedient to their husbands.[18] While this passage does not describe actual family relations, it reflects a Christian ideal. The ideal image of marriage is one of a benignly authoritative husband ruling over a domestically oriented, obedient woman and their children. It informs male attitudes to marriage and particularly how men lament women's disobedience and assert their own rights over their wives' bodies.

The last ninety years or so have been characterized by men impinging on what were formerly women's domains. The earlier power of husbands and *luluna* was more diffuse than that of husbands today. Although women had to be cautious that none of their *luluna* knew anything about their corporeality, legitimate or illegitimate, men did not scrutinize their *luluna*'s lives. On the contrary, the relationship demanded female circumspection. While I am not denying the repressive effects of *luluna* power, the requirements of female discretion allowed women some space for autonomy in the past (Dureau 1998).

Men's present claims to domestic authority are associated with marked changes in women's bodily autonomy, with men now claiming particular authority over their wives' bodies. Women, then, are subjected to more minute scrutiny by their husbands, a scrutiny often coercively focused on their reproductive bodies. Women are, for example, often compelled to accept their husbands' sexual advances.[19] Many described men's angry accusations of infidelity or breach of their wifely responsibilities when they refused intercourse.

Conjugality and Family Planning

Apart from the difficulties entailed in refusing intercourse, women are also dependent on their husbands' approval if they wish to contracept. People hold that men's rights over their wives' fertility are legally protected in the Solomon

Islands. Although there is no explicit law about who can be provided with contraceptives, in practice they are not supplied to unmarried women, nor to married women without their husbands' consent (Lloyd and Winn 1985, cited in McMurray and Lucas 1990, 15; Lovi and Osuga 1998, 301–2). SIPPA advertises its policy as one of providing services to "married couples" and the government nurses employed on the island all said that they were supposed to provide only for married couples with the husband's consent.

Many men readily consent to their wives contracepting. Most of these men cite the discomforts and dangers of pregnancy, childbirth, and lactation; the work involved in rearing younger children; and the ever-increasing physical and financial costs of children. Such solicitude stems from the closeness of particular individual relationships, rather than being informed by notions that reproduction is women's business or that women have rights in their bodies. Many more men resolutely oppose, or refuse to cooperate with, contraception. Their insistence on their rights, coupled with their concerns about fidelity and their consequent opposition to birth control, informs a common suspicion that women might surreptitiously contracept. Indeed, many women do secretly acquire contraceptives through the clinic if they cannot obtain their husbands' agreement. In my experience, the clinic nurses working on Simbo did not inquire too closely about consent, merely asking the woman whether her husband had agreed.

In 1990 the provincial government sponsored a workshop on Simbo, with the objective of discussing future agriculture, health, and welfare services. The family planning session was heavily attended, and most of the senior men appeared. Yet, despite the convener's requests that as many people as possible participate in the workshops and despite this particular session being of interest to them, very few women attended. The only woman who spoke was a young married teacher without any kin on Simbo, who supported the clinic providing instruction in the rhythm method. There were a number of reasons for women staying away. First, it is more common for men to stand up in public forums. Second, many women were busy about child care and domestic duties, as usual. This was the reason most gave for not attending. But, despite such constraints, many women do manage to attend events that they hold to be important, even if they do not speak, and large numbers of women went to the other workshop sessions. Women did regard this session as important: for several days second-hand accounts of its content were recounted and several women asked me for details about the information provided by the facilitator. Although most cited domesticity as the reason for their nonattendance, this does not explain their lower involvement in the family planning session than in other sessions. I think the third and fourth reasons cited were more germane.

As one woman said, "I'd be ashamed to be there with my *luluna*" and another added, "My husband would ask why I wanted/needed to be there, and what would I tell him?" For a woman's husband and *luluna* there would be an obvious reason for her participation in a family planning discussion: a personal intention to use contraception. A male *luluna* could be reminded of her corporeality; a husband who opposed family planning would suspect clandestine contraception. On either count, a woman could be subjected to a beating or haranguing—far better, then, to stay away.

There was a general consensus in the workshop that population pressure was a major problem on Simbo, and there was prolonged discussion about possible solutions. Most agreed that, as well as encouraging island exogamy and off-island residence of all young couples with land rights elsewhere, people must be encouraged to limit family size. But there was arguably little (male) commitment to the now stated ideal of restricting family sizes. Exogamous marriage and off-island residence would permit a continuation of current birthrates. Further, there was a constant counter-theme in the discussions—that solutions to overcrowding should not override male domestic rights in women. In particular, women must not be enabled to seek birth control without their husbands' consent. Samu, a man in his late forties with eight children, the youngest of whom was still suckling at the time, summarized the general feeling. Earlier in the day he had proposed forcing all couples with several children off the island to take up land rights elsewhere and now spoke on family planning:

> Mr. Chairman, I'd like to support limiting family size, because land here on Simbo is so small. But the women must not be allowed to go sneaking down to the clinic without asking their husbands first.

His statement was met with a low murmur of approval.[20]

These attitudes do not have a straightforward relationship to mission or government initiatives. Both have been effective vehicles of local level change, and the churches have been very influential in developing national family planning policy, persisting in the earlier missionary insistence that contraception encourages promiscuity (Lovi and Osuga 1998; McMurray and Lucas 1990, 13–15; O'Collins 1978, 1979). But Tinoni Simbo have not been passive recipients of external agents. Responses to family planning methods are informed by the local politics of reproduction and conceptualizations of the body (Ginsburg and Rapp 1991, esp. 312–13; MacCormack 1988). Thus, premarital and marital fertility rates are both informed by the ways in which the politics and norms of local gender relations are played out in the contexts constructed by the "intersecting interests of states and other powerful institutions such as multinational and national corporations, international development agencies, Western medicine and religious groups" (Ginsburg and Rapp 1991, 312).

McDowell (1988, 243–45) notes that in much of Papua New Guinea men associated contraception with female promiscuity long before conversion or substantial contact with Europe. Although we are talking about very different societies, it is possible that similar correlations were made in the western Solomons. Certainly, it would be simplistic to interpret contemporary male attitudes toward abortion and contraception solely in terms of Christian ideology. Still, Christian rhetoric about promiscuity and male rights in female bodies may have fitted men's preexisting concerns about their wives. With the decline of siblingship and the consolidation of marriage as the major site of gender relations (Dureau 1998), men's interests as husbands have meshed neatly with such norms.

Young Women and Fertility

It is virtually impossible to obtain contraceptives if one is unmarried.[21] SIPPA, as I noted, offers services exclusively to married couples and the belief that this is a legal restriction also determines services offered by the local clinic. There is little possibility of discreet contraception for unmarried women. The nurses are often related to their patients and it is difficult to keep attendance secret. The clinic is a public space, usually crowded with patients, visitors, men congregating around the room in which the radio telephone is housed, and general passersby. While married women with small children are expected to attend the clinic regularly as part of the local maternal and child health services, girls have little reason to go there, unless they are ill.

Although conjugality is now central to gender relations and male *luluna* powers have declined, *luluna* relations remain focal points of premarital sexuality. Most unmarried people conduct their affairs clandestinely, as always, relying on trusted same-sex siblings or close friends in a similar situation, and sometimes confiding in their same-sex parent. The difference today is that the possibility of preventing or terminating pregnancy has been removed. This shift from premarital to conjugal contraception is reflected in the fact that most families now support at least one unmarried daughter and her young child or children.[22] If women with premarital offspring eventually marry other men, their husbands regard these children as irrelevant to contraceptive decision making. Indeed, such children often contribute to men's anxiety about their wives' fidelity, making them less amenable to contraception.

Girls who marry as a result of pregnancy usually do so before giving birth.

When premarital pregnancy precipitates earlier marriage, women embark upon regular childbirth at an earlier age and can potentially bear more children. This consequence of premarital pregnancy should not be overstated, because many other people marry young, anyway. Since the establishment of colonial and church rule, *tabe,* the system whereby parents negotiated their children's marriages, has disappeared. There may always have been a relatively large number of marriages established by virilocal elopement (*pogoso uku,* lit. "carry [and] flee"), but its frequency has increased with the demise of *tabe* and the relative attenuation of male *luluna* powers. Many people claim that people now marry at a younger age, with most elopements occurring when girls are between about sixteen and twenty-one. Certainly, elopement contributes to earlier marriages than would occur if *tabe* was the norm *today:* it is usually the issue of age that precipitates elopements, as parents urge their unheeding offspring to "wait a little, first" until they are older. Most elopements occur when girls are between about sixteen and twenty-one and parental or *luluna* interventions almost never succeed.

Marriage, Reproduction, and Contraception

Everybody is expected to reproduce and those unable to do so are figures of pity.[23] Although adult status is conferred by marriage, marriage is not regarded as properly established until the couple has children and pregnancy is expected within the first year. People who do not have children within two to three years are suspected of infertility. This puts pressure on both parties and early marriage is often associated with inordinate levels of male violence against wives. A number of women told me that persistent severe physical abuse ceased completely when they finally became pregnant. The use of contraception in this interval is therefore unthinkable to men and women. So, young women are eager to start on the cycle of motherhood as soon as possible. Those using or seeking family planning help, then, are definitively women who have married and borne at least one child but usually three or four children. My comments on the efficacy of family planning practices are restricted to them.

Births are usually closely spaced, about two years or less apart. The decline from 8 or more births in the 1930s and 1950s to current numbers of about 5.5 is remarkable. The drop, however, does not approach the reduction in birthrates desired by Simbo women or the government. Contemporary women find maternity burdensome, a complaint stemming from their work burdens and the debilitation wrought by numerous births. They are keen to curb their fecundity, being eager to participate in a range of roles and activities that they see as incompatible with intensive child care requirements (Dureau 1993). They

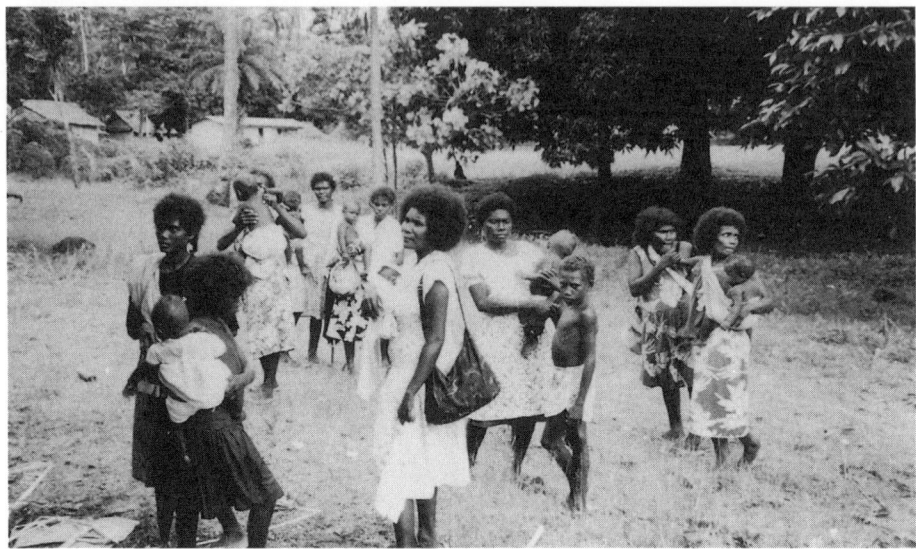

Fig. 9. Women and children waiting for MCH services at the local clinic

do not compare their reproductive patterns with those of women who mothered eight or ten children, so much as express envy of those earlier forebears who reputedly had only two children.

Young and middle-aged women are the first since pacification to visualize controlling their family size. In conducting reproductive surveys, I asked all women how many children they wanted, or had wanted, in their marriages. When I asked this question of those older women with large numbers of children, they often laughed loudly and pointed out that, as something beyond their control, they had had no ideal numbers: "God gave me my children, Christina. It was his liking how many I had."

People are now renegotiating attitudes, practices, and rights in regard to birth control, female bodies, and domestic powers and responsibilities. This situation entails many uncertainties: desired family size,[24] ideal spacing between births, the safety of contraceptive techniques, what factors to take into account, and how to go about implementing their decisions remain contentious issues. The Christian, Pauline ideology of conjugal hierarchy and the politics of domesticity exacerbate the contestation.

The discretion required of women who seek contraception against their husbands' wishes might be seen as conducive to the revival of local contraceptives and abortifacients. Most, however, have been forgotten. Some women do

Mutual Goals? 247

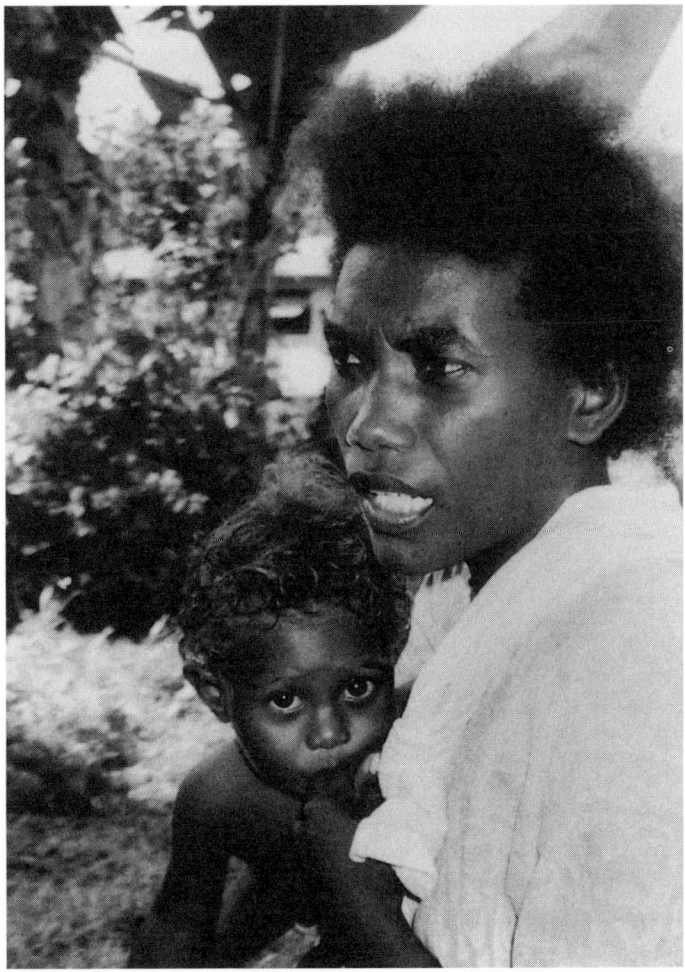

Fig. 10. Vai, suckling her third child while arranging upcoming UCWF activities with neighboring women

resort to the few remembered mixtures, but they are generally regarded as ineffective. Some people maintain that "custom medicine" (*meresana kastom*) never was effective, in contrast to the assumed "real" or "true" strength of Western medicine. Others hold that the real cures have been lost and what is given out now is inauthentic. Finally, some argue that such treatments, which were dependent on invocations to the spirits, are now impotent because of the strength of Christianity.

Although many women and girls claim that there are abortifacient barks and leaves in the bush, virtually all of them said they did not know them or how to process them. Only one person said that she had aborted a pregnancy by drinking the juice of a particular leaf. Perhaps more indicative of the paucity of knowledge, two women had unsuccessfully resorted to drinking excessive quantities of lime juice in attempts to terminate their seventh and eight pregnancies.[25] On three occasions I was discreetly approached by older women who hoped that I could concoct abortifacients for their pregnant daughters;[26] they said that their grandmothers knew how, but they themselves had never learned. But these were all situations of desperation: a young girl fearful of her *luluna*'s response; two women despondent at the prospect of additional dependents; mothers lamenting their children's precocious maternity or shameful incestuous pregnancies. Quite apart from the lack of technical skill, for most people abortion is not an acceptable option. As elsewhere in the Pacific, it is illegal in the Solomons (Pulea 1986, 109–10), and the Christian churches, like early missions, oppose it. It is also regarded as unacceptable on Simbo, most rhetorically and publicly by men, but many women privately say that they could not abort, irrespective of their desire to avoid further births.

Women eager to contracept and willing to evade their husbands' surveillance turn, perforce, to the local clinic or nearby Gizo provincial hospital for the government family planning service. Their family planning goals and intentions thus apparently accord with the national government's strategies to curb population growth. It is ironic, then, that both women and local nursing personnel report continual frustration and lack of success of family planning initiatives. The clinic provides a range of contraceptive techniques imported from Western nations, the most commonly available of which are tubal ligation, Depo Provera injections, oral contraceptives, intrauterine contraceptive devices (IUDs), and condoms. At the local level, where we might expect the synchronization of official service and family planning demand, women regarded all of them as inappropriate.

The clinic and the regional hospital both favor the use of Depo Provera injections. Treatments are effective for several months, and injection time is the only clinic visit required. Yet, while a few women testify to its effectiveness and stress that they have had no problems, most cite a range of side effects. The "needle 'spoils' women's bodies," they say. They cite hot and cold flushes or prolonged chills as well as weakness, severe headaches, abdominal distension and pain, fluid retention, and, in a number of cases, pregnancy (cf. Whittaker, this volume). While some are glad of the amenorrhea that can accompany treatment, others feel that the retention of uterine blood is part of the problem.

Women did not report, or psychosomatically experience, symptoms they may have been warned about in patient literature or instruction provided by health authorities. No attempt was made to inform people of the possible side effects of medications in any of the cases I knew about while living and working on Simbo or Gizo. As far as I could ascertain, Simbo women had not heard of any of the feminist or medical debates about the safety of the drug in Western countries. They were describing their own experiences or those of others they knew. Of the many women on Simbo who had used Depo Provera, most had only one or two treatments before passing on to other measures or abandoning family planning. Many others declined to try the drug because of their observations of its effects on others. Further, a few who suffered no side effects discontinued use because of apprehensions provoked by other women's experiences.

Oral contraceptives are used rarely and, when they are, without great success. There seem to be three reasons for this. First, patient compliance with all Western medication regimes is poor. Many people see medicine as having something of a cumulative effect and do not acknowledge that treatments need to be precisely administered by dosage and timing. Their views here are confirmed by the ways in which medicine often works when taken counter to the clinic staff's instructions—taking only part of a course of antibiotics, for example. The result is a general imprecision about dosages and timing. The second reason for poor compliance stems from the health service's reaction to perceptions of poor compliance (see also Kabeer 1994, 209). The oral contraceptives available tend to be high-dosage hormones, in order to offset the variations in timing in taking medication. The outcome of this, of course, is that side effects are intensified and those women who do take oral contraceptives complain of the same kind of symptoms as those on Depo Provera, with the exception of abdominal pain. Finally, pills are viable only for those women whose husbands consent to the use of contraception. Otherwise, they must be secreted somewhere around the house, leaving the possibility of discovery and its consequences.

IUDs, which require a trip to Gizo Hospital, are also available. Women are reluctant to use them, however; most said they feared for their safety, citing others who have suffered acute or chronic abdominal pain, medical crises necessitating surgical intervention (perforated uterus?), and abdominal infections. The case of one woman who developed uterine cancer while an IUD was in situ was also interpreted as demonstrating their danger. Once again, women were unaware of the Dalkon Shield scandal or any other contention about IUD safety in European societies. In fact, they argued that these side effects are rare elsewhere, but commonplace in the Solomons, and explicitly attributed the differences to what they described as the relative inadequacy of medical personnel in the Solomons and the superiority of European life. Irrespective of the validity of these observations, women act on their belief that they are true. Those who did use IUDs were largely women who had spent some time living in Honiara and had them inserted there.[27]

There is more to this fear of using IUDs than the anecdotal evidence of others. Local conceptualizations of the body inevitably inflect sexuality and reproductivity (MacCormack 1988; Martin 1987; Taylor 1990). I presume that local notions of heat, coldness and menstruation inform reactions to the effects of Depo Provera. Likewise, Simbo women's notion of the danger associated with IUDs conforms to a generalized uneasiness about having anything at all inserted into their bodies. When this is articulated, it is phrased in terms of things getting lost, continuing to rise, and thus not being able to be removed at all or causing damage to other organs. People are formally aware of the uterus as an enclosed space, when questioned directly in such terms. They know of the Western conception model. But there is a countervailing, generally unexplicated, model of the uterus (*lovu koburu*, lit. "baby's mat," the term used for both uterus and placenta) as a temporary construction that is postnatally eliminated from the vagina, an orifice opening into the rest of the abdominal cavity (see also MacCormack 1988, for similar anatomical models in Sierra Leone and Jamaica). The general avoidance of tampons, diaphragms, and IUDs is therefore underlined by a lingering mistrust of their remaining in place and fulfilling only their intended functions.

People also express grave misgivings about tubal ligation. In this case, reluctance is couched in terms of enfeeblement. Verbalization is forceful and direct. Typically:

> No, I'm afraid of that. Everyone who has the "knife" gets sick or weak. Do you know so-and-so? She had it, and look at her now. She's never been well since. She can't go up to the garden any more or carry firewood since she had the operation.

Women also cite cases of postoperative infection, including one woman reputed to have died some years ago. Virtually the only people who have tubal ligations on Simbo are those who had them while living in Honiara or women who acquiesced to surgery after all other measures failed. Of those who had always lived on the island, the lowest number of children born prior to ligation was six.

A number of younger women, although by no means all, have more favorable attitudes to ligation than previous generations. These women, aged below thirty, already have three or four children and want to stop. They do not express fear about the operation or doubts about its desirability but are constrained by a range of other factors: they talk about other women who have been refused the operation by doctors on the grounds of age, about their mothers being antagonistic, about the clinic nurses' opposition, and unease about their husbands, even in cases in which the latter are supportive of the surgery. These women are acutely aware of the disadvantaged position of widows and divorcees who have undergone sterilization. A well-known, possibly apocryphal, tale tells of a mother of six who persuaded medical personnel to perform a ligation without first obtaining her husband's consent. Upon discovering this, he deserted her. The woman was left to care for her children without male help, and with little hope of marrying again and acquiring a male contribution to her subsistence. No man, women point out, would marry a woman who could not have a child.

Men say, "They would be wasting my fluid night after night." Tubal ligation seems to arouse particular male animosity. Men oppose ligation on the grounds of its potential medical consequences and often because they themselves want more children. Beyond these concerns, too, lurks the pervasive fear that their wives, relieved of the risks of pregnancy, will become promiscuous. Many women also believe this. Two of the three women most renowned for the frequency of their adulteries were pointed out as having had ligations. Indeed, one of the two once told me that she opposed the procedure because it induced an "adultery disease" in women. One of these women was widely said to have had the operation in order to facilitate her promiscuity, but the other was reputed to have become a serial adulterer only after the operation. What is interesting here is the suggestion that tubal ligation might *cause* promiscuity.

Given the difficulties associated with female-focused contraception, it might be argued that local contraception should center on more male-focused methods, such as timed abstinence, withdrawal, condom use, or vasectomy. I have noted several reasons for male opposition to female contraception, including the fear of promiscuity, determination to assert domestic authority, and anxiety about medical consequences. If men see local population levels as contributing to resource depletion, their anxieties about their domestic authority and their wives' faithfulness make it difficult to countenance the prospect of contraception within their own marriages. These concerns could presumably be ameliorated if men were to become significant contraceptors. But this possibility is negated by a central disjunction in their perceptions of the problem. Notwithstanding their claims to authority over women's bodies, fertility is generally regarded as a female problem, an assumption that also informs most family planning programs and population policies (Kabeer 1994,

188; see also Jolly, this volume, chap. 9). Even sympathetic men see it as entailing greater burdens for their *wives*. Only in urban areas, where there is much greater dependence on male labor in the wage economy, are Simbo men likely to be supportive of family planning, and here they privilege female-focused contraception. This is hardly unique. Kabeer's brief historical and cross-cultural analysis of family planning programs suggests that "the presence of family-planning programmes has actually discouraged male responsibility in planned parenthood" (1994, 211–12). No Simbo man has ever had a vasectomy, which is usually likened to porcine castration, although family planning staff seem to be enthusiastic about its possibilities. Both women and men acknowledge that men refuse to wear condoms because they "prevent" or "block" men's sexual pleasure (see also Lovi and Osuga 1998, 302).

Even when couples agree to adopt the rhythm method, many men react negatively to women's particular refusals. There is an implication here that they are not committed to their wives' attempts at reducing fertility, that their overt hostility to birth control is replaced by more covert opposition. This may be true of some men, but it is also important to note that sexuality is the major field within which tensions and anxieties about marital fidelity, power, and obedience are played out. The island has long been famed for sexual magic and the purported licentiousness of its people, being known throughout the western Solomons by the "slogan" *tekua kame loia kame* (take one, discard one). Whether or not Simbo people are particularly lascivious, men often accept this characterization in regard to their wives. The results include the anxiety that a wife who regularly declines intercourse may be having an adulterous affair. This leaves withdrawal, which some couples resolve to practice. This tends to be unsuccessful. Women often complain that their husbands "cheat" or sneak on them and ejaculate in their vaginas. They regard this as deliberate rather than accidental. Where the withdrawal fails, men suspect their wives of adultery.

Despite the difficulties involved, women canvas the range of options provided by the local clinic. Either because those options fail or because they heed other women's adverse experiences, they usually relinquish those methods they do try. Many drift into a half-understood use of the rhythm method, sometimes supplemented by male withdrawal. In general, women are eager to adopt "natural" methods of family planning. They argue, first, that they entail no side effects and, second, that they lend themselves to the subterfuge necessitated by men's opposition to contraception. Women say that if they know their fertile periods, they can manipulate the timing of intercourse with their husbands. As Nola explained when she asked me for a pocket calendar:

I will secrete this under my pillow and count my days. Then, if it's a bad day, maybe I can have a fight with my husband and go to my mother's house or my sister's house for a few days. Or I can take one of our small children to bed with me or stay up late talking to kin. Like that, you know. You know, but my husband doesn't. Understand?

Clinic staff, however, are reluctant to teach the rhythm method. The guest speaker at the family planning session mentioned earlier concentrated his efforts on reassuring people about the safety of Depo Provera, tubal ligation, and vasectomy and spoke disparagingly of the method. To my knowledge, none of the staff on Simbo had, themselves, been instructed in it. So, even when women do follow it, the inherent risks are multiplied by faulty calculation and misunderstanding.

Prolonged breastfeeding, the only natural method advocated by the health services, is rejected by Simbo women on the grounds of its recognized unreliability. This issue epitomizes the distance between local people, seeking to maximize their own well-being and that of their families, and the government and SIPPA (representing the International Planned Parenthood Association), which seek to implement population control policies and economic growth incentives through family planning programs (see Griffen 1994, 65–66; Underhill-Sem 1994, 10–11, 13). Although prolonged frequent lactation can reduce female fertility, its effects are highly variable within a population; it is far less reliable under conditions of ample calorie intake, and its effectiveness diminishes markedly after about six months (Bracher 1992; Elia 1985, 153, 186–89; Harrell 1981). Thus, while lactation may be compatible with the goals of curtailing overall population growth, it is unsatisfactory for the individual woman who wants an assurance that *she personally* need not conceive unless and until she chooses to do so. While its failure in a certain number of anonymous cases might be acceptable from the larger perspective, it is not so for the individual facing those consequences (for debates about this point, see Bracher 1992, 1993; Kennedy et al. 1993; Laukaran and Labbok 1993; Millman 1993). Similar incommensurabilities or incompatibilities between population policies and individual welfare attend all the birth control methods offered by the government. Individuals are seeking improvements in their *own* lives, so the specifics of methods, and side effects, are highly relevant. On the contrary, the outlook of planners and developers is directed at the general view, and women's bodies are a means to those ends.

Perhaps I can best capture the constraints and anxieties afflicting contemporary women by a brief account of Mata, a widow in her early thirties with six children:

During her marriage she was twice pregnant on Depo Provera injections and twice in the early months of breastfeeding. Her husband had died about a year before I spoke with her, and, his grave having been cemented, she was eligible to remarry. She is ambivalent about remarriage because, "I've already got six children, and I don't want any more. No man will marry me just for Eroni's [her dead husband] children.[28] And he'd be jealous if I didn't have his baby." As she says, she would be willing to have even one, but the likelihood of successfully restricting it to that number is low given her potential husband's likely reaction to tubal ligation and her previous lack of luck using contraceptive methods. On the other hand [jokingly], "My house is falling down. Where do I sleep? In the cookhouse? And I get cold at night. I've always liked men, you know."

Conclusions

At this point, Simbo women want fewer children because of the workloads and constraints associated with maternity.[29] The number of children they have raised in recent decades has imposed a heavy physical burden on them. While many aspects of their lives have improved as a result of pacification, exposure to missionaries and adoption of Western medicine, the costs have been high and continue to increase. Their labor has increased exponentially, due to the increase in both birth and infant survival rates, the onset of land degradation, and the ever-expanding need for cash.

The failure of family planning policies cannot be attributed to "cultural conservatism." Simbo has a history of enthusiastically adopting novel goods and practices for about two hundred years. In accordance with this "tradition," women are enthusiastic about limiting the size of their families and state their expectations that the government health services assist them in this. So eager are they to do so that many take the risks entailed in evading their husbands' surveillance in order to secure contraceptive services. But the ready availability of a range of unsatisfactory measures offers tantalizing possibilities without providing the means of fulfillment. The more naturalistic means of birth control that women seek are not advocated by the health services on the grounds of their unreliability, thus rendering them more unreliable when they are attempted.

This chapter has not addressed debates concerning the need for population control policies and family planning policies. On Simbo, with its limited land resources, declining productivity, and growing population, it is easy to argue in favor of population reduction, and that issue is debated on the island. The debate is conducted within the context of Islanders' conflicting interests as husbands and wives, with women contesting the prerogatives and powers assumed by men by countering male versions of Christian conjugality with alternative Christian models and challenging men's claims that husbands are authoritative by virtue of long-standing *kastom* (Dureau 1994, chap. 9). Simbo is, as Scheffler (1962, 155 n. 8) noted, in a different context, renowned for its "troublesome women." But these women are not only resisting their husbands: because family planning programs are not necessarily concerned with women's needs and aspirations, Simbo women are also resisting many of the assumptions and implications underlying the services provided.

Dixon-Mueller and Germain argue that the "challenge for the remainder of the 1990s is not only to meet the rising demand for contraception in general, but also to serve better the needs of all women and men who are struggling to regulate their fertility safely, effectively, and with human dignity" (1992, 334). A vital first step is the realization that the former goal cannot be attained without first attending to the second. Certainly, Simbo women, and, I think, western Solomons women in general, will only please the planners when the planners please them.

NOTES

This chapter is based on fieldwork on Simbo between April 1990 and May 1991, and December 1991 and April 1992. As always, my first thanks are to those women and men of Simbo who trusted me with their confidences. This chapter represents a paltry first step toward fulfilling the demands of those who told me to stop asking about "the ways of one day" and write about the "hard lives of Simbo women today." Critical comments by Margaret Jolly, Judith Littleton, Regina Scheyvens, and Yvonne Underhill-Sem have been particularly useful. Thanks for the encouraging remarks of a number of participants at the State, Sexuality, and Reproduction in Asia and the Pacific Conference at the Australian National University, especially Lynette Parker and Mimi Sharma.

1. All personal names are pseudonyms.
2. Men also argue that fishing harvests have declined during this century. This is variously attributed to the loss of pre-Christian incantations and charms and to the Japanese trawlers that are active in Western Province.
3. The vast majority of households eat rice, with or without fish, and noodles at least once or twice weekly. Some households are conspicuous for their daily consumption of "store food." Equally conspicuous are those few impoverished households where store food is never eaten.
4. This excludes those who were born on, or have primary affiliation to, other islands. The New Georgia Group's cognatic descent gives individuals rights on numerous islands, depending upon their genealogical connections.
5. Indeed, for the Solomons as a whole, only the large eastern island of Malaita and the "Polynesian outlier" islands of Tikopia, Rennell, and Bellona suffer from land shortages due to population density. In some places alienation of land for the timber industry also leaves local areas with land shortages.

6. Although Simbo may have a lower or higher rate of population growth than the national average, my crude reproductive data suggest that Simbo women have lower TFRs than the national average. This must be set against the relatively greater provision of medical services in the western Solomons than in the eastern and remote districts. Infant and adult mortality rates may thus be lower. Simbo itself has a clinic and one to three resident nurses. In good weather it is only two to three hours from Gizo Hospital and air services to the main hospital in Honiara. This has undoubted effects on maternal and infant health status, the morbidity of acute malaria, trauma injuries, etc. A comparison: in 1992 a Simbo woman suffered a prolonged labor and, less than twenty-four hours after the onset of labor, was transferred by canoe to Gizo Hospital for a successful cesarean section. The same year a parturient woman from the remote northwestern Shortland Islands was transferred by canoe to Gizo Hospital. By the time a cesarean section was performed she had been in labor for five days, and her baby was stillborn.

7. This number is an estimate based on my own and Rivers's figures. He speaks of the birthrate per marriage, which was particularly low. He seems not to have taken account, however, of the instability that characterized Simbo marriages. While he listed a number of marriages, many people married several times, with two to three marriages over a lifetime common (Rivers 1922, xx).

8. Neither Rivers nor Bennett are explicit about their precise age groups.

9. Bennett's and Hocart's claims about prostitution may be based on misunderstandings of the gifts presented by girls' lovers to their parents.

10. It is difficult to know to what extent accounts of pre-Christian Roviana can be taken to apply to Simbo. The two areas are separated by some distance but have long been closely connected. They were part of a regional economic and military system during much of the nineteenth century and have always had close kinship relations.

11. It is less clear from Green's note whether it was unmarried girls who used the contraceptives. Green refers to "girls" contracepting, which implies so. He sometimes uses *girls*, however, to refer to local women in general.

12. Wood (1990) has chided anthropologists for their generally uncritical acceptance of the efficacy of indigenous contraceptives. In the Simbo case, to the epidemiological factors affecting fertility must be added possible changes to the age of menarche and ovulation. This is difficult to assess. In casual conversation people often suggest that girls now develop breasts and begin menstruating earlier. Recorded age is of little moment on Simbo, so such comments must be treated with caution. They do, however, correspond to the trend toward earlier menarche and ovulation, which is associated with improved nutritional status (Buckley and Gottlieb 1988, 44–46; MacCormack 1982a, 6–8; MacCormack 1982b, 123–24). In the Solomons the colonial and postcolonial control of endemic diseases such as malaria, yaws, and hookworm, which affect nutrition and hematology, may have resulted in an earlier age of menarche and higher rates of ovulation.

13. This chapter is concerned only with that approximate period for which I have oral history and genealogical data, that is, since about the late nineteenth century. I do not doubt that populations may have fluctuated during the nineteenth-century escalation of headhunting in the central and western Solomons.

14. The census of 1930 (BSIP 1930) gives a total Simbo population of 376, but its accuracy is questionable. The results of the census for the protectorate as a whole gave a population of 93,000 instead of the anticipated 150,000. While this was seen as evidence

to support various theories that Solomon Islanders were doomed to extinction (Bennett 1987, 434 n. 86), the conduct of the census itself was also a factor. Letters included with the census report indicate that the high commissioner was dissatisfied with the ways in which data were collected, and he repeatedly demanded more adequate analysis of the material and challenged the competence of the collectors. Although the various district officers were responsible for the collection of data in their own areas, the work was often entrusted to illiterate local people who were supposed to have been taught to use tally sticks. It is unclear how much training or supervision they received or how competent the various district officers were.

15. There are still vague notions that sexuality is depleting for a man. These days it tends to be expressed in terms of a waste of fluid (should no offspring result over a period of time) or of short-term weakness.

16. The United Church of Papua New Guinea and the Solomon Islands, the Methodist Mission's successor, remains the main church on the island, claiming perhaps 85 percent of the population. The Seventh Day Adventist Mission was also established there in 1932 and the Christian Fellowship Church emerged from the Methodist schism in 1961. Both of these were instigated by Simbo men in the face of strong opposition. They remain small, most members being lineally related to their founders. There is also a very small enclave of South Seas Evangelical Church followers, most of them the families of Malaitan men who have married into Simbo and converted to the church after arrival.

17. I continue to struggle with the question of *why* missionaries had such immediate and unquestioned authority. Simbo people had long experience of manipulating outsiders in order to derive maximum benefit without compromising their cultural autonomy. See Dureau 1994 for discussion of these issues.

18. "Wives, submit yourselves to your own husbands as to the Lord. / For a husband has authority over his wife, just as Christ has authority over the church: and Christ is himself the Saviour of the Church, his body. / And so wives must submit completely to their husbands just as the church submits itself to Christ. / Husbands, love your wives, just as Christ loved the church and gave his life for it." This passage, sometimes including verses 26–33, was almost invariably read out at church weddings; it was also selected by the minister on the occasion of the women's inter-island church rally and at the Mother's Day feast held at Lengana, the island's main village; and it was frequently chosen by the various male preachers who conduct services around the island. I have not heard any female preachers cite this passage. Nothing that I was told or observed led me to think, however, that women consciously resisted its injunctions or the usual local interpretations of it.

19. The range of conjugal sexuality is, of course, enormous, yet women regard such behavior as the male norm. This is well reflected in the exceptions: a number of women told me that their husbands were good men, in contrast to other men, because they did not enforce sexual demands on them.

20. Although his own inconsistencies were not lost on the other men. A number of them later commented quietly to me that he himself had married into Simbo and made wry remarks about his larger-than-average family.

21. Cf. Pulea (1986, 94), who argues that, although discouraged, unmarried women are "not prevented from availing themselves of family planning services."

22. Such children are not regarded as illegitimate or a shame on the family. While

one hears occasional disapproving remarks that a particular child has no father, this refers to the lack of input provided by a genitor who has not married in, thus leaving full responsibility on the family. Women, too, remark on the stupidity of young girls who rush headlong into the labors of motherhood. The negative consequences of premarital pregnancy are slighter than they were. Although women continue to be fearful of their *luluna*, the fear of death has changed to one of physical assault. When an unmarried girl admits to pregnancy or sexual misdemeanor, her parents and senior kin rush to ensure that her *luluna* accept a symbolic compensation (*ira*) before they hear about the woman's condition. The *ira* rarely amounts to more than two dollars, a sum that is expected to cover a large number of men. Even on cash-poor Simbo this is an insignificant quantity. The amount is hardly relevant; what is important is its offer and acceptance. More distant *luluna*, exceeding second cousins, may not receive anything, being expected to be placated by that of close *luluna*. Similarly, younger brothers in a sibling set may not receive anything. Having once accepted the money, even if not aware of the reason beforehand, a man or boy is prohibited from taking any further measures against the woman. At times, for various reasons, a man refuses to accept *ira,* but this is uncommon, and in such cases the woman usually manages to keep her distance from the man in question, or he, although refusing the *ira* as a mark of his continuing displeasure, avoids her areas.

23. These fall into one of three categories: the infertile (*egoro*); men whom no woman is willing to marry (*ziru*); and those classified as "disabled" (*qao*). The latter are virtually always precluded from marriage, although not from sexual involvement—all disabled women have one or more children, as do a number of the men. Mobile "disabled" men are regarded as possessing the magic that bestows special sexual prowess, and some are renowned for the number of their lovers. A small number of disabled people do, in fact, marry—usually men, rather later in life than usual, to women who have previously been married and already have a number of children.

24. Many women and men now say they want four children: two girls and two boys (with a firstborn girl, women add). While women seem to mean this and usually begin agitating to end childbearing after having four children, men do not follow up such statements with committed action, and in many cases it appears they are talking about a minimum number. The number four also has somewhat mystical associations in Simbo thought, recurring in death ritual, local cures, and determined efforts to fit the five major lineages and six districts to a configuration of four. For some people, then, it is probably simply an automatically stated number when questioned about quantities.

25. Some women are said to attempt it by taking a high dose of antimalarial medication. This is usually stated, however, when people are commenting on birth defects.

26. Chowning (1988) received similar requests from Kove women.

27. Urban Simbo women tend to limit their family size at an earlier stage than those who continue to live on the island after marriage. Greater susceptibility to economic constraints on large families as well as access to specialist professional reproductive counseling and a widespread belief that medical procedures carried out in Honiara are superior and more efficacious all contribute to this difference.

28. I know of only one occasion in which a man married a woman who was known to have had a tubal ligation. This man had long shown his indifference to reproduction through his determined bachelorhood, although he had a child through a previous informal relationship. There was a general feeling that, given the sexual capriciousness of both of them, theirs would be a short-term liaison.

29. We should be careful of assuming that women simply want to reduce their family size. It is the context within which they are responsible for numerous children that they find problematic. Thus, shifts in the distribution of responsibility, which freed women from some of their workload, could result in less desire to reduce family size. Counts (1988) makes the point that, where women can control the spacing of children, total numbers are not necessarily relevant, and large families may be quite acceptable.

REFERENCES

Bennett, J. A. 1987. *Wealth of the Solomons: A history of a Pacific archipelago, 1800–1978.* Pacific Islands Monograph no. 3. Honolulu: University of Hawaii Press.

Bracher, M. 1992. Breastfeeding, lactational infecundity, contraception and the spacing of births: Implications of the Bellagio Consensus statement. *Health Transition Review* 2 (1): 19–48.

———. 1993. Bellagio revisited. *Health Transition Review* 3 (1): 109–13.

BSIP [British Solomon Islands Protectorate]. 1930. *Census of the population of the British Solomon Islands Protectorate: Records of the Western Pacific High Commission.* Microfilm, National Archives of Fiji, Suva.

Buckley, T., and A. Gottlieb. 1988. A critical appraisal of theories of menstrual symbolism. In *Blood magic: The anthropology of menstruation,* ed. T. Buckley and A. Gottlieb, 3–50. Berkeley: University of California Press.

Cambridge University Library. Fred Green to Rivers, typewritten note (included with letter of 25 Nov 1909?) "MEDICEN [sic] to PREVENT CONCEPTION." Haddon Collection, envelope 12018. Cambridge: Cambridge University Library.

Chowning, A. 1988. Family fertility decisions among the Kove. In *Reproductive decision making and the value of children in rural Papua New Guinea,* ed. N. McDowell, 179–97. IASER Monograph 27. Boroko: Institute of Applied Social and Economic Research.

Counts, D. A. 1988. Kaliai children: Changes in family planning in a West New Britain society. In *Reproductive decision making and the value of children in rural Papua New Guinea,* ed. N. McDowell, 163–77. IASER Monograph 27. Boroko: Institute of Applied Social and Economic Research.

Dixon-Mueller, R., and A. Germain. 1992. Stalking the elusive "unmet need" for family planning. *Studies in Family Planning* 23 (5): 330–35.

Dureau, C. M. 1993. Nobody asked the mother: Women and maternity on Simbo, western Solomon Islands. *Oceania* 64 (1): 18–35.

———. 1994. Mixed blessings: Christianity and history in women's lives on Simbo, western Solomon Islands. Ph.D. diss., Macquarie University, Sydney.

———. 1998. From sisters to wives: Changing contexts of maternity on Simbo, Western Solomon Islands. In *Maternities and Modernities: Colonial and postcolonial experiences in Asia and the Pacific,* ed. K. Ram and M. Jolly, 239–74. Cambridge: Cambridge University Press.

Edge-Partington, T. W. 1907. Ingava, chief of Rubiana, Solomon Islands: died 1906. *Man* 7:22–23.

Elia, I. 1985. *The female animal.* Oxford: Oxford University Press.

Ginsburg, F., and R. Rapp. 1991. The politics of reproduction. *Annual Review of Anthropology* 20:311–43.

Griffen, V. 1994. Women, development and population: A critique of the Port Vila Declaration. In *Sustainable development or malignant growth? Perspectives of Pacific Island women*, ed. 'A. Emberson-Bain, 63–72. Suva: Marama Publications.

Harrell, B. 1981. Lactation and menstruation in cultural perspective. *American Anthropologist* 83:796–823.

Hocart, A. M. 1931. Warfare in Eddystone of the Solomon Islands. *Journal of the Royal Anthropological Institute of Great Britain and Ireland* 61:301–24.

———. N.d.a. Gardens and food plants. MS, Alexander Turnbull Library, Wellington, New Zealand.

———. N.d.b. Relations of the sexes and marriage. MS, Alexander Turnbull Library, Wellington, New Zealand.

Jackson, K. B. 1978. Tie hokara tie vaka black man white man: A study of the New Georgia Group to 1925. Ph.D. diss., Australian National University, Canberra.

Kabeer, N. 1994. *Reversed realities: Gender hierarchies in development thought*. London: Verso.

Kennedy, K. I., et al. 1993. Rejoinder to Bracher. *Health Transition Review* 3 (1): 107–8.

Laukaran, V. H., and M. H. Labbok. 1993. The lactational amenorrhoea method re-examined: A response to Bracher's simulation models. *Health Transition Review* 3 (1): 97–100.

Lovi, A., and K. Osuga. 1998. Solomon Islands. In *Sexually transmitted diseases in Asia and the Pacific*, ed. T. Brown et al., 298–303. Armidale: Venereology Publishing.

MacCormack, C. P. 1982a. Biological, cultural and social adaptation in human fertility and birth: A synthesis. In *Ethnography of fertility and birth*, ed. C. P. MacCormack, 1–23. London: Academic Press.

———. 1982b. Health, fertility and birth in Moyamba District, Sierra Leone. In *Ethnography of fertility and birth*, ed. C. P. MacCormack, 115–39. London: Academic Press.

———. 1988. Lay concepts of reproductive physiology related to contraceptive use: A method of investigation. In *Micro approaches to demographic research*, ed. J. Caldwell, A. Hill, and V. Hull, 441–48. London: Kegan Paul.

Martin, E. 1987. *The woman in the body: A cultural analysis of reproduction*. Boston: Beacon Press.

McDowell, N. 1988. Conclusions: Continuity and change. In *Reproductive decision making and the value of children in rural Papua New Guinea*, ed. N. McDowell, 237–63. IASER Monograph 27. Boroko: Institute of Applied Social and Economic Research.

McMurray, C., and D. Lucas. 1990. Fertility and family planning in the South Pacific. Islands/Australia Working Paper no. 90/10. Canberra: National Centre for Development Studies, Research School of Pacific Studies, Australian National University.

Millman, S. 1993. Promoting breastfeeding as birth control. *Health Transition Review* 3 (1): 101–6.

Nag, M. 1980. How modernization can also increase fertility. *Current Anthropology* 21 (5): 571–87.

O'Collins, M. 1978. Overview of social welfare and family planning programmes in the Solomon Islands. Report prepared for the United Nations Interregional Technical Meeting on Social Welfare Aspects of Family Planning, Manila, United Nations Social Welfare and Development Centre for Asia and the Pacific.

———. 1979. Family planning programmes in Papua New Guinea and Solomon Islands. Australia and New Zealand Association for the Advancement of Science, 49th Congress, Auckland, New Zealand.

Ogan, E., J. Nash, and D. Mitchell. 1976. Culture change and fertility in two Bougainville populations. In *The measures of man: Methodologies in biological anthropology*, ed. E. Giles and J. S. Friedlaender, 533–49. Cambridge, Mass.: Peabody Museum Press.

Pulea, M. 1986. *The family, law and population in the Pacific Islands*. Suva: Institute of Pacific Studies, University of the South Pacific.

Rivers, W. H. R. 1922. The psychological factor. In *Essays on the depopulation of Melanesia*, ed. W. H. R. Rivers, 84–113. Cambridge: Cambridge University Press.

Rosaldo, M. 1980. The use and abuse of anthropology: Reflections on feminism and cross-cultural understanding. *Signs* 5:389–417.

Scheffler, H. W. 1962. Kindred and kin groups in Simbo Island social structure. *Ethnology* 1:135–57.

Scragg, R. F. R. 1969. Mortality changes in rural New Guinea. *Papua New Guinea Medical Journal* 12:73–83.

———. 1977. Historical epidemiology in Papua New Guinea. *Papua New Guinea Medical Journal* 20:102–9.

S.I. [Solomon Islands] Census Office. 1988. *Statistical Bulletin No. 3/88. Solomon Islands Census Report 1: Population by sex, age and ward: Final results*. Honiara: Census Office.

Taylor, C. C. 1990. Condoms and cosmology: The "fractal" person and sexual risk in Rwanda. *Social Science and Medicine* 31 (9): 1023–28.

Underhill-Sem, Y. 1994. Blame it all on population: Perceptions, statistics and reality in the population debate in the Pacific. In *Sustainable development or malignant growth? Perspectives of Pacific Island women*, ed. 'A. Emberson-Bain, 1–15. Suva: Marama Publications.

Wood, J. W. 1990. Fertility in anthropological populations. *Annual Review of Anthropology* 19:211–42.

CHAPTER 9

Infertile States: Person and Collectivity, Region and Nation in the Rhetoric of Pacific Population

Margaret Jolly

> In the future we will weep for our empty country, our empty families and our empty hearts. We need people not family planning.
> —Josephine Abijah, Papua Besena politician

> The woman is like the fountain . . . she is the source . . . she is the mother, the creator. A man is either made or destroyed by the woman: she may choose if there is a new life; she may take the herbs to prevent pregnancy; she may prevent a child from surviving after birth; she may prevent her husband from becoming generous; she may adopt any children and provide for other children. The woman who knows her husband well may do a variety of things to make or destroy him.
> —Bernard Narokobi, Papua New Guinea politician and lawyer

The epigraphs to this chapter represent two indigenous voices from Papua New Guinea, both expressing fears about "fertility control" in the days just before and after that state became independent in 1975. The first voice, Josephine Abijah, was one of very few women who rose briefly to national prominence as a politician. Though a leader of the separatist movement Papua Besena, she invokes the shared idea of "our empty country" to oppose family planning. Bernard Narokobi, still a major figure in the politics of Papua New Guinea, speaks of a rather more intimate threat from women; he sees them as both creators and destroyers of life, potentially nurturing or harming their children and husbands. It is in the space between these female and male voices, between the evocation of a national and a personal "state," that I situate this chapter.

My title "Infertile States" expressly condenses the image of a person not reproducing—through infertility, abstinence, contraception, or abortion—and the image of a nation-state pursuing zero population growth or replacement levels of fertility. Through this play on words I highlight the problematic relation between gendered persons and collectivities in contemporary discussions of fertility, family planning, and population in the Pacific. What concerns me here are the changing contours, the "borders of being," that construct the reproductivity of male and female persons in relation to each other and to collectivities that range from parochial local or kinship groups to the borders of islands, nation-states, and regions. This is not just a matter of an increasing scale of reproductive horizons. Historical processes have to varying degrees transformed the "partible persons" of the recent Pacific past (see Strathern 1988; cf. Jolly 1992) into reproductive "individuals" and created contests between local, national, regional, and global interests and investments in human fertility.

Such contests are particularly focused on the reproductive bodies of women, rather than men. This is a critical shift from the indigenous regimes of the Pacific, where men were construed as vitally involved in the practices and politics of fertility. Today family planning debates are often represented as a contest between the reproductive policies of nation-states and the desires and interests of individuals, or canonically, as Robinson (this volume) depicts it, between "government agency" and "women's agency." There is no doubt that in certain countries, such as China and India, there is a violent collision between the antinatalist policies of states and the desires of many women (and men) for more children (see Ram and Sigley, this volume). In both countries there is abundant contemporary evidence of blunt coercion and forcible persuasion in programs of contraception and sterilization. In other states, present and past, there has been an equally violent contradiction between pronatalist state policies and women's desires to restrict their children through abortion, infanticide, abstinence, or contraception (see Ginsburg and Rapp 1995). But, even in those countries where the contest between individual and state interests seems stark and violent, women's agency and government agency can appear more complicit. The capacity of women to "choose" can be expressly celebrated and aligned with the desires of nation-states and international agencies to "control," in explicit opposition to the desires of men, overt or imputed. This is the shape of reproductive politics in the contemporary Pacific, a shape that molds and constrains the choices of all, women and men.

In this chapter I speak in very general terms about how the Pacific is portrayed in present and past discourses about "population." This regional designation—like the subregional labels "Melanesia," "Polynesia," and "Micronesia"—embraces not just many far-flung islands but enormous cultural and linguistic diversity, deriving from the ancestral navigations of both Austronesian-speaking and Papuan-speaking peoples (see map 3). Such diversity is often captured through language statistics and atlases—Papua New Guinea has 700 and Vanuatu 110 extant indigenous languages. Such indigenous diversities were compounded by a complicated history of colonization by Spanish, Portuguese, British, French, German, American, Japanese, and Australian powers. Some Pacific islands, like New Caledonia and French Polynesia, are still not sovereign states, while all are subject to the neocolonial influences of aid and development agencies, emanating especially from erstwhile colonizers. My focus is on the independent nations of the southwest Pacific—Papua New Guinea, the Solomons, Vanuatu, and Fiji—countries about which much has been written by anthropologists, historians, demographers, and development economists. My origin point, or *stamba*, to use a Bislama or pidgin concept, is my earlier ethnography and colonial history of Vanuatu.[1] But from that ground I navigate to other places, making connections across this vast ocean (see Hauʻofa 1998). By privileging Oceanic connections, I sometimes occlude not just cultural particulars but embodied specificities. Along with the differences between genders, which are foregrounded, there are other differences—of age, ethnicity, religion, region, and class—which are, perforce, backgrounded here.[2]

This chapter navigates several spatio-temporal zones and diverse academic and policy literatures on fertility in the Pacific. Perhaps I should chart my course. I start with a critical consideration of the contemporary "specter" of overpopulation. This dominates the discourses of demography, development economics, and policy making. I then juxtapose this with the recent "ghost" of Pacific depopulation, a problem that engaged not just Pacific peoples but innumerable foreign advisors—missionaries, colonial officials, and biomedical practitioners—in the late nineteenth and early twentieth centuries. In talk of both overpopulation and its precursor, depopulation, women are seen as the more natural "targets" of government concern and intervention. The tropes of "improving" and "emancipating" mothers prevail in both colonial and postcolonial epochs. This often promised freeing women not just from tradition but also from the strictures of indigenous male domination, a rhetoric that elided those past powers women had as mothers, sisters, and daughters and which marginalized men in the modern regimes of fertility.

The next section of the chapter moves deeper into the past, in a review of indigenous or ancestral regimes of fertility. I argue that the fertility of human beings, "nature," and the cosmos were powerfully connected in indigenous Oceanic models and that value and power inhered not in uncontrolled fecundity but controlled nurture, growth, and health. Moreover, as is obvious in the anthropology of male cults, fertility was not, naturally, "women's business." Men were everywhere vitally involved in the reproduction of human life and indeed often dominated women, individually and collectively. From a consideration of the privileged centrality of men in the anthropological literature on

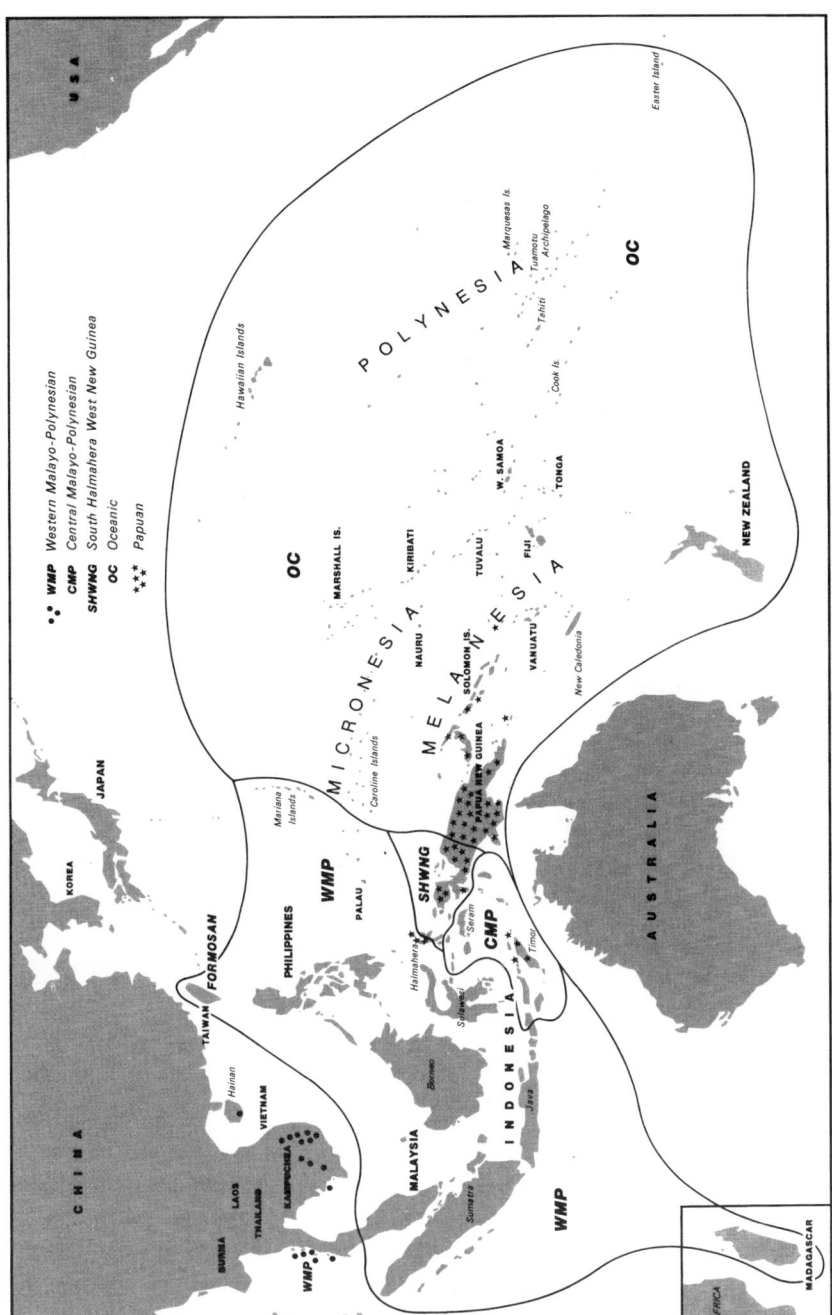

Map 3. The geographical distribution and classification of languages (and approximate Papuan Languages) across the Asia and Pacific regions, showing subregions of Melanesia, Polynesia, and Micronesia

fertility cults, I move on to ponder their virtual absence in the demography of contemporary family planning. Men are rarely the preferred targets of demographic research and government programs and until very recently have been often extruded from "family planning," except as its presumed opponents. The chapter concludes with a review of the difficulty of both embracing men and empowering women in contemporary global projects of "choice" in population and development.

The Specter of Overpopulation

In contemporary demographic and economic discourse, the Pacific islands, like many regions of the developing world, are seen as dangerously "torrid zones." Although the demographic "excesses" and the economic insufficiencies of these tiny, insular states are never seen to approach the enormity of the problems posited for the huge continents and the "masses" of India or of China, their leaders are still regularly regaled by foreign advisors and international agencies for their failure to implement successful family planning and to keep populations within the viable limits imposed by the scarce resources of land and sea, of private and state infrastructure. Any perusal of national plans and regional statements, of policy prescriptions and academic analyses of the contemporary Pacific, yields the specter of overpopulation. So, an influential analysis and projection of the future of the Pacific, self-consciously presented as a "doomsday scenario," portrays rapid population growth as foundational to its nightmare vision. Its cover proclaims: "By 2010, population growth in the Pacific islands is careering beyond control: it has doubled to 9 million." There are rather more refined demographic analyses inside the covers, but they are framed by Calick's journalistic rhetoric thus:

> In *taim bilong tumbuna*—the days of old, in Tok Pisin—island populations were constrained by disease and national disaster. . . . But times are changing. . . . Migratory opportunities are diminishing . . . in parts . . . arable land is running short. Life cannot continue as it is now lived. So much is clear. (1993, 2)

> Children are, of course a great blessing. But in the not too distant past, the sense of blessing was always enhanced by the awareness that many did not survive long. Today, as *Pacific 2010* makes graphically clear, the region's population growth is careering, albeit happily for now, beyond control. Already the next generation's options are thereby diminished. (8)

We might ponder that curious caveat—"careering, albeit happily for now." But the aim of the book is plain. It aspires not just to substitute a utopic vision of the island Pacific as paradise with a dystopic vision but also to avert the nightmare by sound policy initiatives, by encouraging not just family planning but economic restructuring. South Pacific leaders are enjoined to take bold action "before looming disasters impose their own grim patterns on the next generation and beyond" (Calick 1993, 11). And, along with providing the "factual tools needed to focus choices" for leaders, this commentator stakes his faith in the emergence of a more mature island capitalism, since "research has tended to show that successful family planning programmes have coincided with the emergence of a self-confident middle class" (8).

There are many elements of his past and future telling that are problematic. His view of the ancestral past, the *taim bilong tumbuna,* as a time of unrestrained fecundity controlled only by natural disaster, disease, and infant mortality is dramatically at variance with the pervasive evidence of indigenous "family planning" through herbal contraceptives, abortifacients, infanticide, and most particularly patterns of abstinence and heterosexual sequestration (McDowell 1988; and see later discussion). Calick's future prognostications are comparably gross. There is no denying that population growth is high in *some* countries and *may* outstrip the potential of states to provide adequate schooling and health services, particularly in Papua New Guinea, the Solomon Islands, and Vanuatu (Gannicott 1993, 15ff.). In some islands and regions there *is* a lack of arable land, and migrants to town ultimately risk being cut off from ancestral places and being rendered landless (see, e.g., Simbo in the Solomons, Dureau, this volume). But the demographic problems are far more diverse and complicated than such pronouncements herald. In the same volume McMurray warns of the "short history of census taking and population monitoring in most of the Pacific" and thus the "considerable uncertainty about population growth prospects in the region" (1993a, 49). Although persuaded of the population problems of several island states, McMurray cautions that, rather than focusing exclusively on overall population growth, trends in school enrollments, labor force, and urbanization are equally crucial to demographic projections and national plans (1993b, 63). Morever, I argue, contra Calick, that island capitalism may generate not so much a mature, self-confident, and demographically disciplined middle class as increased poverty in both rural and urban regions and unstable demographic patterns, given uncertain and insecure futures.

National plans of the several independent states of the southwest Pacific have in the last ten years or so moved from a relaxed attitude to population to a new urgency about family planning for the nation. For example, in Vanuatu, in the Second National Plan of 1987–91, there was adjudged to be "no particularly urgent problem related to the growth, size and movement of population" (Vanuatu, National Planning and Statistics Office 1988, 149; cf. Booth 1985; and Vanuatu, National Planning and Statistics Office 1986). But in the Third Plan of 1992–97 a national reduction of births was, rather, seen as the "only viable policy measure" (Vanuatu, National Planning and Statistics Office 1992, 7; see also Gannicott 1993, 14). Similar shifts transpired in the national plans of Papua New Guinea and the Solomons, where, despite some oscillations, there has been a government policy of curbing population for about a decade and where broader population policies have been developed (see McMurray and Lucas 1990).

The Port Vila Declaration issued by all regional leaders of the Pacific in 1993, preparatory to the International Conference on Population and Development in Cairo in 1994, expressed shared official opinion (South Pacific Commission 1994a). This declaration was published as part of a South Pacific Commission document, which offered population profiles for all Pacific island states (see figs. 11 and 12) and a regional analysis that stressed both the connectedness of the "sea of islands" (see Hauʻofa 1993) and their diverse demographic and development trajectories. The overall tone of this publication is more measured than Calick's rhetoric in *Pacific 2010*. It warns that "smallness" does not mean that population issues are unimportant or minimal (South Pacific Commission 1994a, 3), but it is cautious about gross generalizations, insisting on subregional differences and on differences between and within countries. It notes that the population of the whole region has been growing steadily at 2.3 percent each year, but that this regional average masks the subregional differences between Micronesia at 3.5 percent, Polynesia at 1.5 percent, and Melanesia at 2.3 percent. It shows how population pyramids for Melanesia, Micronesia, and Polynesia differ (see fig. 13), although noting that all have the "broad base and concave shape which are the sign of youthful populations with considerable potential for future population growth" (1994a, 7).

The subregional differences are in some degree due to differential patterns of out-migration, but there are also significant differences in total fertility rates (see fig. 14), with Nauru and the Federated States of Micronesia highest at 7.5 and 7.2, respectively, and the Commonwealth of the Northern Mariana Islands the lowest at 2.4, with Papua New Guinea, the Solomons, and Vanuatu all over 5 (1994a, 8). The reasons for such marked differences are "not yet fully understood": in some contexts "fertility is declining amidst low and stagnating contraceptive prevalence rates," while remaining stable where contraceptive prevalence has increased (1994a, 9). It applauds the large reductions in infant mortality rates across the Pacific, but notes that other aspects of maternal and

DEVELOPMENT STATISTICS

PACIFIC ISLAND POPULATIONS

From the Pacific Island Population wall chart, produced by the Population/Demography Programme.
South Pacific Commission, PO Box D5, Noumea, New Caledonia

	Last census	Population at last census	Land area (km²)	Population density (people/ km²)	Population doubling time (years)	Sex ratio (males/100 females)	Median age	Infant mortlity rate (c)	Life expectancy at birth males (d)	Life expectancy at birth females (d)
Fiji	1986 (a)	715 375	18 272	44	35	103	20.2	16 (1994)	72 (1995) (e)	75 (1995) (e)
PNG	1990 *	3 607 954 (b)	462 243	9	30	112	18.2	82 (1991)	52 (1991)	51 (1991)
Solomon Islands	1986	285 176	28 370	14	20	103	15.8	38 (1986)	60 (1986)	61 (1986)
Vanuatu	1989	142 419	12 190	14	25	106	17.6	45 (1989)	62 (1989)	64 (1989)
Kiribati	1995 *	77 658	811	97	50	98	19.9	65 (1990)	58 (1990)	63 (1990)
Tonga	1986 (a)	94 649	747	120	139	101	18.1	8 (1991-94)	70 (1996) (e)	74 (1996) (e)
Samoa	1991	161 298	2 935	56	139	110	18.2	22 (1991-94)	70 (1996) (e)	74 (1996) (e)

* Provisional results; census still in progress.
a These countries and territories conducted a census in 1996, for which the results are not yet available; Fiji (25/8), Tonga (30/11)
b This figure excludes the population of North Solomons Province (Bougainville), estimated by Hayes (1993) at 155 000 at the time of the 1990 census. If this figure was added to the census total, the PNG population would have been 3 762 954. A mid-year population estimate for 1996 on this basis would mean a PNG population of 4 319 800.
c Infant mortality rate (IMR): the number of deaths to infants under 1 year of age for each 1 000 live births.
d Life expectancy at birth: an estimate of the average number of years a person can expect to live.
e These figures are based on recent estimates prepared by the SPC Population/Demography Programme.

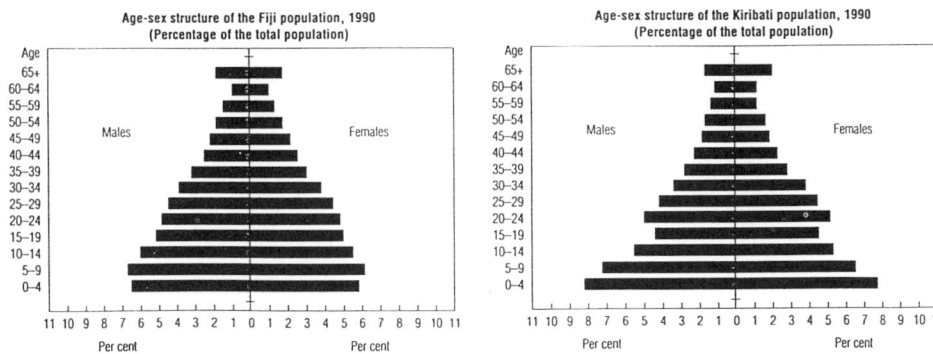

Fig. 11. Pacific Island populations, wall chart. (South Pacific Commission 1994b)

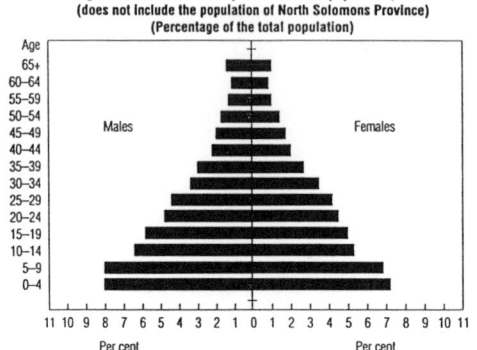
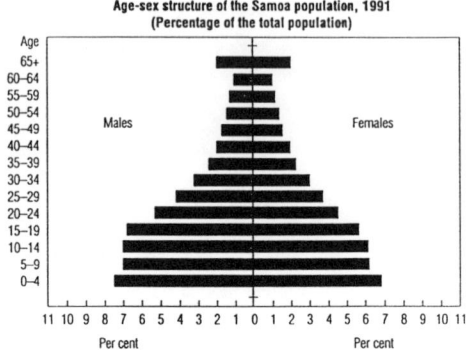
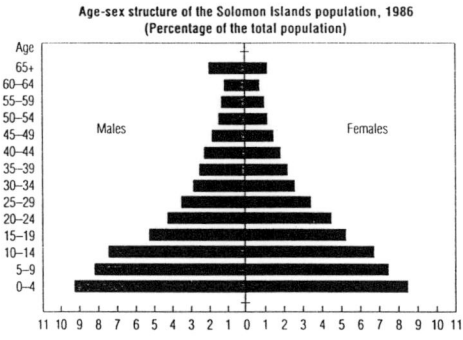
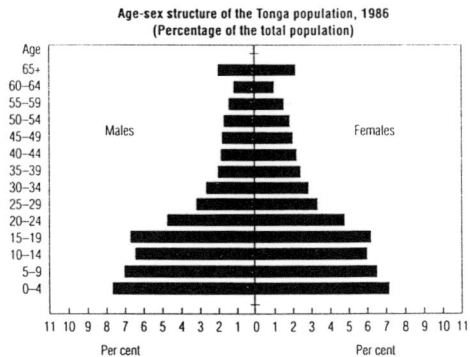
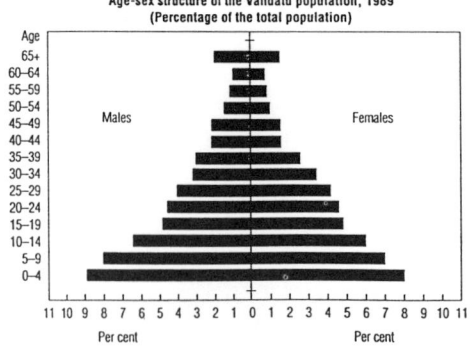

DEVELOPMENT
STATISTICS

Fig. 12. Pacific Island populations, wall chart, cont'd. (South Pacific Commission 1994b)

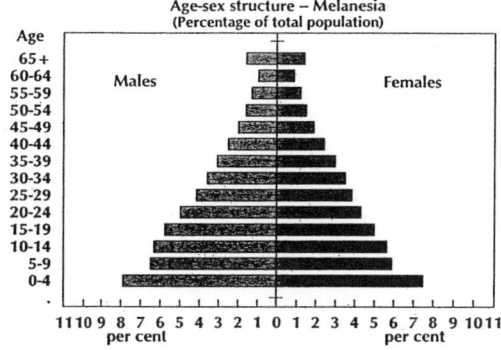
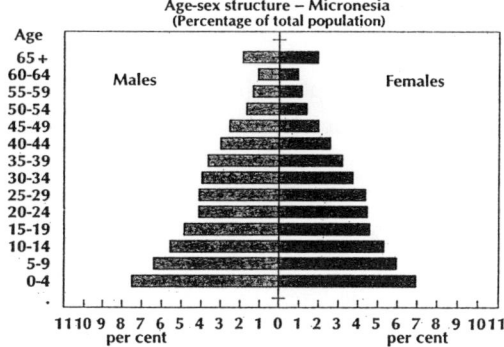
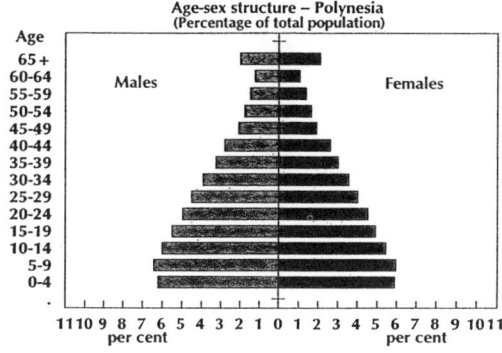

Fig. 13. Population pyramids for Melanesia, Micronesia, and Polynesia compared. (South Pacific Commission 1994a, 7)

child health have been disappointing, in particular "family planning." It stresses the crucial importance of developing programs that go beyond present models.

> Most programmes in the region emphasise safe motherhood in a traditional family context; they ignore the rights of unmarried women and adolescent girls and the role of men. This severely limits the effectiveness of such programmes and prevents the achievement of broader population and development objectives aimed at slowing rapid and unsustainable population growth. (South Pacific Commission 1994a, 9)

The regional analysis commissioned for the Port Vila meeting raised compelling and critical questions. But these were still framed by a neo-Malthusian specter of overpopulation. "Should the current trends continue the Pacific islands' population will double in 30 years time from its present 6.7 million people to around 13.5 million people with the fastest growth occurring in towns and cities" (1994a, 15). And despite the accumulated uncertainties of projections about the future, the report concluded that population issues are of utmost and singular urgency for island governments, which, if unattended, "develop a momentum of their own" (1994a, 15) that will undo other national development efforts. Yet many of the questions posed raised large doubts about the capacities of states to effect such changes. Still, in the final declaration, Pacific leaders assumed that with due international assistance and aid they *did* have the power to formulate and implement such population programs. Their concluding statement supported gender equality, the empowerment of women, and the need for increased male involvement in family planning programs (1994a, 47). But it insisted on the salience of tradition and community and on the *family* context of family planning, since the family "sits at the nexus of tradition and modernity" (1994a, 48). Ultimately, they argued, "family planning is a means of improving the quality of family life and not an end in itself" (1994a, 48).

In a critique of this declaration and existing government programs Griffen acknowledges gender-sensitive additions to official population policies. But for her the focus is still narrowly on *control* of fertility, and despite token references to the empowerment of women and gender equality women are still imaged as the targets of family planning. There is still a narrow view of family planning in the context of maternal and child health, rather than a broader focus on sexual and reproductive knowledge and behavior embracing men as well as women and young, single people as well as married couples (Griffen 1994, 68–69). The *family* in *family planning* is unduly restrictive. Moreover, population growth is singled out as the main cause of contemporary problems (such as ecological degradation, unemployment, and urban crime). In her view, the notion of sustainable development deployed did not address deeper questions such as the regional constructions of alternative forms of "development," the place of "culture," and "tradition" in such processes and the ecological damage of uncontrolled capitalist growth (emanating from extractive industries like logging and mining in particular). Moreover, although the declaration does allude to the ecological consequences of high technology and growth in allusions to global warming and nuclear testing, I note that they are quarantined to an "outside." "The causes of such changes have their origins far from our region and are beyond the control of our countries and territories" (South Pacific Commission 1994a, 47). Unsustainable development within is, rather, equated with high population growth, which alone seems to threaten "the quality of life."

Such conclusions conform to what Underhill-Sem (1994) has characterized as "blame it all on population." Her critique, like that of Griffen, appeared in a collection of papers by Pacific women, pointedly called *Sustainable Development or Malignant Growth?* Underhill-Sem (1994, 2–3) attests, echoing the preparatory papers for Port Vila, that crude indicators of regional demography, such as infant mortality, total fertility rate or life expectancy, vary dramatically across the region. Moreover, she claims that the pervasive use of ethnological categories to label subregions on the basis of assumed cultural similarity—Melanesia, Polynesia, Micronesia—tends to reinscribe the centrality of culture as an obstacle in changing population patterns, whereas more sophisticated comparative demography is looking *across* such borders, at the complex interaction of environmental, economic, social, and political forces.

She is cautious about accepting higher claims for a regional growth rate, in part because of the uncertainties of much demographic data, noted earlier, but also because the demographic dominance of Papua New Guinea means that it exerts an undue influence on the regional average. In 1994 it claimed 60 percent of the region's population of 6.7 million. At the opposite extreme, the tiny island of Niue had only 2,267 in 1989 and was declining by 5.3 percent primarily because of out-migration. She finds more plausible the earlier estimate of a regional average of 2.1 percent (South Pacific Commission 1993; Underhill-Sem 1994, 4). Moreover, she notes that in many countries the problem is not high density, but *low* density, particularly in remote rural areas, which suffer from small markets and expensive, infrequent transportation. High density in urban areas is patently an issue in the Marshall Islands, but elsewhere, she contends, rapid rates of urbanization appear to be slowing. Underhill-Sem is not attempting to deny the problems of fast population growth in certain contexts.

She predicts continuing high growth in countries such as Vanuatu, the Solomons and Papua New Guinea, where high fertility rates and a youthful population, coupled with low out-migration, will generate strong pressures on resources and on the services of health and education throughout the next decade at least. But, rather than placing her faith in a global theory of a demographic transition to low fertility, she insists that fertility will only fall when couples *want* to reduce their family size (cf. Caldwell 1982; Greenhalgh 1995). So long as the economic value of children remains high and the ideal of a small family is not accepted, high population growth in such countries will continue (Underhill-Sem 1994, 8). Both women *and* men need to be convinced of the need to have fewer children.

On certain islands and in certain countries high population growth coupled with low economic growth *may be* a problem. But what Underhill-Sem observes is a tendency to project a doomsday vision, which both exaggerates the problem and assimilates diverse experiences to a homogenous fate (cf. Fry 1997). Uncritical acceptance of the wisdom that slower population growth will improve economic growth and "journalistic scaremongering" do not, in her view, help to discern the determinants and conditions of growth in the region. Aid projects and policies that "instruct family planning workers to tell their clients (most of whom are women) about the problems of rapid population growth and how they have a responsibility to limit the number of children they have for the benefit of the country or the world" (Underhill-Sem 1994, 13) will, she attests, continue to be unpersuasive (cf. Dureau, this volume). The emphasis should be on more intimate local needs and messages made more responsive to the diverse local patterns of fertility, mortality, and migration. Her claim is both strengthened and complicated if we juxtapose this specter of overpopulation in the Pacific present with the ghost of depopulation in the recent past.

The Ghost of Depopulation

In the late nineteenth and early twentieth centuries this contrasting specter haunted both Islanders and Europeans engaged in the development work of the colonial period—in mission stations, plantations, district offices or medical aid posts. There is a poignant historical dimension to the chronic failures of family planning programs in the contemporary Pacific. For, as Spriggs has observed,

> Aid agency concerns over low participation in family-planning programmes in much of Island Melanesia and alarm at what are some of the highest population growth rates in the world must be balanced by an

appreciation of the history of the islands and the perception of the inhabitants that they are but a tiny remnant of the populations that once lived on them. Older people alive today remember when rates of population decline and the effects of diseases, such as tuberculosis, were such that they were told by visiting Europeans that they would all be dead within a few years. (1997, 262)

The nature and scale of the demographic catastrophe that beset the Pacific has been much debated (see A. Bushnell, 1993; O. Bushnell 1993; Denoon 1995; McArthur 1967; Rallu 1991; Stannard 1989), but in many places depopulation was precipitous and disastrous. For instance, as Spriggs attests, on the island of Aneityum in the south of Vanuatu, population plummeted from 3,513 in 1858 to 272 in 1924, and then to 186 in 1941. It marginally recovered, from the 1960s, but was still at the last census count 94 to 97 percent below estimates of the pre-contact figure (Spriggs 1997, 257–61; see fig. 14). This is probably the worst case of decline in the southwest Pacific. But throughout the islands of Fiji, Vanuatu, the Solomons, and Papua New Guinea people suffered the successive scourges of influenza, measles, dysentery, whooping cough, diphtheria and the lingering effects of venereal diseases, which not only claimed lives but had persisting sequelae in reduced fertility. It was not without cause that the English anthropologist Bernard Deacon spoke of the people of Southwest Bay in Malakula as "a vanishing people" (1934) before he himself succumbed to blackwater fever (a fatal complication of malaria). He, like the German ethnographer Felix Speiser, was in Vanuatu at a time when the population had fallen to its nadir and their texts are replete with a sense of malaise and despair, captured by the voice of a woman from Port Olry Santo, recorded by Speiser, "Why should we go on having children? Since the white man came they all die" (recorded in 1911–12, but first published in 1923) (Speiser 1990[1923], 50).

Thus, suggests Spriggs, "scepticism of the value of limiting births would seem perfectly reasonable on many islands in the region when their recent history is remembered" (1997, 263). Echoing Spriggs, I argue that the specter of overpopulation in the Pacific present needs to be juxtaposed with the ghost of depopulation that haunts the recent past. Older Pacific people, women and men, often express disquiet and consternation about a reversal of demographic experience and of foreign advice over the course of a few generations. Moreover, present prophecies of overpopulation often blur indigenous and exogenous sources of the contemporary problems of "family planning." First, insofar as they see many of the obstacles to family planning as to development in general as cultural or traditional, they tend to portray ancestral or indigenous regimes of fertility as unconstrained and excessive, even "natural" (see Robin-

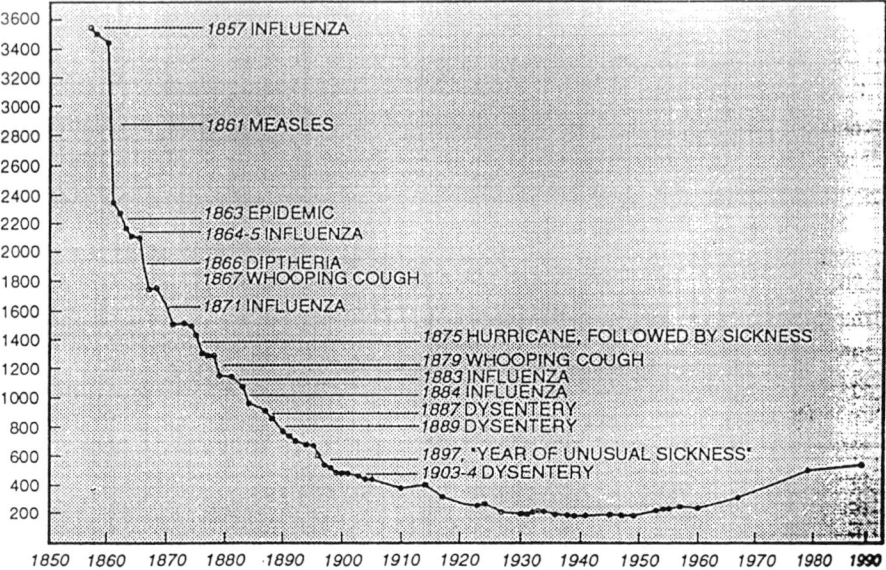

Fig. 14. Population decline and recovery on Aneityum Island, Vanuatu, 1850–1990. (From Spriggs 1997, 257, fig. 9.2.)

son, this volume). They tend to forget indigenous forms of "family planning," and in particular the crucial significance of birth spacing, through postpartum abstinence and protracted breastfeeding in many of the islands of the southwest Pacific. Second, they often de-emphasize the effects of foreign penetration and colonial control on local demographic regimes or portray them only in biologistic terms. The crucial effects of introduced diseases, medical techniques, and drugs are typically admitted. But the Christian reformation of sexuality and conjugality and colonial state projects to curb depopulation from the late nineteenth to the twentieth century were equally critical in the historical origins of contemporary overpopulation. These are rarely so privileged in demographic analysis (but see Dureau 1993, 1998, this volume; Jolly 1998).

As Hunt has so persuasively argued for Zaire (previously the Belgian Congo, and now the Independent Republic of the Congo), the problem of "too many children too quickly," both for parents and for the nation as a whole, is not the "innocent and inescapable outcome of 'modernization'" (1997, 308). Such contemporary problems are in part due to a concerted colonial effort to "combat the prejudices which separate the spouses" (1997, 307), to reduce birth intervals and increase the birthrate. This was part of a colonial project to remake African women in the image of European mothers, through maternal and infant health programs such as those of the Congo (evocatively called *gouttes de lait,* or "drops of milk"). Belgian women used the image of suckling, of giving milk to promote their benevolent maternalistic projects on behalf of African women. Sometimes they espoused the breast, sometimes the bottle, but more constant was their vision of a modern mother, the fulcrum of a stable monogamous family whose life was disciplined in both work and love. Familial discipline did not embrace postpartum abstinence, however, which was portrayed as a primitive ordeal that no civilized African should suffer. Colonial concern for the dying out of Africans was both compassionate and strategic, motivated by the threat of a declining labor force in the Congo as elsewhere in Africa and the Pacific (Hunt 1997, 287ff.).

As I have argued elsewhere (Jolly 1998), the colonial concern for the "dying out" of Pacific peoples had strategic interests beyond the threat of a declining labor force. Labor was a problem, but, as is most obvious in the case of Fiji under the British, the colonial state had other less instrumental concerns in establishing their "rule": namely, the promotion of a novel concept of "population" that connected the bodies of persons and the state (see Foucault 1980; cf. Reed 1997). Importantly, for much of the colonial period, indigenous Fijians were thought inappropriate for work in the plantations of the colonies, and indentured laborers were transported from other colonial sites, particularly from India but also from the islands of the southwest Pacific—from Vanuatu, the Solomons, and Papua New Guinea. Yet, despite the fact that Fijians were for the most part exempted from such labor, the colonial concern was not for the wretched mortality of the indentured laborers (see Kelly 1991; Lal 1985), but with the depopulation of the native races. Indeed, the *Report of a Commission of Enquiry into the Decrease of the Native Population,* more commonly dubbed the *Decrease Report* (1896), was—as its title betrays—devoted solely to indigenous Fijians. This is an extraordinary document for several reasons: its length, comprehensiveness, and influence; the zealousness with which it investigated the many alleged causes of depopulation; the range of submissions from colonial officers, missionaries, anthropologists, settlers, as well as indigenous Fijians; and, finally, because many of its recommendations were implemented (see Jolly 1998; Lukere 1997). It canvassed a wide range of causes for the "decrease," typically marshaled in opposed columns as indigenous and exogenous. On the side of indigenous causes were listed: abortion and infanticide, warfare and head-hunting, polygamy, early marriage, sexual depravity, unsanitary habits, native narcotics, the communal system, and, most important, unskilled midwives and mothers. On the side of the exogenous the catalogue included: introduced diseases, the labor trade, new foods, alcohol, new firearms, and European clothes. Also named were those "psychological causes," attributed to European contact, "general insouciance of the native mind" and "growing disinclination to bear children" (see table 4). Perhaps most singular is the fact that the commissioners' conclusions drew on indigenous testimony—albeit mainly the voices of high-ranking Fijian men.

Fijian men named a cause that was rarely admitted by outsiders: the deleterious effects of Christian conversion on conjugal behavior. In their view the celebration of monogamy promoted a relation between husband and wife that was too intimate. Husbands and wives were not only sharing a bed but were resuming sexual relations too early after the birth of a child. The commissioners reported "the fixed belief of the Fijians that incontinence impairs the quality of the mother's milk" (Decrease Report 1896, 145). The cohabitation of the parents during the suckling period was thought thereby to cause *dabe*—a sickness in the child, signs of "attenuation," accompanied by an "enlarged abdomen and general debility" (1896, 146). "Native witnesses" suggested that in the past babes were suckled from twelve to thirty-six months or even longer, and that "the feeling of the most intelligent natives" was that cohabitation should best be avoided for a year after birth—to avoid impoverishing the milk or the woman falling pregnant again before the infant was weaned. The commissioners adjudicated that

> So long as the village *bure ni sa* [the communal men's house] existed and the husband and wife lived in different houses, each under the surveillance of persons of their own sex, secret cohabitation was impracticable. It was made still less possible by the custom of young mothers of leaving their husband's house and going to live with their relations for a year after the birth of a child; but since the *bure* system has been abandoned, and an imitation of European life substituted for it, husband and wife no longer separate during the period of lactation, but rather give their parole to public opinion to preserve the abstinence prescribed by ancient custom. The health of the child is jealously watched by the other villagers for signs that the parents have failed in their duty. (1896, 146)

The commissioners endorsed the practice with their own pragmatic logic—given the lack of stamina of the Fijian mother, her poor nutrition, and the lack of local breast milk substitutes, they perceived its benefits and satirized those missionaries who saw the isolation of the nursing mother as "absurd and superstitious." But their instrumental recuperation of the practice was rendered difficult by the additional discovery that adulterous affairs by the new father could also cause *dabe*. Thus, "in Namosi, where lactation was continued

TABLE 4. Alleged Deleterious Influences and Causes of Depopulation and Racial Degeneracy

Attributed to Influence of, and Contact with Europeans	Held to Be Unconnected with Advent to Europeans but Inherent in the Native Life and Culture
1. Changed habitat	Insanitary native dwellings and domestic habits
2. Concentration of houses and villages	Decentralization
3. European clothing	
4. Unsuitability of European food	Quality and supply of native food and drinking water
5. Recruiting system and segregation of sexes on plantations	
6. Abolition of native communal system and authority of chiefs	Native communal system and power of chiefs
7. Alcohol	Native narcotics (Kava drinking, betel chewing, etc.)
8. Introduced diseases, endemic and epidemic	Native endemic diseases, and diseases of children tending to permanently injure health
9. Obstacles to marriage and female postponement of marriage, due to European control or interference	Obstacles to marriage in native marriage customs and child marriages
10. Influence of penal laws against fornication (where enforced, as in Fiji)	Sexual depravity inherent in native life and customs
11. Abolition of native warfare	Native warfare
12. Abolition of head-hunting	Head-hunting
13.	Infanticide, abortion, and prevention of conception
14. Increase of infant mortality under new conditions	Infant mortality as result of native customs, unskilled midwifery, work during pregnancy, etc.
15. Abolition of polygamy	Polygamy and condition of women
16.	Consanguineous marriages, and in-breeding
17. Psychological causes, including general insouciance of the native mind and growing disinclination to bear children	

Source: Decrease Report 1896.

280 Borders of Being

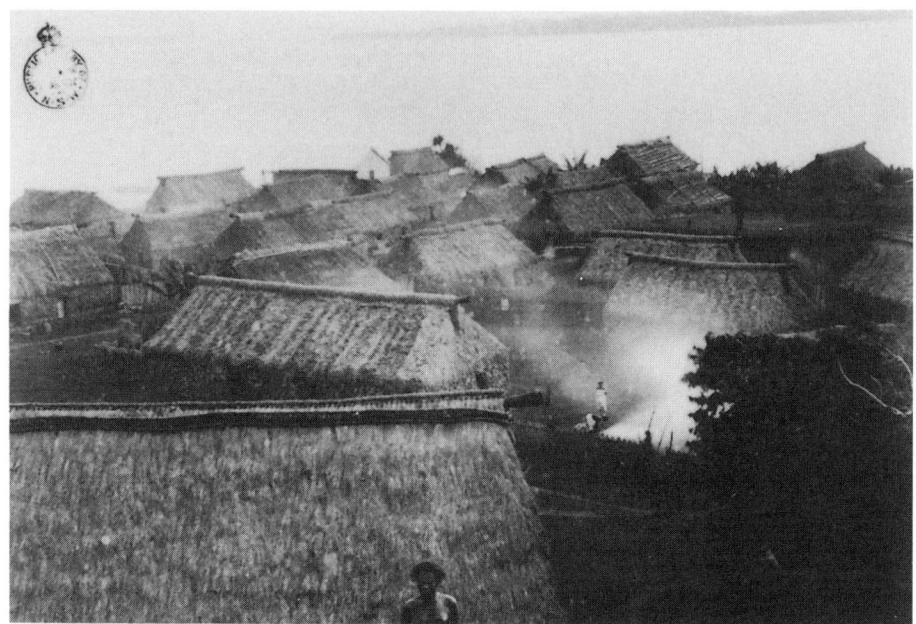

Fig. 15. Indigenous patterns of housing on Bau, Fiji (original caption was "Roof Tops of Bau"). (From A. J. Webb, *Illustrated History of Fiji*, 1885 [Mitchell Library, Sydney, ML ref. Q998.8/W], 22.)

for three years, a man who had 'an intrigue with another woman,' caused his child to sicken with *dabe,* or in exquisite translation of local idiom 'alien thigh-locking'" (1896, 146). The commissioners ultimately concluded that "retrogression is now impossible" and that the only feasible remedy is the "use of milk from the lower animals" (148)—a remedy that, of course, portended even more infant malnutrition and death (cf. Manderson 1982, 1984).

Dabe was only one cause mooted for the "decrease" of Fijians, and indeed, as we will see the decline of sexual segregation, postpartum probably led to a dramatic increase in population as birth intervals narrowed. As both Lukere and I have documented elsewhere in much greater detail (Jolly 1998; Lukere 1997), although the report assiduously sifts a wide variety of causes for depopulation, the ensuing practical action of the Fijian colonial state effectively fixates on mothers, castigates their "insouciance," and implements a series of surveillances and projects of sanitation and reform that are directed more at mothers than at fathers, more at women than at men. Fathers were the target of state intervention but in a way that tended to construct them as the "auxil-

Infertile States 281

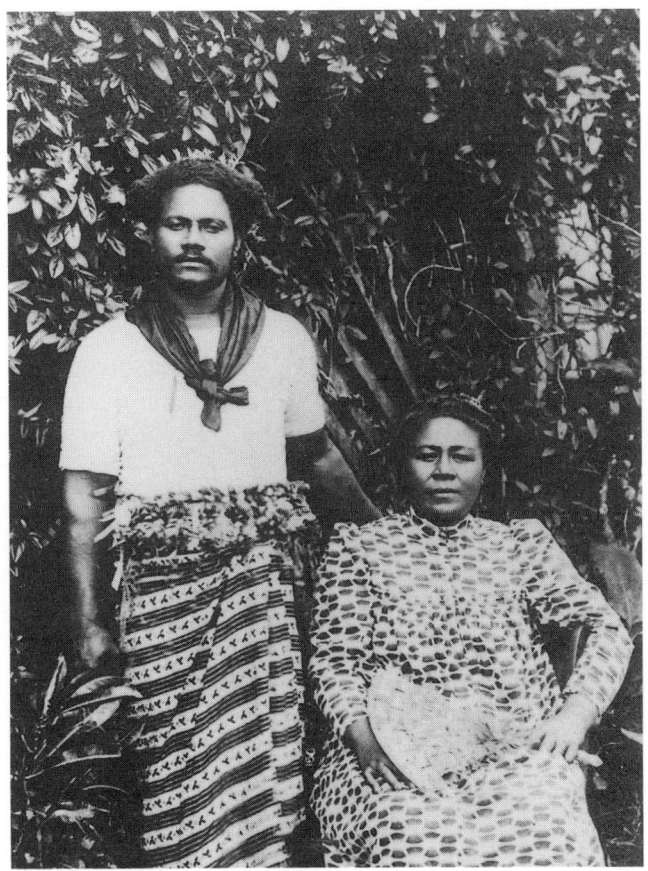

Fig. 16. High-ranking Fijians in European-style clothing after Christian conversion (original caption was "High Fijians"). (From photo album of W.C.F., *Views of Fiji* [Mitchell Library, Sydney, ML ref. F988.8/1A2].)

iaries," responsible primarily as "providers" for their pregnant wives, who should not have to work, and especially not perform hard manual labor (see Lukere 1997). The state project of repopulation at times distanced itself from that of Christian missionaries with its zealous promotion of monogamous, nucleated couples, an "imitation of European life" in lieu of the "ancient custom" of sexual segregation. But the colonial state also promoted a new model of gender relations that privileged heterosexual conjugality over the gendered collectivities of kinship of lineages and clans, in which women were sisters and daughters as much as wives and mothers (cf. Dureau 1998; Weiner 1995). Collectivities of lineages and clans were deployed in the projects of state control over population but in a way that construed them as supremely dominated by the interests of men, and especially high-ranking or senior men. So, in the first decades of the twentieth century, Fijian chiefs were drafted into surveillance of the reproductive behavior of married couples in their regions and enjoined not only to investigate infant deaths but to reward fecund fathers with baby bonuses (Lukere 1997). Such colonial projects of repopulation in Fiji, as elsewhere, betray a pervasive tendency to privilege female interest in the new "choices" afforded by monogamous marriage but to evacuate female interest from the ancestral collectivities of lineages and clans (cf. Jolly 1994a).

Thus ensues a cliché of many colonialist and developmentalist discourses, whereby *tradition* is construed as in male interests and *modernity* in female interests and the choice of the female person is privileged, in the negotiations between them (see Jolly 1997). This is especially clear in the way in which, in missionary and colonial officials' ruminations about "Melanesian marriage," arranged unions are regularly seen to force the bride more than the groom and bride wealth is viewed unambiguously as a "price," which renders the woman like an object or an animal (see Jolly 1994a). Foreign interventions, and especially those projects of reform of family and fertility that were the particular concern of Christian missions, were habitually represented as primarily in the interests of women, and often against the interests of men. So, especially in Vanuatu, the Solomons, and Papua New Guinea, where women were often portrayed as "beasts of burden" or "slaves" of their menfolk, Christian missionaries deemed their projects recuperative "to save the girls for brighter and better lives" (Jolly 1991; Jolly and Macintyre 1989; Langmore 1989). I am not denying that many of the indigenous cultures of this region evinced strong patterns of gendered hierarchy and male domination. What I am arguing is that the imputation of an alliance between foreign interests and female interests in such programs of "improvement" was a pervasive feature of colonial discourses and continues to saturate present discourses of development, particularly apropos fertility and reproductive politics.

But the impact of Christian missions and other colonial forces on gendered hierarchy and on familial life is, as Christine Dureau (1994, 1998, this volume) demonstrates, so lucidly for Simbo in the western Solomons, a process replete with paradox and irony. Although the situation she depicts for Simbo is distinctive, her portrayal of "mixed blessings" for women can be more generally applied, especially in the sphere of fertility and reproduction. She argues that, for Simbo, one form of inequality has been replaced by another: control of women's sexuality and fertility has passed locally from brothers to husbands, and husbands' powers are to some extent enshrined both in Christian sermons

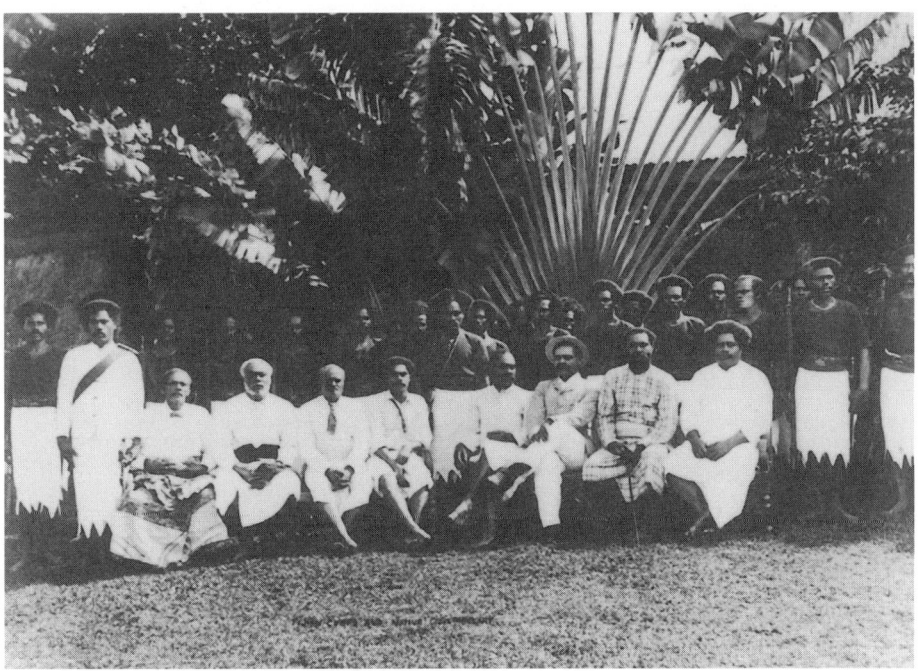

Fig. 17. "Fijian Chiefs and Native Constabulary" (original caption). (From photo album of W.C.F., *Views of Fiji* [Mitchell Library, Sydney, ML ref. F988.8/1A1].)

and state laws. Island demography in 1900 is very hard to reconstruct, but she contends that it was most likely one of low fertility, coupled with high mortality, especially of infants and mothers. McMurray (1993c), too, suggests very high rates of mortality in the Solomons in the late nineteenth and early twentieth centuries due to the combined effects of introduced disease and endemic diseases—of malaria, yaws, tuberculosis, and leprosy. But, whereas she opines that "Solomon Islanders have probably always tended to have large families" (McMurray 1993c, 91) and that growth was checked primarily by high mortality, Dureau suggests that large families were *not* characteristic of the pre-Christian past and believes cultural constraints on fertility were as crucial as biological ones.

Based on both genealogical and oral historical data she suggests a past ideal of two children per woman—one to carry and one to guide while escaping raids in war. This ideal may have been difficult to realize, not just because of late menarche and irregular ovulation, coupled with high rates of infant mortality, but because of indigenous patterns of sexual sequestration and abstinence. Married couples were enjoined to abstain for protracted periods, not only after the birth of a child but during the phases of fishing and warfare when men lived in large communal houses and stayed celibate, lest by losing semen they lost potency. Since married women were probably struggling to realize their ideal of two children, herbal contraceptions, abortifacients, and infanticide were likely more important to those women who conceived either before or beyond marriage. Contraception then was "women's business," and Dureau argues that women were, in reproductive affairs, autonomous of their husbands. And yet this indigenous regime of reproduction was surely a manifestation neither of women's collectivity nor their unfettered autonomy. Birthing, alone or assisted by other female kin (see Dureau 1993, 1998), was seen as dangerous and defiling, both according to oral testimony of living Simbo women and foreign ethnographers' accounts of that era. Moreover, although husbands exerted little influence over their wives' fertility, brothers were vitally interested in the sexuality and fertility of their sisters. Their own survival and success in bonito and head-hunting expeditions was thought to depend on their sisters' sexual continence. A woman who had sex with someone other than her husband could be killed by her *luluna* (her brother, real or classificatory). Thus, I would argue that women's autonomy in bearing or not bearing babies was ultimately eclipsed by philosophies of growth and fertility that privileged the violent control and the spiritual transcendence of men (cf. Biersack 1995).

On the basis of intensive genealogical and oral historical research, Dureau further suggests that the impact of Christian missions dramatically increased both the ideal and the actual number of live children per woman. This was not just through the corporeal effects of medicalizing childbirth or introduced drugs but due to a novel Christian celebration of conjugal intimacy and husbands' rights. "Pacification" by the British in 1900 meant not just the end of warfare but the end of those communal houses that were the repository of ancestral skulls and the site of a group's regeneration. The message of Methodism was heard and uncommonly heeded soon after (Dureau 1994). Ancestral practices that constrained fertility were challenged by missionaries—not just contraception, abortion, and infanticide but also protracted breastfeeding, postpartum abstinence, and long periods of ritual renunciation. In stressing the spiritual superiority of a monogamous, more nucleated family, missionaries also insisted on the conjugal rights of men as husbands. Although the ancestral vitality of the brother's interest in the sexuality and fertility of his sister and the contemporary strength of men's corporeal claims as husbands may be violent and extreme on Simbo, there are elements of this pattern that are common throughout the southwest Pacific (see Jolly and Macintyre 1989).

Such projects of reform were not just colonial impositions. Although both women and men on Simbo often proclaim that certain aspects of parenting today are because "the missionaries told us" Christianity has here, as elsewhere, been indigenized (see Barker 1992; White 1991). Throughout the Pacific, people talk of passing from the "time of darkness" to the "time of light," and in this process new gendered values of sexuality, conjugality, and parenthood were and are promoted. Such values are today being advanced in the second wave of conversions in the Pacific, in the burgeoning influence of evangelical and charismatic churches throughout the islands of the southwest and in the interior of Papua New Guinea. The family values espoused can be discerned from a booklet entitled *Marriage: The Melanesian Way*, published in Wewak by Christian Books Inc. (Fountain 1984). This details the bad aspects of "traditional marriage"—polygamy, the bride-price, and arranged marriage—and perceives the underlying problem as "the lower status of women" (1984, 11).[3] It also attacks the falsity of indigenous beliefs—that menstrual blood is polluting, that several acts of intercourse are needed to make the baby, and that the "man not have intercourse with his wife during pregnancy and breastfeeding. All these beliefs are false and come about because of an inadequate understanding of how conception takes place" (1984, 13). Such misconceptions create tensions that can be averted not just by accurate information about "the biology of sex and child-birth" but, more reliably, by forming marriages between individuals based on "love and mutual respect" (1984, 17). Christian marriage promises a new, more individuated kind of person in relation to collectivities and transformed relations of sexuality and fertility between women and men. But at this point we need to look more closely at this imagined past of traditional marriage and beyond to what I have telegraphically called "ancestral regimes of fertility."

Taim Bilong Tumbuna: By Ancient Custom?

Offering *any* portrait of ancestral fertility is fraught with the dangers of recuperation through reconstruction. Anthropologists are, perhaps justly, often accused of both romanticizing the ancestral past of Pacific *kastom* and of denying the radical effects of foreign intrusion. There is, as Shelley Mallett (1995) has consummately argued, a particular tendency to exoticize and dehistoricize in the literature on "conception" beliefs in Melanesia. She highlights how in recent conversations with women and men on Nuakata Island (the Massim, Papua New Guinea) her own questions were saturated with presumptions—derived from her prior reading of Massim ethnographies and her "commonsense" of Western philosophical precepts. This discursive frame included ancient debates on "virgin birth" in the Trobriands or, in her phrase, "insubstantial paternity" (cf. Wolfe 1999); the substantialist fixations of most anthropological theories about Melanesian conception, and Western premises about how the conjugation of egg and sperm determined not just sexed individuals but gendered identities (Martin 1991). Mallett (1995) acknowledges how all this shaped her faltering questions, such as "How is the baby made?" Rather than proffering either a canonical Melanesian or a biomedical model in reply, her interlocutors, like Mona, insisted that babies were, ultimately, the result of divine agency, the work of God (cf. Dureau, this volume). Although menstrual blood and being with a man matters, it is "God who makes matter," "God who forms the baby." Initially frustrated by such replies, Mallett asked if Mona's mother believed something different, and in response Mona recounted the second creation story in Genesis! In stressing biblical rather than indigenous knowledge, Mona stressed shared rather than different cultural understandings (1995, 55). Heeding Mallett's example, we must in reconstructions of a Pacific or a Melanesian past, of ancestral patterns of fertility be aware of how pasts are made presents, in contemporary debates about fertility and population.[4] Contemporary Pacific women and men negotiate a confluence between different and sometimes contesting ancestral, Christian, and biomedical understandings of conception and pregnancy, nurture and growth.

Let me evoke the potency and the contemporaneity of such contests through an image of a powerful and dangerous fertility stone from south Pentecost, Vanuatu. Carved from sandstone in a Janus form it is modeled with the characteristic anthropomorphic features of "ancestors," more widely known from the carved faces of wooden *slitgongs* from the neighboring and culturally cognate island of Ambrym. Such stones are still planted in gardens to make tubers (yams and taro) grow and swell.[5] In the traditionalist villages of this region they are the particular preserve of indigenous priests of agricultural fertility, who initiate the several phases of gardening, clearing, planting, weeding, harvesting, and who must during these dangerous days abstain from sexual relations. They bury the stone to secure a bountiful harvest for all. Its face is benign, almost smiling. The fingers rest on a swollen stomach, perhaps corpulent and satiated with food or swollen with a baby. In Sa, the indigenous language, the expression *ni mkup* is similarly ambiguous—signifying either a stomach stretched with food or a fetus. But, despite the palpable mimesis between making crops and babies grow, this like many other fertility statues, stones, flutes, and bullroarers from the southwest Pacific are not supposed to be seen by women. Indeed, a woman's ability to conceive and bear children is thought to be imperiled if she so much as gazes at one. When stones such as these were displayed in 1996 in a superb exhibition of the arts of Vanuatu in Port Vila, *Spirit blong bubu i kam bak* (The spirits of the ancestors have returned), women were excluded from the partitioned space where they were

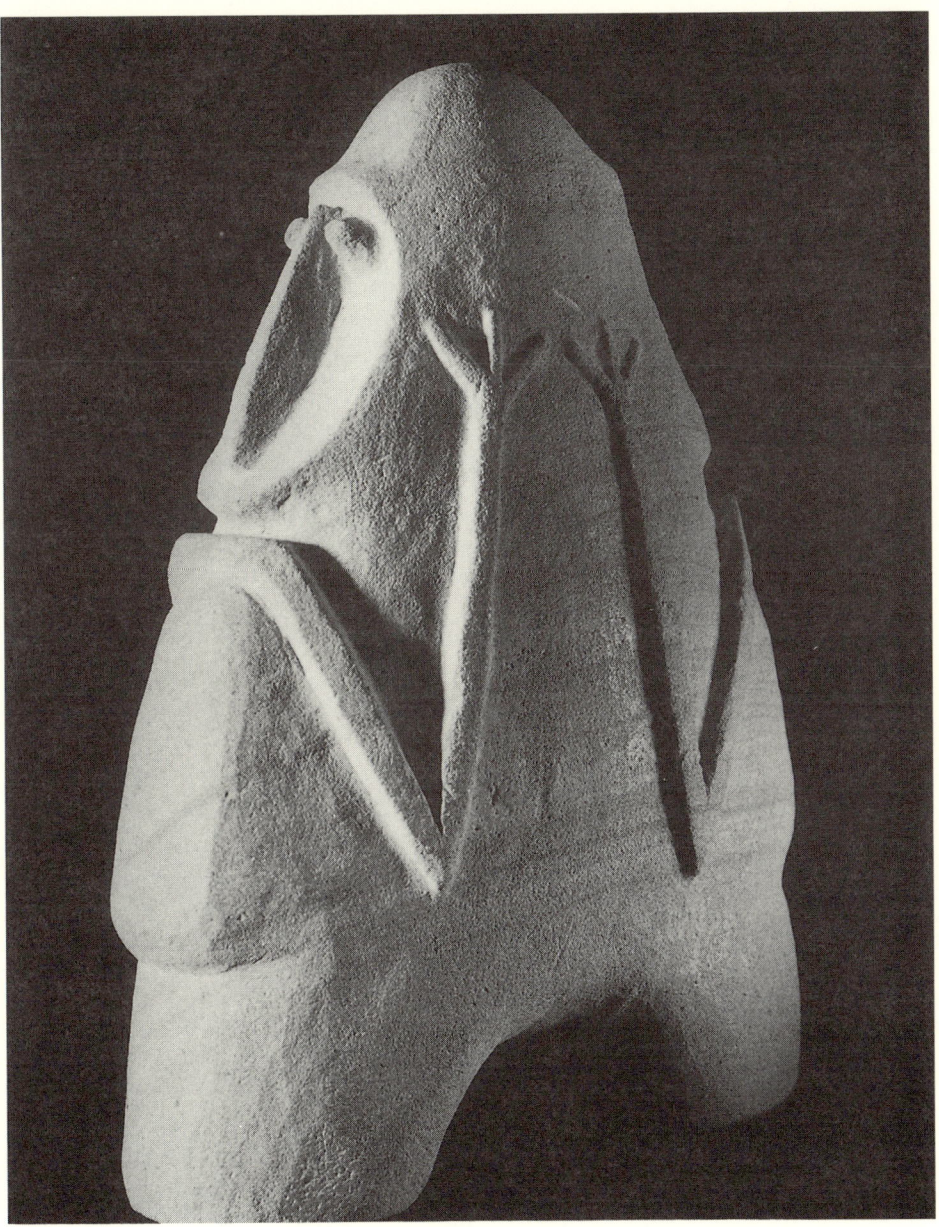

Fig. 18. Sandstone sculpture in Janus form, with ancestral faces, used to ensure the fertility of crops in south Pentecost, Vanuatu. (In the author's collection; photograph by Bob Cooper.)

displayed, and a male guard was permanently posted outside.[6] Although several leaders of evangelical churches objected to the entire exhibition as recuperating and disseminating the "arts of the devil," most indigenous women and local women's organizations calmly signaled their acceptance of the fact that such stones should be sequestered, since they were powerful and dangerous to their persons.

As well as evoking a cultural political contest about the power of the ancestors projecting into the present, such objects embody the three dimensions of ancestral, indigenous fertility I now highlight—first, the intimate connection between human and ecological fertility; second, the celebration of controlled fertility through abstinence; and, third, the problematic relation of women and men in negotiating their respective powers of fertility. Let me consider these dimensions, first in very general terms and then through the lens of the ethnographic literature on "male cults" in Melanesia.

Ancestral regimes of fertility like contemporary family planning programs posited a connection between person and collectivity, but the nature of these categories, their gendered connection and the very conception of fertility or reproduction differed. In the Pacific past human fertility was intrinsically connected to the fertility and growth of other living things: life, growth, and health bore witness to ancestral or divine blessing just as famine, sickness, and death portended the opposite. Whereas in contemporary debates in developed countries we struggle to integrate population with ecology in models of "sustainable development," indigenous Pacific constructs routinely linked the fertility of humans with that of nature through cosmogenetic conceptions, evoked in narratives, rites, and objects.

Throughout the southwest Pacific the fertility of persons was inherently related to the fertility of the world, and especially to those parts of the natural world that were planted and nurtured like human persons. From many isolated islands and remote valleys we know of the intimate connections perceived between growing pigs or crops—yams, taro, sweet potato, or extracting sago—and growing babies. Such links have been typically interpreted as metaphoric—the womb is likened to the *bilum*, or basket, used to carry crops (see Strathern 1981; cf. MacKenzie 1991). Pigs were thought to "mirror" the ways in which women and men reproduced (Jolly 1984). But the concept of metaphor depends on the prior separation of semantic fields, and in many languages human and natural fertility were in fact perceived as a single domain. So, among the Sa speakers of south Pentecost, Vanuatu, with whom I lived in the 1970s, the vernacular notion of *lo sal* (inside the road or path) denotes the process of regeneration that connects birth, circumcision, marriage, and death with the rites of growing crops, nurturing and then sacrificing pigs, and, in the past, killing people. The growth, fertility, and sexuality of the human body are linked with root and tree crops—taro with women, yams with men, and coconuts with both (Jolly 1994b, 68, 167–68). Coconut juice, likened both to mother's milk and to semen, is poured onto babies as a tonic for their growth and future fertility. But sacrifice and death is also required to make things grow. Pigs are still sacrificed to the ancestors to secure the health of the living and the growth of crops. Until the late 1920s, enemies were killed in war to propitiate ancestors while cannibal feasts revitalized the strength not just of male warriors but all men and women of the victorious group.

Despite tremendous linguistic and cultural diversity throughout the Austronesian- and Papuan-speaking regions of the southwest Pacific and the variable nature and intensity of growing crops and raising pigs, there *was* a constant in that human fertility was connected to broader notions of fecundity, which was seen to have both originated in and be guaranteed by ancestral power. Such ancestors might be so remote from the living as to constitute primordial deities, or be so close as to be little more than the embodiments of the named dead, but their benevolent or malevolent relation to this world was everywhere witnessed. Divine, ancestral powers were seen both as the ultimate cause of a successful harvest or drought and famine and of healthy babies or the blights of barrenness and death in childbirth.[7] Both men and women were typically seen to attain mature, adult identity only when they became fathers or mothers. Infertility, usually traced to the mother rather than the father, was much lamented but regularly assuaged by pervasive practices of adoption. More generally, classificatory kinship practices, though diverse, celebrated collective modes of generation and nurture rather than privileging the elementary relation of mother, father, and child.

Yet, despite the pervasive ideals of fecundity and growth, these were not valued as uncontrolled, as the wild, untrammeled forces of either nature or human nature (cf. MacCormack and Strathern 1980). Throughout the region there was a pervasive stress on the *control* of human fertility. This was, as I have already suggested, often through abstinence and celibacy. Prolonged, frequent breastfeeding was sustained in most islands and often linked with protracted postpartum abstinence, through the widespread notion that semen soured or spoiled breast milk (Marshall 1985, 159–62, 167–68, 181–83). Sexual sequestration and celibacy was also characteristically enjoined in phases of agriculture, hunting, fishing, and warfare as well as during the extended rituals of male initiation or fertility cults. So, again illustrating from my ethnographic research with the Sa speakers of Vanuatu, there were long periods of abstinence (*palan*) in the lives of both women and men. *Ni mpal* (I abstain) is an expression used for both fasting and sexual continence. Sexual abstinence is typically accompanied by restrictions on eating certain foods, foods that are marked by the gender of their contexts rather than their consumers. When a baby is born, both mother and father (and classificatory "mothers"and "fathers") eat only taro, and not yams, for twenty days afterward. The parents refrain from sexual intercourse for two to three years after the birth, or as long as the infant suckles. If the child is a boy, they refrain from sex again for several months after his circumcision at about age five and eat only yams for this period. Eating taro would debilitate him, while having sex would cause the circumcision sores to fester and stink. Couples are also enjoined to abstain from sex during the planting and harvest of yams and taro and during the rites of killing pigs and the land dive.[8]

Elsewhere I have argued that the stress on birth spacing and on periodic sexual abstinences or renunciations was not so much a negative proscription as a positive, productive injunction, ensuring health and well-being (Jolly 2001a). The widespread postpartum taboo on conjugal sexuality was expressly to space children as one spaces taro in a garden so that the child or tuber grows and swells, with sufficient sustenance. Along with avoiding the contamination of semen, it was thought that if a woman had a baby on the breast and one in the belly at the same time, then neither would thrive. The locus of such control was not foremost an individual exercising choice (cf. Strathern 1988, 272–73) but, rather, a collectivity, a local group or a lineage that through such cyclical renunciations ensured both the replacement of persons and the perpetuation of an ancestrally ordained order.

But—as well as abstinence—indigenous contraceptives, abortifacients, and infanticide are widely reported not just for Vanuatu (see Jolly 2001b) but throughout the region, and these were more under the control of women and, it is often claimed, used against the wishes of husbands and male-dominated groups (see Narokobi et al. 1980, qtd. earlier). So, McDowell (1988, 10) reports the almost universal presence of contraception, abortion, and infanticide throughout Papua New Guinea, although all were progressively outlawed by the Christian churches from the late nineteenth century and made illegal by the colonial state and then the independent state from 1975. Contraceptives were usually derived from the bark of trees, but also used were vines, bamboo shoots, betel nuts, and various peelings, leaves and petals. Some techniques involved not internal ingestion, but application to the outside of the body—stinging nettles rubbed on the abdomen or spells recited over plants such as taro or pandanus, whose uprooting or decay were supposed to simulate the infertility desired by the woman.[9] The reasons adduced for contraception frequently included avoidance of the pain and discomfort of childbirth or limiting family size, but women also mentioned the desire not to lose their beauty or avoid being tied to an undesirable husband. Contraceptives were also used to prevent children being born of premarital or extramarital liaisons (16–17). The reasons for abortion were rather similar, but abortion was often the preferred solution if conjugal sex had taken place during a prohibited period or a child had been conceived in an illicit union (15–16). Infanticide was also widely practiced in the past. Twins, abnormal babies, or those born of illicit or incestuous unions were especially at risk. In some parts of Papua New Guinea, and elsewhere in the region, female infanticide was more common than male (see McArthur 1974; McDowell 1988, 18–19). Frequently mentioned as a reason for infanticide, especially in the Highlands and the Sepik regions, was anger or revenge toward the husband and the desire to spite or subvert the strength of his group (McDowell 1988, 18–19; and see Narokobi et al. 1980, 36). Yet, although women did have some autonomous control over reproduction and could flout the desires of husbands and other male kin, fertility was not seen to be exclusively or even primarily their concern and responsibility, a fact that is obvious from even a preliminary perusal of the extensive literature of the anthropology of male cults.[10]

The Anthropology of Male Cults

Most of the ethnographic literature on fertility in the southwest Pacific is about not women or birth, which is rarely depicted and analyzed (see Byford 1999), but the elaborate rituals of male cults (see Allen 1967; Herdt 1981, 1987; Jolly 2001a) or, in more recent parlance, fertility cults (e.g., Whitehead 1986). Yet, although birthing is rarely foregrounded, the relation between women's birthing and male cults has long been debated, with a suite of theories suggesting that they mimic women's natural reproductive capacities, a mimesis variously attributed to male anxiety, envy, or sheer antagonism. Whereas the work of the late Annette Weiner (1976, 1982, 1988, 1995) stressed the centrality of women in reproduction, both corporeal and social, in the matrilineal Trobriands, in many other parts of Papua New Guinea—in the Highlands and the Sepik, for instance—it is men who vaunt their centrality in the processes of reproduction. There is a tendency for Western observers to read this as male posturing, as dubious claims to spiritual transcendence, on the presumption that mothers are made by nature, and fathers by culture.

This presumptive dichotomy of the biological bedrock of maternity as against the cultural construction of "insubstantial paternity" has been most powerfully criticized by Marilyn Strathern (1988). She has probably been the most fervent deconstructionist for the Pacific of the view of gender as grounded in sex, in the biology of male and female natures (but see Butler 1993; Martin 1987). Both in analyzing gender relations in Melanesia and in discerning the impact of the new reproductive technologies in the "West" she posits a theory of gender that does not presume the "facts" of sexual difference. For Melanesia she posits, in opposition to a "Western" model of an individual defined by the edges of the body, a notion of a "partible person," composed of both masculine and feminine aspects and formed by multiple authorship, of debts to others. She detects how ethnographers have imposed Euro-American theories of conception, gestation, and nurture onto Melanesian materials. This is nowhere clearer than in her critique of Herdt's analysis of male cults (1981, 1987). When Sambia or Baruya men say that breast milk is in fact transformed semen, ingested from the husband in intercourse and fellatio, or that it is men, not women, who make babies, can we simply dismiss this on the basis of our own folk or scientific theories? Strathern suggests that Euro-American conception theories imply that the baby more naturally "belongs" to the mother, that it is an extension of her proprietorial body. For Sambia and Baruya, she avers, the maternal body is, in local understandings, a paternal body (Jolly 1992, 144; Strathern 1988, 314–18).

Strathern's deconstructive exercises are scintillating but depend on a rhetorical strategy that constructs Melanesia and the "West" as antithetical and which ultimately denies their historical relation in the course of colonialism and postcolonial development projects. Even such understandings of bodies and persons characteristic of those in the interior Highlands of Papua New Guinea have been in conversation with Western models—imported by Christian missions, by state officials, and by development agents since the "first contacts" of the 1930s. She thus marginalizes the very processes that constitute my central questions—if and how the "partible persons" of ancestral collectivities are slowly being remade into modern "individuals," invested with the new sexual antagonism of reproductive interests, mobilized by nation-states and international agencies. This process not only has the potential to interpellate a new individuated subject but to cast male and female interests as perforce opposed in the politics of fertility. In the ethnography of male cults we view a world in which homosocial, even homosexual, male desires and interests transcend heterosexuality and domesticity, through cosmogenetic narratives of fertility and a masculinist mythopoesis of life and death. By contrast, the demography of family planning is firmly focused on the daily practices and life projects of the conjugal couple (and especially the wife) but attempts to link these to the broader collective visions of nation-states and international agencies promoting urgent messages, to save the nation and the planet. Such global prophecies have in some Pacific sites encountered more parochial doomsday visions, with the advent of evangelical Christianity and the termination of male cults.

Several observers of the Highlands of Papua New Guinea witness that with the end of male cults there has not been that reduction of sexual hostility and male domination that earlier theorists such as Langness (1967) might have predicted but, rather, a shift to new forms of strife between men and women. Meggitt (1989) suggested that the end of pollution beliefs and avoidance practices had generated greater sexual violence and rape among the Mae Enga. Later ethnographers reported not just worsening relations between women and men but, indeed, indigenous theories of a wasting world, which connected notions of human malaise and cosmic degeneration. So, Clark (1997) documented Huli men's perceptions that the end of the bachelor cult had rendered young men less healthy, their skin flabby and dull, their bodies emaciated and shrinking.[11] Women, and especially those who do not conform to the novel Christian models of the good wife and mother, are perceived by men as hungry for sex and money. They are labeled *pamuk,* promiscuous, loose women, even prostitutes. They, rather than their male partners or clients, are seen as the source of sexual promiscuity and venereal diseases, including HIV/AIDS, spreading along the new roads of modernity and state penetration. Money is perceived as hot and dirty, as polluting as was women's "bad blood" before. So Clark (1997) charted a transformation of a misogynist mythopoetics from an older sexual antagonism predicated on collective segregation and celibacy to a newer sexual antagonism based on the violent exercise of sexual self-interest on the part of both women and men (see also Knauft 1997 and Tuzin 1997). Money here is linked to undisciplined and deviant sexuality and fertility, not the consoling image of middle-class restraint that Calick (1993) imagines.

A recent but controversial national study of sexual and reproductive knowledge and behavior in Papua New Guinea (National Sex and Reproduction Research Team and Jenkins 1994) suggests that the Huli pattern of increasing promiscuity, spreading venereal diseases, increasing sexual commerce, and mounting sexual violence is not unique. This report aspires to bring together the aims of combating HIV/AIDS and enhancing "family planning." It again insists that sexual and reproductive health programs need to engage men as well as women and to be accessible to adolescents, single people and those in sexual liaisons beyond the normative conjugal couple or "family." Novel sexualities and fertilities in the southwest Pacific pose urgent problems for planners of families and of states. But how far is the female and family focus of most family planning projects adequate to the task?

The Demography of Contemporary Family Planning in the Pacific

While men are central to the huge literature on male cults or fertility rituals in Melanesia, they are much less visible in the demographic literature and the contemporary policy and practice of family planning in the Pacific. We can perhaps discern the reasons for this in the important pioneering work by scholars such as Agyei (1988) and McDowell (1988) in Papua New Guinea. Both recognized the indigenous prevalence of family planning, but posed questions about the changing relation of men and women in reproductive decision making, and the changing "value of children." Ultimately both saw men as *the* problem in the implementation of modern contraceptive practice.

William Agyei, a Ugandan demographer who worked in Papua New Guinea in the early 1980s, was despite his commitment to a global theory of demographic transition in the Third World sensitive to local beliefs and practices of fertility. His study, based on a survey of several thousand men and women in both villages and towns, reported perduring and pervasive patterns of breastfeeding and sexual abstinence, everywhere seen as ensuring the welfare of mother and child. Although breastfeeding persisted for an average of about twenty-one months in rural and urban areas, abstinence was recorded as being rather briefer in towns.[12]

This survey revealed fertility that was "high by world standards" and documented that, although both rural and urban respondents favored "large" families, the rural ideal was about six and the urban ideal about four for *both* men and women, regardless of whether they lived in villages or towns. Agyei found that the majority of *both* men and women wanted large families. But, unlike men, women could see the advantages of smaller families in having enough land and money, food and clothes. Children were desired to support their parents in old age but also to contribute to the wealth and strength of the extended family. Not only husbands but male-dominated local groups, lineages, and *wantoks* (communities of people speaking the same language) were implicated in urging women to have more children. Desire for fewer children was seen to arise especially from women's education and from the perceived pressures of the cash economy, especially in town.

Knowledge about contraceptives was, he found, high in both urban and rural areas, but practice was predominantly in traditional methods such as breastfeeding, abstinence, and "village medicine," with little use of modern methods—the pill, injection, loop, condom, the ovulation or rhythm method. Usage of such modern methods was rather higher in urban than rural regions, a difference Agyei imputed to easier access. He noted that women could not attain contraceptives from hospitals or clinics without their husbands' consent and that single women or adolescents were obliged to go to private doctors, possible only in towns (Agyei 1988, 99–102). Modern contraceptives were not used because of perceived dangers to mothers and children and because of husbands' disapproval (1988, 103).

Although Agyei thought that negativity about modern methods was the result of "ignorance" and "cultural conservatism," on the part of men particularly, he also discerned that some women were hostile because they feared diminished control over their own fertility. He brushed aside such obstacles, however, and placed his faith in nationwide education programs based on indigenous methods. He vaunted the Breastfeeding Promotion Programme as the "pivot on which the formulation of policy hinges" (1988, 119), since breastfeeding not only promoted infant nutrition but, if frequent enough, had an anovulatory effect. But methods other than abstinence were needed, especially for those urban, highly-educated women who were not able to breastfeed for long. Yet, paradoxically in his view, breastfeeding was also an obstacle, since it consolidated practices of sexual abstinence and obstructed "the serious use of modern contraception to space births" (1988, 120). Breastfeeding and abstinence needed to be complemented by "modern" family planning services. The main obstacle he discerned on the path to modernity was not so much women's reluctance but male opposition. Women's fears and anxieties about modern methods were construed as "ignorance," and women were assumed to tolerate increased state control over their fertility in exchange for more autonomy from men.

This perception of women securing greater reproductive autonomy from men through an alliance with the forces of modernity and the state is advanced in more radical feminist terms by McDowell and her coauthors (1988). In her introduction she also insisted on the prevalence of indigenous family planning and queried the relevance of the theory of demographic transition to Papua New Guinea and in particular arguments advanced about the changing "value of children" on the evidence of peasant societies in Asia and Africa. In Papua New Guinea she noted boys did little work at all, and so compulsory schooling and capitalist transformations in agriculture would not necessarily radically transform the "value" of male children. She asserted that rural women wanted "to plan their families, space their children and often limit the number of children they bear (even if their husbands do not agree)" (1988, 7).

Unlike Agyei she stressed the gap between the reproductive interests and ideals of women and men. Despite the ethnographic diversity displayed in the collection she edited she found a uniformity in that "women often desired fewer children than men, and men never wanted fewer than women" (1988, 12).

She derived this difference from collective (masculinist) concerns about group strength rather than the individuated rationality of the conjugal couple. Many children and large groups were seen to secure security in a hostile and changing world, and family planning projects were seen by some as tantamount to ethnocide. At the most extreme were the "Baby Gardens" of the Hahalis Welfare Society in Buka, where free sex and unrestrained fertility were promoted both as anticolonial practice and ethnic recuperation—the foundation of Bougainvillean strength vis-à-vis the rest of Papua New Guinea (McDowell 1988, 239–40). Although some female politicians, like Josephine Abijah (*Post-Courier* 1974, qtd. earlier), opposed family planning, McDowell saw group concerns about vitality and security as preeminently male affairs (1988, 238–42). But coupled with this image of an expansionist male-dominated collectivity was the image of the jealous, anxious husband. Family planning was seen by many Papua New Guinean men as posing the threat of female promiscuity and of adultery (see also Dureau, this volume). Yet, whereas a woman did not need her husband's approval to abort or contracept in the past, now a woman who wanted to avail herself of modern methods must first ask her husband's permission. Like Agyei, McDowell placed her faith in effective family planning programs, in clinics with good supplies of contraceptives, expert staff, and education to allay the "fears and anxieties," especially of the rural and uneducated (1988, 7).

And yet a decade later family planning programs in Papua New Guinea, as elsewhere in the southwest Pacific, continue to disappoint those who desire to restrict population. In part, this derives from the economic and political insufficiencies of these small states. Despite the ardor and largesse of international donors and agencies committed to population control, these are poor countries and health services in Papua New Guinea, the Solomons and Vanuatu are rapidly deteriorating rather than improving. Moreover, as Dureau argues for the Solomons (this volume), the seeming mutuality of women's and government goals are regularly confounded by inadequate health services, which, if they have supplies at all, fail to deliver the forms of contraception women desire. But we might also ask how far disappointments are due to sexual and reproductive issues still being promoted in the context of maternal and child health. This is clear in the chronic coupling of those very acronyms MCH/FP—maternal and child health and family planning. How far, we might ask, is male hostility not only presumed but perpetuated by the very character of family planning services? Little research or practice focuses on men and fertility since women are, it seems, the more natural parents and thus the natural targets of family planning programs.[13]

Indeed, some demographic analyses not only describe but prescribe an emancipatory desire for women to "free" themselves from the reproductive controls of men, as an expression of a modernist sensibility. One of the important, accumulating effects of missionary and colonial state projects in the region was to focus attention and responsibility for parenting on women as mothers (see Jolly 1998). Although men as husbands were credited with power over their wives, this power was typically constructed as more distant or "auxiliary" to the intimate power women exerted as mothers. Many contemporary family planning programs perpetuate, and even amplify, this tendency to construct having and not having babies as "women's business." So, the residual power of a husband to veto the contraceptive choices of his wife is often seen as the recalcitrant persistence of indigenous misogyny or, as in Agyei's analysis, "cultural conservatism." Yet this conjugal veto probably owes more to Christian and colonial doctrines of the husband/father as the head of a monogamous, nuclear family than it does to ancestral models of fertility.

It is crucial to empower women in their sexual and reproductive lives, but the process whereby they, rather than men, are the targets of family planning tends both to extrude men from the process and exempt them from a sense of responsibility or mutuality in deciding if and when to have babies. Of course, mutuality is a mirage in households dominated by male interests. And the reproductive desires of single women and men may diverge as much as those of married couples. Yet we might ponder how the very structure of contraceptive services, with their familial but female focus, compounds such gendered tensions and conflicts. In the southwest Pacific, as elsewhere, be they the objectified targets of states and international agencies or the subjects who choose, it is women who are typically privileged as the natural locus of fertility in the globalizing rhetoric and practice of population politics.

Conclusion

In the introduction to this volume I discussed some of the more general, theoretical problems with the notion of choice in the arena of global reproductive politics, and in particular the International Conference on Population and Development held in Cairo in 1994. What relevance does this have for the Pacific? As with all international conferences the pressing questions are how far the resolutions will be effectively implemented. A research project sponsored by the Asian-Pacific Resource and Research Centre for Women (ARROW) in the Asia-Pacific region found few concrete changes in the eight countries surveyed and claimed that population policies remained "demographic centred and target-oriented in terms of quantifiable goals, rather than people centred development" (ARROW 1996, 1). Although no new national policies had been developed, there had at program level been a

> widespread shift conceptually from family planning and maternal and child health to a concern with broadening reproductive health, to include youth and older women and a range of services dealing with sexually transmitted diseases and reproductive cancers. But sexuality education, services for adolescents and innovations to "increase men's responsibility for reproduction and sexual health" were still missing. (1996, 2)

We might ask, how can the dual aims of empowering women and embracing men in the new global reproductive politics be achieved? They are not necessarily mutually exclusive. But their combination may prove particularly difficult in the Pacific. "Empowering" women might, as in many other times and places, be interpreted as an attack on traditional culture from new foreign agencies, albeit those representing international rather than imperial interests. But, as we have witnessed in the regional debates on human rights, the universal or international is too often blithely equated with *Western* and often opposed, particularly by Pacific men, as a new form of foreign or imperial intrusion (see Jolly 1996b).

Indigenous regimes of fertility in the Pacific were predicated on conjoint and collective processes of reproduction. They did not thereby entail consensual or harmonious relations between men and women, but *both* were vitally involved. Although making children entailed the separation of women and men as much as their conjugation, these "separate spaces" were not thereby spaces of reproductive freedom or autonomy. Indeed, to read such stories into these ancient sites risks writing recuperative feminist romances. It projects into the past not just the Western, capitalist ideal of individuated subjects but the consoling fiction that indigenous women were poised to liberate themselves from the control of indigenous men. Such a stress on the resistant agency and the particular emancipatory promise of women in breaking the bonds of tradition or male domination has a long history in the colonial discourses of the southwest Pacific, from the earliest travelers' tales, through missionary tracts, to the edicts of colonial and contemporary population projects.[14]

The engagement of missionary and colonial state officials with population had important, if paradoxical, effects. They focused on mothers as the agents of *de*population. Early "family planning" to *re*populate similarly occurred in the context of maternal and child health. Both Christian missions and colonial states rewarded fathers for robustly insisting on their conjugal rights, but missionaries and states alike also vaunted women's agency to escape the yoke of tradition and male domination. The long history of family planning in maternal and child health clinics run by missions or government will need to be reconceptualized if men are not to continue to view these as sites where women "sneak off" to pursue their own selfish interests—for fewer children or better sex.

The new global rhetoric of choice again privileges women and again risks entrenching the assumption that men are *by their nature* hostile to such choices, and especially choices to have fewer children. Of course, many men *are* hostile to family planning, or they may publically support family planning but privately resist it. Some men *do* oppose their wives' desires for fewer children. But the divergent interests of husband and wife, men and women, are also entangled in contests between local, national, and global interests, which often *construct* their desires and interests as irrevocably opposed.

NOTES

I thank Heather Booth, Bronwen Douglas, Deb Foskey, Greg Fry, Peter Larmour, Lisa Law, Shelley Mallett, Julie Park, Fiona Paisley, Penelope Schoeffel, Philip Setel, Christine Sylvester, Andrea Whittaker, and Jimmy Weiner for comments and criticisms of this essay in its successive drafts. I am especially grateful to Heather for her critical demographic insights, and to Bronwen and Deb for pushing me to distinguish more carefully the notions of agency and of choice. I thank my coeditor, Kalpana Ram, for suggesting ways in which my own voice could better be heard amid the din of debate. I am also grateful for both the kind comments and the constructive criticisms of the two anonymous readers commissioned by the press. Not all the good suggestions could be effected in this version, which, because it eschews a linear journey on a huge terrain of place and time, may induce a vertiginous sense in the reader. Jimmy Weiner and Shelley Mallett are probably correct in thinking this should have been a book!

1. In Papua New Guinea, the Solomons and Vanuatu, pidgin languages are the dominant lingua franca between indigenous people. The pidgin of Papua New Guinea is called Tok Pisin, and that of Vanuatu is called Bislama. All these variants of pidgin are, despite lexicons derived from English, French, German, and Portuguese, Austronesian languages according to their grammar.

2. Given the particularistic cast of much of my other writing, I trust the reader might indulge and even appreciate my generalizing purpose here.

3. This booklet does in fact allude to some of the positive aspects of traditional marriage—the fact of there being little divorce—and even concedes that bride wealth strengthened the bonds of marriage through strengthening the relations of groups. But it also notes that bride wealth has, with the advent of the cash economy, become more like a price.

4. Mallett (1995, 1997) also suggests apropos indigenous understandings on Nuakata that conception is not a privileged moment in making babies. Compare Underhill-Sem (2000).

5. Such stones are reported on many islands throughout the archipelago—including Pentecost, Ambrym, Malo, and Malakula. Speiser includes natural lumps of stone and coral and those fashioned from soft tufa or sandstone in his category of amulets. As well as their uses in the growth of root and tree crops and pigs, and in causing rain or sun, he notes that such stones were also used both in causing and protecting against illness and sorcery attacks (Speiser 1990 [1923], 310–14; pl. 84). This intimate connection between creative and destructive aspects of sacred power has been noted by many commentators on Vanuatu (see Douglas 1989; Jolly 1996a). See also photographs of such stones in the museum collections in Paris and Basel as reproduced in *Arts of Vanuatu* (Bonnemaison et al. 1996, 164–67).

6. They were on public display to both men and women in the Basel display of the exhibition in 1997, but due deference was given to their dangerous power by sequestering them in a kind of alcove, which was demarcated with a blowup of a historical photograph taken by Speiser depicting a woman and a child sitting on the edge of the fence enclosing a men's communal house on Malakula.

7. This is not to deny the importance of notions of witchcraft, sorcery, and magic, the destructive and creative powers attributed to the living. But such powers were seen to emanate ultimately from the manipulation of divine sources of power in a realm beyond, though still in quotidian connection to the lived world.

8. This ritual, held in association with the yam harvest, has been much written about and photographed and is today an important tourist spectacle. It is acknowledged to be the inspiration for the Western craze of bungee jumping (Jolly 1994b).

9. See the specific techniques for contraception, abortion, and inducing sterility discussed by many contributors to McDowell 1988 (60–61, 89–90, 108, 156, 183). By comparison, in south Pentecost, Vanuatu, a distillation made from the petals of red hibiscus was made to induce menstruation or procure abortion. Walter and Bourdy (1986) attest to a wide variety of indigenous contraceptive techniques in Vanuatu and suggest only marginal acceptance of modern forms of family planning. Yet Osteria's survey records that those relying on "modern methods" of contraception varied from about 13.7 in the Northern District to about 27.1 in the urban areas. (1984, 114, table x-1)

10. Weiner argued for the Trobriands that it is women who generate intragenerational continuity and perpetuate the cycles of regeneration through their focal place in birth and death rituals. Men by contrast are marginal as fathers, contributing nurture and food rather than substance, and preoccupied with ephemeral rather than eternal matters (cf. Mosko 1985, 209–12). Weiner has been criticized by Strathern (1981) for the way she tended, especially in her earlier work, to identify women with their reproductive bodies and failed to concede the differences between women in the varied reproductive regimes of the region, witness the Melpa of the Highlands, studied by Strathern (1972, 1988).

11. This relates to the ancestral ideas about bachelors' beauty and glamor. Boys must ingest semen so that they grow and become stronger, healthier, and more beautiful than women—with shiny, taut skin, developed musculature, and magnificent hair (e.g., Biersack 1987, 1995; Herdt 1987, 139–55).

12. He reported that the average in rural regions was 21.4 months for men and 20.2 months for women, while in urban areas it was 19.5 months for men and 16.6 months for women. He does not comment on the intriguing fact that women reported shorter periods of abstinence than men.

13. In a rare recent exception Setel focuses on fertility in the male life course in his paper on the coastal Boiken of East Sepik Province, Papua New Guinea. Men often talk of "someone to take my place," by which they mean not only children as replacements in a corporeal, genealogical, or demographic sense but in perpetuating a man's place in ownership and control of natural resources and in perpetuating networks of debt and exchange. Men are seen to be vitally interested not just in the production of their own children but the broader business of social reproduction. Men's adult social identity as much as women's is attained through bearing or adopting children, not so much as one's individual descendants but to ensure the growth and strength of collectivities—local groups or lineages—in the variable local politics of exchange. Setel argues that for men fertility was still primarily testament to collective clan strength, rather than an expression of individual virility. "For Waviö men, sexuality lay at the centre of a cultural paradox: it was dangerous to one's health and masculinity while simultaneously fundamental to the attainment and maintenance of manhood" (Setel 2000, 233–34). But Setel also tries to situate this in the context of historical change. Although many aspects of the men's cults, the *tambaran,* here have been abandoned as elsewhere in the Sepik (see Tuzin 1997), the practices of gender segregation and of abstinence—and, indeed, the pervasive values of fertility as cosmology—continue "to inform notions of reproduction, gender and personhood." Christianity, here too, has afforded the greatest challenges, more strongly through the new charismatic churches, such as the Assemblies of God, rather than the older established congregations of Catholicism. With this second wave of conversions to evangelical Christianity comes anew the challenge to expose not just the illusions of male cults but the falsity of traditional beliefs about conception and pollution and the horror of women's subordination (Tuzin 1997).

14. I do not want to imply that this trope of emancipation accomplished such a liberatory effect on women. As Bronwen Douglas insists (pers. comm. 1998), missionary projects objectified women and subordinated rather than freed them. Moreover, women who did show undue "freedom" even vis-à-vis their husbands were castigated, unless this freedom entailed a movement toward the mission from a heathen husband. But the promise of improvement and of emancipation through enlightenment is a dominant trope and one that links colonial projects of "civilization" and contemporary projects of "development."

REFERENCES

Agyei, W. K. A. 1988. *Fertility and family planning in the Third World: A case study of Papua New Guinea.* London: Croom Helm.
Allen, M. R. 1967. *Male cults and secret initiations in Melanesia.* Melbourne: Melbourne University Press.
ARROW [Asian-Pacific Resource and Research Centre for Women]. 1996. Women's and gender perspectives in health policies and programmes. *ARROWs for Change* 2 (3): 1–12.
Barker, J. 1992. Christianity in western Melanesian ethnography. In *History and tradition in Melanesian anthropology,* ed. J. Carrier, 144–73. Berkeley: University of California Press.

Biersack, A. 1987. Moonlight: Negative images of transcendence in Paiela pollution. *Oceania* 57:178–94.

———. 1995. Heterosexual meanings: Society, economy, and gender among Ipilis. In *Papuan borderlands: Huli, Duna and Ipili perspectives on the Papua New Guinea highlands*, ed. A. Biersack, 231–63. Ann Arbor: University of Michigan Press.

Bonnemaison, J., et al., eds. 1996. *Arts of Vanuatu*. Bathurst, N.S.W.: Crawford House Publishing.

Booth, H. 1985. *Fertility and mortality in Vanuatu: The demographic analysis of the 1979 census*. Pacific Population Paper no. 1. Noumea, New Caledonia: South Pacific Commission.

Bushnell, A. F. 1993. "The horror" reconsidered: An evaluation of the historical evidence for population decline in Hawai'i, 1778–1803. *Pacific Studies* 16 (3): 115–62.

Bushnell, O. A. 1993. *The gifts of civilization: Germs and genocide in Hawai'i*. Honolulu: University of Hawaii Press.

Butler, J. P. 1993. *Bodies that matter: On the discursive limits of "sex."* New York: Routledge.

Byford, J. 1999. Dealing with death, beginning with birth: Women's health and childbirth on Misima Island, Papua New Guinea. Ph.D. diss., Australian National University, Canberra.

Caldwell, J. C. 1982. *Theory of fertility decline*. London: Academic Press.

Calick, R. 1993. A doomsday scenario? In *Pacific 2010: Challenging the future*, ed. R. Cole, 1–11. Canberra: National Centre for Development Studies, Research School of Pacific Studies, Australian National University.

Clark, J. 1997. State of desire: Transformations in Huli sexuality. In *Sites of desire, economies of pleasure: Sexualities in Asia and the Pacific*, ed. L. Manderson and M. Jolly, 191–211. Chicago: Chicago University Press.

Deacon, A. B. 1934. *Malekula: A vanishing people in the New Hebrides*, ed. C. H. Wedgwood. London: G. Routledge and Sons.

Decrease Report. 1896. *The report of a Commission of Enquiry into the decrease of the native population*. Suva, Fiji: Government Printers.

Denoon, D. 1995. Pacific Island depopulation: Natural or un-natural history? In *New countries and old medicine: Proceedings of an international conference on the history of medicine and health, Auckland, New Zealand, 1994*, ed. L. Bryder and D. A. Dow, 324–39. Auckland: Pyramid Press.

Douglas, B. 1989. Autonomous and controlled spirits: Traditional ritual and early interpretations of Christiantiy on Tanna, Aneityum and the Isle of Pines in comparative perspective. *Journal of the Polynesian Society* 98 (1): 7–48.

Dureau, C. M. 1993. Nobody asked the mother: Women and maternity on Simbo, western Solomon Islands. *Oceania* 64 (1): 18–35.

———. 1994. Mixed blessings: Christianity and history in women's lives, Simbo, western Solomon Islands. Ph.D. diss., Macquarie University.

———. 1998. From sisters to wives: Changing contexts of maternity on Simbo, Western Solomon Islands. In *Maternities and modernities: Colonial and postcolonial experiences in Asia and the Pacific*, ed. K. Ram and M. Jolly, 239–74. Cambridge: Cambridge University Press.

Foucault, M. 1980. *The history of sexuality: An introduction*, vol. 1. Trans. R. Hurley. New York: Vintage Books.

Fountain, O. 1984. *Marriage: The Melanesian way.* Wewak, P.N.G.: Christian Books Melanesia, Inc.

Fry, G. 1997. Framing the islands: Knowledge and power in changing Australian images of "The South Pacific." *The Contemporary Pacific* 9 (2): 305–44.

Gannicott, K. 1993. Population, development and growth. In *Pacific 2010: Challenging the future,* ed. R. Cole, 12–42. Canberra: National Centre for Development Studies, Research School of Pacific Studies, Australian National University.

Ginsburg, F., and R. Rapp, eds. 1995. *Conceiving the new world order: The global politics of reproduction.* Berkeley: University of California Press.

Greenhalgh, S., ed. 1995. *Anthropology and demographic inquiry.* Cambridge and New York: Cambridge University Press.

Griffen, V. 1994. Women, development and population: A critique of the Port Vila Declaration. In *Sustainable development or malignant growth? Perspectives of Pacific Island women,* ed. 'Atu Emberson-Bain, 63–72. Suva, Fiji: Marama Publications.

Hauʻofa, E. 1993. Our sea of islands. In *A new Oceania: Rediscovering our sea of islands,* ed. E. Waddell, V. Naidu, and E. Hau'ofa, 2–16. Suva: University of the South Pacific and Beake House.

———. 1998. The ocean in us. *Contemporary Pacific* 10 (2): 392–410.

Herdt, G. 1981. *Guardians of the flutes: Idioms of masculinity.* New York: McGraw-Hill.

———. 1987. *The Sambia: Ritual and gender in New Guinea.* New York: Holt, Rinehart and Winston.

Hunt, N. 1997. "Le bébé en brousse": European women, African birth spacing, and colonial intervention in breast feeding in the Belgian Congo. In *Tensions of empire: Colonial cultures in a bourgeois world,* ed. F. Cooper and A. L. Stoler, 287–321. Berkeley: University of California Press.

Jolly, M. 1984. The anatomy of pig love: Substance, spirit and gender in South Pentecost, Vanuatu. *Canberra Anthropology* 7 (1–2): 78–108.

———. 1991. "To save the girls for brighter and better lives": Presbyterian missions and women in the south of Vanuatu: 1848–1870. *Journal of Pacific History* 26 (1): 27–48.

———. 1992. Partible persons and multiple authors. A review of Marilyn Strathern's *The gender of the gift. Pacific Studies* 15 (1): 137–49.

———. 1994a. Colonial visions and postcolonial revisions: Families, family law and the allure of universalism. Keynote address to Anthropological Society of New Zealand Conference, Auckland, 22–24 August.

———. 1994b. *Women of the place: Kastom, colonialism and gender in Vanuatu.* Chur: Harwood Academic Publishers.

———. 1996a. Devils, holy spirits, and the swollen God: Translation, conversion and colonial power in the Marist Mission, Vanuatu, 1887–1934. In *Conversion to modernities: The globalization of Christianity,* ed. P. van der Veer, 231–62. New York and London: Routledge.

———. 1996b. *Woman ikat raet long human raet o no?* Women's rights, human rights and domestic violence in Vanuatu. In *The world upside down: Feminisms in the antipodes,* ed. A. Curthoys, H. Irving, and J. Martin. *Feminist Review* 52:169–90.

———. 1997. Woman-nation-state in Vanuatu: Women as signs and subjects in the discourses of *kastom,* modernity and Christianity. In *Narratives of nation in the*

South Pacific, ed. T. Otto and N. Thomas, 133–62. Amsterdam: Harwood Academic Publishers.

———. 1998. Other mothers: Maternal "insouciance" and the depopulation debate in Fiji and Vanuatu, 1890–1930. In *Maternities and modernities: Colonial and postcolonial experiences in Asia and the Pacific,* ed. K. Ram and M. Jolly, 177–212. Cambridge: Cambridge University Press.

———. 2001a. Damming the rivers of milk? Fertility, sexuality and celibacy in Vanuatu and Fiji. In *Gender in Melanesia and Amazonia: Essays in comparison,* ed. D. Tuzin and T. Gregor. Berkeley: University of California Press.

———. 2001b. From darkness to light? Epidemiologies and ethnographies of motherhood in Vanuatu. In *Birthing in the Pacific: Between tradition and modernity,* ed. V. Lukere and M. Jolly. Honolulu: University of Hawai'i Press.

Jolly, M., and M. Macintyre, eds. 1989. *Family and gender in the Pacific: Domestic contradictions and the colonial impact.* Cambridge: Cambridge University Press.

Kelly, J. 1991. *A politics of virtue: Hinduism, sexuality and countercolonial discourse in Fiji.* Chicago: University of Chicago Press.

Knauft, B. 1997. Gender identity, political economy and modernity in Melanesia and Amazonia. *Journal of the Royal Anthropological Institute* 3 (2): 233–59.

Lal, B. 1985. Kunti's cry: Indentured women on Fiji plantations. *Indian Economic and Social History Review* 22:55–71.

Langmore, D. 1989. The object lesson of a civilised, Christian home. *Family and gender in the Pacific: Domestic contradictions and the colonial impact,* 84–94. Cambridge: Cambridge University Press.

Langness, L. 1967. Sexual antagonism in the New Guinea Highlands: A Bena-Bena example. *Oceania* 37 (3): 161–77.

Lukere, V. 1997. Mothers of the Taukei: Fijian women and "the decrease of the race." Ph.D. diss., Australian National University.

MacCormack, C. P., and M. Strathern, eds. 1980. *Nature, culture and gender.* Cambridge: Cambridge University Press.

MacKenzie, M. A. 1991. *Androgynous objects: String bags and gender in central New Guinea.* Chur: Harwood Academic Publishers.

Mallett, S. 1995. Bearing the inconceivable. In *Work in flux,* ed. E. Greenwoood, K. Neumann, and A. Sartori, 41–57. Melbourne: Department of History, University of Melbourne.

———. 1997. Conceiving cultures: Person, place and health on Nua'ata, Papua New Guinea. Ph.D. diss., La Trobe University.

Manderson, L. 1982. Bottle feeding and ideology in colonial Malaya: The production of change. *International Journal of Health Services* 12 (4): 597–616.

———. 1984. "These are modern times": Infant feeding practice in Peninsular Malaysia. *Social Science and Medicine* 18 (1): 47–57.

Marshall, L. B., ed. 1985. *Infant care and feeding in the South Pacific.* New York: Gordon and Breach.

Martin, E. 1987. *The woman in the body.* Boston: Beacon Press.

———. 1991. The egg and the sperm: How science has constructed a romance based on stereotypical male-female roles. *Signs* 16 (3): 485–501.

McArthur, N. 1967. *Island populations of the Pacific.* Canberra: Australian National University Press.

———. 1974. Population and prehistory: The late phase on Aneityum. Ph.D. diss., Australian National University.

McDowell, N., ed. 1988. *Reproductive decision making and the value of children in rural Papua New Guinea.* IASER Monograph 27. Boroko: Institute of Applied Social and Economic Research.

McMurray, C. 1993a. Population projections, 1990–2010: An introduction. In *Pacific 2010: Challenging the future,* ed. R. Cole, 43–49. Canberra: National Centre for Development Studies, Research School of Pacific Studies, Australian National University.

———. 1993b. Papua New Guinea. In *Pacific 2010: Challenging the future,* ed. R. Cole, 50–64. Canberra: National Centre for Development Studies, Research School of Pacific Studies, Australian National University.

———. 1993c. Solomon Islands. In *Pacific 2010: Challenging the future,* ed. R. Cole, 91–104. Canberra: National Centre for Development Studies, Research School of Pacific Studies, Australian National University.

McMurray, C., and D. Lucas. 1990. Fertility and family planning in the South Pacific. Islands/Australia Working Paper no. 90/10. Canberra: National Centre for Development Studies, Research School of Pacific Studies, Australian National University.

Meggitt, M. 1989. Women in contemporary central Enga society. In *Family and gender in the Pacific: Domestic contradictions and the colonial impact,* ed. M. Jolly and M. Macintyre, 135–55. Cambridge: Cambridge University Press.

Mosko, M. 1985. *Quadripartite structures: Categories, relations, and homologies in Bush Mekeo culture.* Cambridge: Cambridge University Press.

Narokobi, B., et al. 1980. *The Melanesian way: Total cosmic vision of life.* Boroko: Institute of Papua New Guinea Studies.

National Sex and Reproduction Research Team, and C. Jenkins. 1994. *National study of sexual and reproductive knowledge and behaviour in Papua New Guinea.* Monograph no. 10. Goroka: Papua New Guinea Institute of Medical Research.

Osteria, T. S. 1984. *Report on the maternal and child health survey of Vanuatu.* Port Vila: Ministry of Health.

Post-Courier (Papua New Guinea), 20 May 1974. Interview with Josephine Abijah.

Rallu, J.-L. 1991. Population of the French overseas territories in the Pacific past, present and future. *Journal of Pacific History* 26 (2): 169–86.

Reed, A. 1997. Contested images and common strategies: Early colonial sexual politics in the Massim. In *Sites of desire, economies of pleasure: Sexualities in Asia and the Pacific,* ed. L. Manderson and M. Jolly, 48–71. Chicago: University of Chicago Press.

Setel, P. 2000 "Someone to take my place": Fertility and the male life-course among coastal Boiken, East Sepik Province, Papua New Guinea. In *Fertility and the male life cycle in the era of fertility decline,* ed. C. Bledsoe, S. Lerner, and J. I. Guyer, 233–56. Oxford: Oxford University Press.

South Pacific Commission. 1993. *South Pacific Economies Statistical Summary (SPESS),* no. 13. Noumea, New Caledonia: South Pacific Commission.

———. 1994a. *Pacific Island populations: Report.* Prepared by the South Pacific Commission for the International Conference on Population and Development, 5–13 September 1994, Cairo. Noumea: South Pacific Commission.

———. 1994b. Pacific Island population wall chart. Noumea: Population/Demography Programme, South Pacific Commission.

Speiser, F. 1990 [1923]. *Ethnology of Vanuatu: An early twentieth century study*, trans. D. Q. Stephenson. Bathurst, N.S.W.: Crawford House Press.

Spriggs, M. 1997. *The Island Melanesians*. Oxford: Blackwell.

Stannard, D. E. 1989. *Before the horror: The population of Hawai'i on the eve of Western contact*. Honolulu: Social Science Research Institute, University of Hawai'i.

Strathern, M. 1972. *Women in between: Female roles in a male world; Mount Hagen, New Guinea*. London: Seminar Press.

———. 1981. Culture in a net bag: The manufacture of a subdiscipline in anthropology. *Man*, n.s. 16:665–88.

———. 1988. *The gender of the gift: Problems with women and problems with society in Melanesia*. Berkeley: University of California Press.

Tuzin, D. 1997. *The Cassowary's revenge: The life and death of masculinity in a New Guinea Society*. Chicago: University of Chicago Press.

Underhill-Sem, Y. 1994. Blame it all on population: Perceptions, statistics and reality in the population debate in the Pacific. In *Sustainable development or malignant growth? Perspectives of Pacific Island women*, ed. 'A. Emberson-Bain, 1–15. Suva, Fiji: Marama Publications.

———. 2000. (Not) speaking of maternities: Pregnancy and childbirth in Wanigela, Oro Province, Papua New Guinea. Ph.D. diss. University of Waikato, Hamilton, NZ.

Vanuatu, National Planning and Statistics Office. 1986. *Report of the Vanuatu urban census 1986*. Port Vila: Government of Vanuatu.

———. 1988. *Second National Development Plan, 1987–1991*. Port Vila: Republic of Vanuatu.

———. 1992. *Third National Development Plan, 1992–1996*. Port Vila: Republic of Vanuatu.

Walter, A., and G. Bourdy. 1986. Pregnancy and confinement in Vanuatu: Methodological notes and preliminary results. Anthropology Work Paper no. 6. Port Vila: ORSTOM.

Weiner, A. 1976. *Women of value, men of renown: New perspectives in Trobriand exchange*. Austin: University of Texas Press.

———. 1982. Sexuality among the anthropologists, reproduction among the informants. *Social Analysis* 12:52–65.

———. 1988. *The Trobrianders of Papua New Guinea*. New York: Holt, Rinehart and Winston.

———. 1995. Reassessing reproduction in social theory. In *Conceiving the new world order: The global politics of reproduction*, ed. F. D. Ginsburg and R. Rapp, 407–24. Berkeley: University of California Press.

White, G. 1991. *Identity through history: Living stories in a Solomon Islands society*. Cambridge: Cambridge University Press.

Whitehead, H. 1986. Varieties of fertility cultism in New Guinea. *American Ethnologist* 13 (1–2): 80–99, 271–89.

Wolfe, P. 1999. *Settler colonialism and the transformation of anthropology: The politics and poetics of an ethnographic event*. London and New York: Cassell.

Contributors

Kamla Bhasin is a founder of Jagori, the Women's Resource and Training Centre in Delhi. She works with the United Nations and is active in the women's movement in South Asia. She has written several books and essays on women, media, education, and development and on gender training. She writes songs for social movements and for children. She is the coauthor, with Ritu Menon, of *Borders and Boundaries: Women in India's Partition* (1998).

Christine M. Dureau is a Lecturer in Social Anthropology at the University of Auckland, New Zealand. After earning her Ph.D. degree at Macquarie University, she was a Postdoctoral Fellow in Pacific History in the Research School of Pacific and Asian Studies at the Australian National University. She has conducted field and archival research on gender, Christianity, and changing worldviews among Simbo communities in the Solomon Islands. She is currently working on an ethnographic history of Fijian missionaries and on a project on nineteenth-century Methodist missionary approaches to evolution. With Morris Low she coedited the volume *The Politics of Knowledge: Science and Evolution in Asia and the Pacific*, a special issue of *History and Anthropology* (1999).

Anne-Marie Hilsdon is a Senior Lecturer in the School of Social Sciences at Curtin University, Perth, Western Australia. She has carried out research on gender, sexuality, and militarism in the Philippines. Her major publication is *Madonnas and Martyrs: Militarism and Violence in the Philippines* (1995). She has a chapter on sexual violence in the Philippines, to appear in *ReOrienting the Body* (ed. Freda Freiberg and Vera Mackie). Forthcoming is the coedited book, *Gender Politics and Human Rights*, to be published by Routledge. Her current research is about Maranao Muslim women in the Philippines.

Margaret Jolly is Professor and Head of the Gender Relations Centre in the Research School of Pacific and Asian Studies, the Australian National University. She has published extensively on women in the Pacific and especially Vanuatu, on the Cook voyages, on gender in colonial history, and on the politics of tradition. Her major publications are *Women of the Place: Kastom, Colonialism and Gender in Vanuatu* (1994); *Women's Difference: Sexuality and Maternity in Colonial and Postcolonial Discourses* (1994); *Family and Gender in the Pacific* (1989), with Martha Macintyre; *Sites of Desire, Economies of Pleasure: Sexualities in Asia and the Pacific* (1997), with Lenore Manderson; and *Maternities and Modernities: Colonial and Postcolonial Experiences in Asia and the Pacific* (1998), with Kalpana Ram.

Ritu Menon is an independent scholar and publisher. She is coeditor of *Against All Odds: Essays on Women, Religion and Development from India and Pakistan* (1994) and guest editor of *Interventions* 1 (2), a special issue on Partition (1999). She has written extensively on women and violence, alternative media, and publishing in the developing world. She is the coauthor, with Kamla Bhasin, of *Borders and Boundaries: Women in India's Partition* (1998).

Lynette Parker is a Senior Lecturer in the School of Asian Studies at the University of Western Australia, Perth. She earned her Ph.D. degree in Anthropology at the Australian National University and then a Postdoctoral Fellowship in the Research School of Pacific and Asian Studies of the Australian National University. She has completed extended anthropological fieldwork in Indonesia, mainly in Bali. Her main publications are on the anthropology of gender and education in journals such as *Indonesia* and the *Journal of the Royal Anthropological Institute* and on fertility in Bali in a forthcoming book entitled *ReOrienting the Body* (ed. Freda Freiberg and Vera Mackie). She is currently completing a book on Balinese villagers' perceptions of their incorporation into the nation-state of Indonesia.

Kalpana Ram is an Australian Research Council Research Fellow, affiliated with Anthropology and Comparative Sociology, Macquarie University, Sydney. She has published on gender, caste, and class in contemporary India as well as more general theoretical essays on feminism, anthropology, and issues of postcolonialism and modernity. Her major publications are *Mukkuvar Women: Gender, Hegemony and Capitalist Transformation in a South Indian Fishing Community* (1991); *Maternities and Modernities: Colonial and Postcolonial Experiences in Asia and the Pacific* (1998), with Margaret Jolly; and *Migrating Feminisms: The Asia/Pacific Region*, special issue of *Women's Studies International Forum* (1998), with J. Kēhaulani Kauanui. Her current research is on spirit possession as a way of rethinking issues of culture and gender in relation to postcolonial modernity and the state in contemporary India. She is also working on the transformations of Indian dance and aesthetics in nationalism both within India and in the overseas Indian diaspora.

Kathryn Robinson is currently a Senior Fellow in Anthropology, Research School of Pacific and Asian Studies at the Australian National University. She is an anthropologist who has worked mainly in South Sulawesi, Indonesia. Her research has been concerned with aspects of contemporary women's social participation in Indonesia, including women's political activism, the relation of women to government programs, and international female labor migration. She has published extensively on the Soroako nickel mine and on Sulawesi traditional architecture and has, with Mukhlis Paeni, edited a series of books on the anthropology of South Sulawesi. Her major publications include *Stepchildren of Progress: The Political Economy of Development in an Indonesian Mining Town* (1986), and *Living through Histories: Culture, History and Social Life in South Sulawesi* (1998), with Mukhlis Paeni.

Gary Sigley is a Lecturer in the School of Asian Studies at the University of Western Australia. He earned his Ph.D. degree at Griffith University, where he carried out research on government and population in China, investigating the historical emergence of "the population" and "the family" as objects of government. He is currently working on a book entitled *Governing Chinese Bodies: Population, Reproduction and the Civilising Process in Contemporary China*.

Andrea Whittaker is currently a Research Fellow at the National Centre for Epidemiology and Population Health at the Australian National University. She was previously an Australian Research Council Postdoctoral Fellow and then Research Fellow with the Gender Relations Centre. She is a medical anthropologist who has conducted research on health and illness both in Thailand and Australia. Her ethnographic study of women's health was recently published as *Intimate Knowledge: Women and Their Health in North-East Thailand* (2000).

Index

ABC, 36, 48–50
abduction, 11, 60, 68–73, 75, 77, 118
  abducted person, 70, 72
  Abducted Persons (Recovery and Restoration) Bill, 75
  resistance, 77
  widows, 77
Abdurochim, 184
Abijah, Josephine, 262, 296
abortion, 9, 17, 18, 20, 36, 38, 46, 53, 89, 92, 93, 144, 163, 197, 208, 210, 211, 213, 219, 220, 222, 225, 237–39, 244, 248, 263, 277, 284, 290, 291
  abortifacients, 20, 220, 224, 237, 246, 248, 267, 284, 290
  herbal, 208
abstinence, 20, 21, 46, 47, 263, 267, 276–78, 284, 288–90, 294, 295
Abu-Lughod, L., 7, 8
Aditjondro, G., 185
AFP (Armed Forces of the Philippines), 155, 166, 168, 169, 171
Africa, 263, 277, 286, 295, 298, 299
agency, 1, 10, 13, 17, 18, 22, 24, 25, 28, 36, 43, 52, 55, 94, 96, 98, 107
  denial of, 52
Aguilar, D. D., 158
Agyei, W. K., 294–97
Akhtar, F., 44
Akhtar, Hanum, 90
Alexander, P., 45
Allen, M. R., 291
All-India Women's Conference (AIWC), 105
All Pakistan Women's Association (APWA), 75

Alsa Masa, 168, 169, 171
Alter, J., 105
Ambrym Island (Vanuatu), 286
Anagnost, A., 23, 24, 100, 108, 109, 132
ancestors, 286, 288, 289
  ancestor group, 180
  ancestral spirits, 210
ancestral, 2, 21, 25, 263, 264, 267, 275, 282, 284–86, 288, 289
ancien régime, 130
Anderson, B., 6, 155
androgynous, 162, 173
Aneityum Island (South Vanuatu), 263, 275
Ani, 232
anticolonial, 10, 82, 100, 106
antinatalist, 12, 17, 18, 20, 26
Archavanitkul, K., and A. Pramualratana, 211
Arditti, R., R. Duelli Klein, and S. Minden, 9
Arellano, L. B., 167
Aristotle, 107
ars erotica, 135
Arya Samaj, 76
asexual, 160
Asia, 7, 10, 21, 28, 295
Asian-Pacific Resource and Research Centre for Women (ARROW), 297, 298
Asian societies, 157
Asia-Pacific, 2
Astawa, I. B., Soegeng Waloeyo, and J. E. Laing, 178, 189
Augustin, P. C., 172
Aunt Bunlaai, 220

311

312 *Index*

Aunt Kaew, 221
Aunt Naam, 214
Aunt Som, 208
Aunt Thii, 220
Aunt Uay, 222
Aunt Wii, 212
Aunt Yii, 221
Australian (later New Zealand) Methodist Mission, 239
Austronesian, 263
Ayurvedic, 214
Azad Kashmir, 69
azas keluargaan (family foundation, Bahasa Indonesian), 14

baap (a Buddhist sin, Thailand), 219
babaylan (Bisayan, Philippines), 158
Bacani, M. K., 16
bachelor system (*danshenzhi*, China), 125
Bagchi, J., 12
Bahawalpur State (Pakistan), 73
Bali (Indonesia), 4, 14, 15, 18–20, 46, 178, 179, 185–91, 194–96, 198
  Denpasar, 185, 186
  Gianyar, 195
  Karangasem, 195
  Klungkung, 184, 195
  nation-state, 179, 190
  PKK (Family Welfare Organization), 14
  ritual, 195
  state, 194, 195
Baluchistan (Pakistan), 69
Bangkok (Thailand), 19
Bangladesh, 12, 90
banjar (Balinese community organization), 15, 16, 180, 190, 191, 192, 193, 194–96
Bankowski, Z., J. Barzelatto, and A. M. Capron, 53
Barker, J., 285
Barlow, T., 141
barrios (villages, Philippines), 157, 165, 167, 171, 172
Barry, C., 160, 163, 173
Baruya (Papua New Guinea), 292
Basu, A., 68, 86

BBC, 48
beatas (nuns, Philippines), 158
bebas (free, Indonesia), 187
Bello, W., 155
Belo, J., 180
Bendesa, I. K. G., and I. M. Sukarsa, 184
Bengal, 58
Bennett, J. A., 237–39
Bernet Kempers, A. J., 180
Bhabha, H., 6, 155
Bhasin, K., 58
Biersack, A., 284
Bihar (India), 71
biomedical, 9, 16, 25
biopolitics, 123, 130, 132
  Chinese, 132
bio-power, 208
birth, 159, 172, 190, 235, 239
birthing, 225
birthrate(s), 106, 110, 208, 225, 243, 276
births, 237, 245
birth spacing, 276, 290
birth workers, 110
bishops, 165, 167, 173
BKKBN (Badan Koordinasi Keluargaan Berencana Nasional, Indonesia), 189–91
Bobbio, N., 107
body-and-soul relationship, 160
Boon, J., 180
Booth, H., 268
borders, 11
Boserup, E., 42
boundaries, 76, 77
Boycott, R., 36
Bracher, M., 253
Brahman, 180
Branson, J., and D. B. Miller, 182
Brassika (east Bali), 178, 180, 182, 184
Bray, D., 123
breastfeeding, 21, 93, 225, 240, 253, 254, 276, 284, 285, 289, 294, 295
bride-price, 18, 210
brides of Christ, 160
Brinkgreve, F., 180
Brown, D., 205
Buddhism, 19, 219, 224, 157

merit, 209
popular, 209
Buhay, H., 162
Bushnell, A., 275
Bushnell, O., 275
Butler, J. P., 292
Byford, J., 291
Byrne, L., 173

CAFGUs (Civilian Armed Forces Geographical Units) Philippines, 168
Cairo conference, 53
Calcutta, 71
Caldwell, J. C., 38, 196, 274
Calick, R., 266–68, 293
Campbellpur (India), 69
capital, 164
capitalism, 171
Caplan, P., 22
Cardinal Sin, 163
Carter, A., 111
Cartier, M., 127
Cass, A., 159, 165, 166, 168
caste, 2, 11, 15, 23, 82, 83, 97–99, 102, 106, 109, 111, 112, 180, 184–86, 196
  endogamous, 15
Cathcart, S., 170
Catholic Church, 156
Cebuano, 157
celibacy, 12, 13, 156, 158, 162, 163, 173, 237, 240, 241, 289, 293
  celibates (*dushenzhuyizhe,* China), 125
Charoenchai, A., and E. Thongkrajai, 216
Chatterjee, P., 6, 7, 12, 22, 82, 99, 100, 102
Chaturachinda, K. et al., 219
Chayovan, N., P. Kamnuansilpa, and J. Knodel, 216
Chen Qingliang, 126
Chen Shaoyu, 127
Chen Yiyun, 134
Chi Guifa, 137
childbearing, 12, 130, 191, 196, 211–13, 234
childbirth, 14, 39, 46, 121, 129, 130, 138, 141, 180, 191, 212, 225, 245, 262, 275, 276, 278, 280, 284, 285, 288–91, 295
  medicalization, 284

child care, 67, 159, 172, 182, 187, 198, 225, 242, 245
childlessness, 210
child rearing, 8, 119
children, 182, 186, 197, 210–13, 216, 235, 237, 242, 246, 251
  of abducted women, 76
  good-quality, 129
China, 4, 5, 17, 22, 37, 100, 108–10, 120–24, 132, 137, 140, 141, 263, 266
  Cultural Revolution, 142
  elite, 119
  "five goods" movement, 142
  government, 145
  Great Leap Forward, 119, 142
  Manchu, 132
  one-child family policy, 9, 17, 23, 37, 109, 124, 129
  People's Republic, 118, 127, 128, 133
  post-Mao, 23
  Qing dynasty of Song, 132, 140
  Sung dynasty, 120
Chinese Eugenic Society, 135
Chinese family, 118, 142
  basic cell of society, 123
  filial respect and piety, 24
  governmental discourse on, 119, 120
  governmentalization of, 142
  ideal, 124
  li (authentic rituals), 120
  modern, 121
  nuclearization of, 120
  premodern, 122
  private, 121
  public, 121
  sociological discourse, 121
  su (vulgar familial traditions), 120
Chinese Marxism/Marxist, 129, 143
Chintana, P., 211
Chirawatkul, S., 215
choice, 18, 21, 24–26, 28, 84–88, 90, 91, 94, 95, 102, 108
  globalization of, 26
Christian(s)/Christianity, 11, 12, 75, 76, 154, 157, 173, 241, 244, 248, 255, 276, 278, 282–86, 298, 290, 293, 297
  Pauline ideology, 246

church, 166, 167
circumcision, 288, 290
citizenship, 1, 4, 6, 13, 15, 61, 76–78, 84, 99, 103, 111, 112, 154, 156, 157, 159, 161, 164, 166, 169–73
  citizen(s), 1, 82, 96, 99, 104, 109, 154, 196, 224
  citizen-subjects, 10
  gender, 76
  notions of, 6
Clark, J., 293
class, 2, 7, 8, 11, 19, 23, 82, 83, 91, 93, 97, 98, 112, 120, 143, 157, 171, 197, 206, 208, 216, 217, 264, 267, 293
clerics, 167
Cohen, P. T., 217, 218
colonial, 2, 4, 5, 44, 62, 101–3, 110, 158, 166, 170, 245, 264, 274, 276, 277, 282, 284, 296–98
  colonialism, 292
  state, 280, 281, 290, 298
colonization, 156, 264
communalism, 102
communism/communist, 122, 156, 205
  Communist Party of China (CPC), 118
Community, 76, 79
Community Development Program, 205
Concerned Citizens for Justice and Peace (CCJP, Philippines), 164
Confucian, 23, 24, 118, 119
  elite, 120
  esthetics of conduct, 120
  neo-Confucianism, 119, 132
conjugality, 241, 244, 255
Conly, S. R., and J. J. Speidel, 38
Connor, L., 182
consciousness, 155
contraception, 9, 16, 18, 19, 21, 36, 38, 39, 41, 43, 46, 47, 50, 54, 92, 93, 98, 104, 105, 108, 130, 134, 178, 179, 183, 187–91, 194, 196–98, 203, 206, 208, 209, 211, 212, 214, 217, 223, 232, 235, 237, 239, 240, 242–45, 249, 252, 255
  choice, 22, 85
  diaphragm, 188
  herbal, 267, 284
  hormonal implants, 22
  indigenous forms of, 20
  medicines, 209
  nontechnological methods, 87
  Norplant, 19
  side effects, 89
  State-sponsored technologies, 111
  technologies, 19, 25, 87, 88, 89, 94, 216, 225, 234, 235
  tubal ligations, 19
convents, 158, 159, 170
corporeality, 19, 20, 23, 235, 238, 241, 243
Corrêa, S., and R. Petchesky, 27, 28
Corrêa, S., with R. Reichmann, 27
Covarrubias, M., 179, 180, 186
critical consciousness, 164
Croll, E., 129
Cunningham, C. E., B. Yoddumnurn, and W. Ratanasupa, 206
custom medicine, 247

Dalkon Shield, 249
Das, V., 1, 10, 83
dating (*lianai*, China), 136
datu (indigenous leaders, Philippines), 170
Daughters of Mary of the Assumption, 156
Davin, D., 123, 141, 142
Davis, D., and S. Harrell, 120
Deacon, B., 275
death, 141
De Beer, P., 205
Delhi, 70
Demaine, H., 205, 207
democracy, 77, 85, 98, 99, 108, 112, 156
  liberal, 156
  participatory, 85
  secular, 77
demographic transition, 274, 294, 295
demography, 5, 25, 38, 82, 84, 86, 92, 99, 179, 180, 196, 239, 264, 266, 273, 283, 292, 294
Denoon, D., 275
Department of Rural Development, 212
Depo Provera, 19, 46, 50, 214, 223, 224, 248–50, 253, 254
Desak Putu Parmiti, 184

desexualized, 163
Deshpande, S., 100
development, 2, 18, 20, 23, 37–42, 46, 48, 64, 82, 96, 100, 102, 103, 108–10, 129, 155, 160, 162, 164, 188, 194, 203, 205–7, 210, 218, 225, 244, 264, 266, 268, 272–75, 282
   agencies, 9, 292
   assistance, 37
   economic, 82
   holistic, 92
   interventions, 37
   sustainable, 53, 273, 288, 292
developmentalism, 85, 100, 105, 107
devil worship, 239
Dikötter, F., 122, 132
Ding Juan, 136
discourse(s), 5, 7, 38, 39, 43, 48, 52, 54, 82–84, 91–93, 96, 118, 132, 134, 141, 142, 143, 171, 205–7, 210, 216, 218, 224, 263, 264, 266, 282
   Chinese governmental, 124
   Confucian, 119
   development, 282
   economy of pleasure, 134, 143
   emancipatory, 43
   family, 118, 120
   governmental, 123, 124, 135
   of liberation, 171
   medicalized, 132
   official, 132
   official Chinese, 137
   population, 39
   Third World, 38
   Western political, 119
divorce, 9, 16, 118, 125, 134, 163, 182, 210
Dixon-Mueller, R., and A. Germain, 255
domestic service, 159
Dong Jian, 138
Donzelot, J., 121, 122, 124
drugs, 220
Dureau, C., 4, 15, 18–21, 43, 45, 238, 239, 241, 244, 254, 267, 274, 276, 281–84, 286, 296
Dussel, E., 172

East Bengal, 71
East Punjab, 66
East Punjab States Union (PEPSU), 70
Ebrey, P., 119, 120
economic inequality, 232
economy of pleasure, 137, 142
economy, 60, 62, 64, 65, 78, 92, 100, 103, 104, 106, 107, 129, 163, 164, 179, 183–86, 198, 204, 207, 210, 238, 252, 294
Ecumenical Association of Third World Theologians (EATWOT), 157
Edge-Partington, T. W., 237
Edmondson, J. C., 178
educating (*jiaohua*), 119
education, 27, 97, 129, 132, 134, 138, 144, 154, 183, 185, 186, 196–98, 205–7, 210, 225, 240, 274, 289, 294–96, 298
Eighth Five Year Plan, 85
Elia, I., 253
eligible couples (ElCos, Bali), 190
elite, 155, 163, 164, 205, 217, 218
elopement, 180, 245
El Salvador, 167
Elshtain, J. B., 156
embodiment, 1, 8, 26, 159, 160, 162, 163, 172, 173, 216, 235
employment bureau, 65
empowerment, 9, 18, 25, 27, 203, 217, 224, 272
endemic raiding, 237
endogamy, 180
Engels, 126
epidemiology, 236, 237
Escobar, A., 2, 54, 100
ethnicity, 7, 11, 18–20, 23, 99, 111, 120, 143, 206, 216, 217, 225, 264
ethnic Lao, 204, 206, 217, 218
ethnic purity, 76
ethnographic research, 204, 236
ethnography, 4, 264, 292
eugenics, theory of, 5, 23, 24
Eurocentric, 157
European mothers, 277
evacuation centers, 168
evangelical church(es), 285, 288
Evans, H., 134

exogamy, 243
exploitation, 159

Fabella, V., 155, 157–61, 163, 172
familial harmony, 123, 133, 144
family, 1, 6, 13, 14, 23, 179, 182, 183, 187, 194, 196, 211, 213, 222, 235, 236, 240, 241, 246, 272, 274, 277, 282, 284, 291, 293, 294, 297
  abnormal, 125
  basic cell of society, 119
  communal living unit (*shenghuo danwei*, China), 123
  Confucian, 118
  "eugenic" confines of, 126
  feudal, 118
  historical entity, 125
  modern, 121
  nuclear, 126
  as object, 122
  productivity, 123
  rituals, 186
  social welfare, 119
  state, 14
  traditional, 121
  values of, 6
family planning, 10, 16, 18, 20, 22, 25, 37, 39, 41, 44, 50, 52–54, 82, 90, 93, 94, 97, 98, 104, 105, 108, 111, 129, 130, 134, 140, 178, 179, 188–91, 194, 196–98, 203, 204, 206–8, 211–13, 217, 218, 224, 225, 234, 242, 243, 245, 248, 249, 252–55, 263, 266–68, 272, 274–76, 293–99
  community participation, 207
  indigenous, 295
  maternal and child health, 298
  programs, 41, 47, 50, 272, 274, 288, 296, 297
  status of women, 42, 43
  Voluntary Acceptance of Family Planning (India). *See* Gandotra, M. M., and N. Das Voluntary Health Service (India), 89
Family Planning Association of India, 96, 98
Fanon, F., 155, 170

fecundity, 12, 15, 179, 180, 183, 197, 234, 237, 245, 264, 267, 289
female status, 92, 93
feminism, 4, 12, 15, 25, 27, 39, 40, 42, 43, 47–50, 52, 53, 84, 92, 98, 105, 110, 154, 158, 172, 249, 295, 298
  ecofeminism, 44
  feminist, 59, 156
  feminist theology, 160, 161
  new wave, 36
  second-wave, 36, 48
feminization, 162
fertility, 2, 4, 5, 9, 15, 16, 19, 20, 25, 26, 36–49, 52–55, 84, 86, 90, 93, 111, 178–80, 189, 196, 198, 203, 208, 209, 211–14, 218, 224, 225, 234, 238, 239, 241, 243, 251–53, 255, 262–64, 268, 274, 275, 282–86, 288, 289, 291–97
  concept of natural, 45
  control, 5, 18, 21, 38, 272
  cults, 266, 289, 291
  decline, 42
  indigenous forms/regimes of, 18, 21, 298
  rates, 39, 268, 274
  statues, 286
  stone, 286
feudal, 137–39, 144
  feudal patriarchy, 133
  feudal states, 6
Fiji (southwest Pacific), 5, 240
Fijians (southwest Pacific), 277, 278, 280
Filipino, 154, 155, 158, 162–64, 173
FINRRAGE (Feminist International Network of Resistance to Reproductive and Genetic Engineering), 43
Firestone, S., 48
First World, 5, 17, 54
forcible conversions, 72
Foucault, M., 101, 107, 130–32, 208, 277
Fountain, O., 264, 285
Franklin, S., 17
Freedman, R., and B. Berelson, 178
Friere, P., 164
Fry, G., 274

Gabriela, 157

Gaitskell, D., and E. Unterhalter, 13
Gallop, J., 49
ganbu (cadres, China), 141
Gandhi, Indira, 50, 88, 94
Gandhi, M., 12, 22, 105
Gandhi, S., 88
Gandotra, M. M., and N. Das, 95, 96
Gannicott, K., 267
Gao Yulan, 138
Gebara, I., 156, 164
Geertz, H., and C. Geertz, 180
Gellner, E., 6
gender, 1, 2, 5–7, 10, 12, 27, 83, 98, 112, 120, 143, 154, 158, 159, 163, 171, 195, 203, 209, 210, 219, 236, 238, 244, 263, 264, 272, 281, 282, 285, 286, 288, 290, 292, 297
 citizenship, 5, 12
 nationalism, 5
genealogies, 237
Georgia, 238
Germain, A., 219
Ghosh, D., 103, 104
Ginsburg, F. D., 17
Ginsburg, F. D., and R. Rapp, 9, 240, 243, 244, 263
global, 2, 5, 8, 9
goblins (*brujas y duendes*, Philippines), 158
Goddess theology, 160
Golley, L., 37
governmentality, 26
 alliance and sexuality, 130
Grandmother Sian, 212
Grandmother Sow, 209
Great Leap Forward, 119
Greenhalgh, S., 38, 39, 111, 274
Green Revolution, 184, 187
Griffen, V., 253, 272
Grovijahn, J. M., 167
Guerrero, M. C., 158
Gujarat (India), 69
gynecology, 204, 218

Handwerker, L., 8, 9, 109, 110, 134, 140
Hanks, J. R., 208
Han Lei, 138

Harrell, B., 253
Harrison, P., 178
Harvey, D., 38
Haryana, 59
Hasan, Z., 84
Hauʻofa, E., 268
Havanon, N., J. Knodel, and W. Sittitrai, 213
health, 204–6, 208, 213, 214, 217, 218, 235, 239, 249, 254
Hegel, 102
Heng, G., and J. Devan, 6
herbal medicines, 221
Herdt, G., 291, 292
Hill, H., 178, 180, 183, 188, 191
Hilsdon, A., 4, 12, 13, 28, 158, 159, 172, 173
Hindu, 11, 12, 23, 69, 71, 72, 111, 191
 consciousness, 75
 dharma, 11, 75
 Hinduism, 157
 Hindus, 10, 58, 59
History of Sexuality, The (Foucault), 130
Hitavada (Nagpur, India), 61
HIV/AIDS, 27, 49, 197, 293
Hobart, M., 206
Hobbes, 107, 108
Hobsbawm, E. J., 6
Hocart, A. M., 235, 236, 238
Honiara (Solomon Islands), 250
Honig, E., and G. Hershatter, 136, 142
hormonal abortifacient RU486, 43
hormones, 249
hot medicines, 221
Hsiao Kung-Chuan, 122
hu (household, China), 125
Huang San, 128
Hugo et al., 185
Hu Jin, 136
Hull, T., 178, 191
Hull, V., 194
human rights, 13, 28, 156, 166, 170, 298
humoral, 19
humoral balance, 214, 215
Hunt, N., 276, 277
Hunter, I., 131
Hunter, T. M., 180

318   Index

hybridization, 121
hypogamy, 180

identities, 4, 7, 59, 61, 78, 84, 98, 99, 111, 141, 159, 172, 180, 194, 198, 204, 205, 286
imagined communities, 1, 8
incest, 134, 219
India, 4, 13, 37, 50, 58, 60, 62, 63, 66, 68, 70, 74, 75, 77, 82–86, 94, 97, 100, 104, 107, 108, 110, 263, 266, 277
   community, 63, 77
   Constituent Assembly of, 65, 68, 69, 71–73
   democracy, 95
   Emergency, 22, 86, 94, 95, 98, 99, 108, 109, 111
   family planning, 22
   gender, 77
   gender and state, 79
   independence, 59, 87
   Ministry of Relief and Rehabilitation, 62
   nationalism, 7
   nation-state, 104, 106
   Partition, 1, 4, 5, 58
   postcolonial state, 82
   post-Partition, 75, 77–79
   poverty, 111
   state, 61, 63, 70, 72, 82, 84, 85, 101, 107, 111
India and Pakistan, partition of, 10
Indian Health Activists, 90
indigenous medications, 238
Indonesia, 4, 14, 22, 37, 39, 43–45, 50, 54, 178–80, 184, 191, 194
   family planning program, 16
   Hari Ibu (National Mother's Day), 14
   Hari Kartini (national holiday), 14
   National Women's Congress, 14
Indonesian National Family Planning Board, 178
industrialization, 185
infanticide, 237, 238, 263, 267, 277, 284, 290, 291
infant mortality, 237, 239, 267, 268, 273, 283

infant mortality rates, 92, 179, 183, 191
infertile women, 9, 17
international agencies, 263, 272, 292, 296, 297
International Conference of Population and Development (ICPD), 26, 53, 268, 297
internationalization, 185
International Planned Parenthood Federation (IPPF), 38, 43
intimacy, 163
intrauterine devices (IUDs), 179, 188, 189, 191, 195, 196, 206, 214, 216, 217, 220, 248–50
in-vitro fertilization (IVF), 43, 46
IPSR, 203
Irvine, W., 215
Isaan (northeast Thailand), 19, 25, 203–6, 210, 218, 221
Islam, 11, 72, 76, 156, 157
Iveković, R., 76

Jacka, T., 123
Jackson, K. B., 237
Jamaica, 250
Jayawardena, K., 15
Jefferey, P., R. Jefferey, and A. Lyon, 8
Jeffrey, R., 92
Jenkins, C., 293
Jin, Y. T., 159, 161
Johnson, K. A., 143, 144
Johnson, S., 26, 27
Jolly, M., 4–6, 8, 17, 18, 20, 21, 25, 28, 45, 54, 252, 263, 276, 277, 280, 282, 288–92, 297, 298
Jolly, M., and M. Macintyre, 282, 284

Kabeer, N., 249, 251, 252
Kandiyoti, D., 7
Kane, P., 123, 127, 129
Kang Youwei, 122
Kantor Statistik, 188
kastom (tradition, Bislama, Vanuatu), 255, 285
katalonan (Tagalog, Philippines), 158
Katoppo, M., 161
Katrak, K. H., 12

kauban (working together for the people, Philippines), 161
Kazuko, O., 118
Keller, S., 63
Kelly, J., 277
Kennedy, K. I., et al., 253
Kerala (India), 92
Keyes, C. F., 204–6, 209, 210
Khamphee prathom chindaa (Thai Book of Genesis), 221
Khon Kaen Public Health Office, 211
Kirsch, T., 209
Kishwar, M., 12
Kligman, G., 17
Knauft, B., 293
Knodel, J., and N. Chayovan, 212
Knodel, J., A. Chamratrithirong, and N. Debavalya, 203, 209
knowledge(s), 83, 86, 190, 234, 248, 272, 286, 293, 294
　indigenous, 133
　object of, 101
　practice, 120, 132
　production of, 83
　sexual, 128
　textual, 4
　various forms of, 120
Krannich L., and C. R. Krannich, 203
Kristeva, J., 77, 78
Krongkaew, M., 204

labor, 15, 41, 42, 44, 45, 52, 62, 65, 93, 184, 185, 196, 210–12, 235, 239, 241, 267, 277, 281
　indentured, 277
　plantation, 239
Ladipo, O. A., 219
Lady Hardinge Medical College (Delhi, India), 65
Lake, M., 14
Lal, B., 277
land, 243
　ritual, 237, 238
Langmore, D., 282
Langness, L., 293
Laos, 204, 205
Latin America, 157, 163, 164, 167, 172

Laukaran, V. H., and M. H. Labbok, 253
Leech, M., 77
Lee Park, S. A., 158
Leftist movements, 155
lesbian, 163
Liang Zhongtang et al., 123
liberal, 83, 89, 94, 108, 121
　liberalism, 85, 86, 105
　liberalist democracy, 163
　values, 105
liberation, 128, 131, 133, 140, 154, 161, 162, 165
liberation theology, 154, 156–58, 163, 172
lineage, 1. *See also* family
Liu Guangren, 124
Liu Xianming, 127
Liu Zheng, 123
Li Xingchun, 138
Li Yinhe, 132
Lloyd, G., 110
Lloyd and Winn. *See* McMurray, C., and D. Lucas
Lock, M., and P. A. Kaufert, 9
Locke, 107, 108
London, B., 205
lo sal ("inside the road or path," south Pentecost, Vanuatu), 288
love (*qingai*), 138
Lovi, A., and K. Osuga, 242, 243, 252
Lovric, B., 180
Lukere, V., 277, 280–82
luluna (opposite sex classificatory siblings, "brothers" (female speaker), Simbo, western Solomon Islands), 20, 238, 241, 243–45, 248, 284
Lumad peoples (Philippines), 170
lust (*xingyu*, China), 138

MacCormack, C. P., 243, 250
MacKenzie, M. A., 288
Madonna, 13
magic, 208, 252
mai-baap (India), 75, 77, 79
malaria, 237
Malaysia, 4, 13, 17, 22
male cults, 264, 288, 291–94
Mallett, S., 285, 286

Malthusian notion, the, 38
Mananzan, M. J., 158, 159, 161, 162, 164
Mananzan, M. J., and S. A. Park, 159, 162, 172
Manderson, L., 214, 280
Manderson, L., and P. L. Rice, 8
Manila, 156
Mao, 24, 141
marriage, 11, 24, 69, 72, 118, 119, 126, 127, 129, 130, 134, 137–40, 160, 180, 182, 197, 210, 212, 213, 238, 241, 245, 254, 277, 282, 284, 285, 288
  child, 11
  public, 128
Marriage Law (China), 128
Marshall, L. B., 289
Marshall Islands (Pacific), 273
Martin, E., 235, 250, 286, 292
martyrdom, 167
Marxism, 154
  Marxist, 125
Maryknoll Sisters, 156
masculine, 167
masculinist, 162
Mason, K. O., 42
massage doctors, 219
masses, 164
maternal and child health (MCH), 19, 21, 110, 211, 239, 272, 296, 298, 299
maternal death, 219
maternal desire, 224
maternal God, 161
maternal health, 106, 130
maternity, 12, 13
matrilineal, 18, 210, 291
matrilocal, 238
Ma Xiaonian, 137
Maxwell, N. E., 217
McArthur, N., 275, 291
McClintock, A., 13, 156
McDowell, N., 237, 244, 267, 290, 291, 295, 296
MCH/FP (maternal and child health and family planning), 296
McMurray, C., 267, 283
McMurray, C., and D. Lucas, 242, 243, 268

McNeil, M., I. Varcoe, and S. Yearley, 9
McNicoll, G., 178
medicalization, 225
medical treatment(s), 198, 239, 240
Meerut (India), 71
Meggitt, M., 293
Meier, G., 178
Meijer, M., 127, 128
Melanesia (Pacific), 263, 268, 273, 274, 282, 285, 286, 288, 292, 294
Menon, R., 4, 58
Menon, R., and K. Bhasin, 1, 4, 10, 15, 23, 67, 71, 73, 77, 155
menstruation, 209, 214, 215, 221, 250
Methodist Mission, 240
Micronesia (Pacific), 263, 268, 273
midwives, 209, 212, 220, 225, 277
Mies, M., and V. Shiva, 44, 45
Miller, D. B., and J. Branson, 180
Miller, J., 131
Mindanao, 156, 157, 163, 165, 171, 172
Ministry of Labour in Bombay and Delhi (India), 65
Ministry of Relief and Rehabilitation (India), 74
Minson, J., 121, 131
miscarriage, 213
missionaries, 4, 5, 239, 240, 243, 248, 254, 264, 277, 278, 281, 282, 284, 285, 297, 298
  Methodist, 20
missionary, 44, 165, 243
MNLF (Moro National Liberation Front, Philippines), 12, 155
Mobile Development Units (MDUs), 205
mobilization of emotions, 6
models of choice, 10
modernity, 82, 109–11, 206, 272, 282, 293, 295
Molineaux, D. J., 163
monkhood, 209
monogamy, 277, 278, 281, 282, 284, 297
morbidity, 219
Morgan, 126
Morsy, S. A., 9
mor tahan (army-trained medics who sell their services, Thailand), 220

mortality, 27, 42
Mougne, C., 208, 213
Muecke, M. A., 210
Mulholland, J., 221
Muslim(s), 8, 10, 12, 23, 58, 59, 71, 72, 73, 75, 76, 111
　non-Muslims, 73

Nag, M., 240
Narayana, G., and J. F. Kantner, 87–89, 91, 92, 94, 96–98, 107
Narkavonnakit, T., 219, 220
Narokobi, B. et al., 262, 291
National Democratic Movement/National Democratic Front (Philippines), 12, 164
National Economic and Social Development Board (NESDB, Thailand), 206–8, 211
nationalist struggles, 157
nation-states, 204, 206. *See also* state
Nauru (Pacific), 268
Nehru, R., 61, 62, 64, 74
neocolonial, 264
neo-Malthusian, 38, 53, 272
New Caledonia (Pacific), 264
New Georgia Group (Solomon Islands), 235, 236
New People's Army (NPA, Philippines), 12, 154, 155
NGOs (nongovernment organizations), 18, 91, 207
Nichter, M., and M. Nichter, 221
nineteenth century, 158
Niue Island (Pacific), 273
Nuakata Island (the Massim, Papua New Guinea), 285
nuns, 5, 12, 13, 154, 156, 158–71, 173
nurse midwives, 110

O'Brien, M., 48
O'Collins, M., 243
Oduyoye, M., and M. R. A. Kanyoro, 158
Oey-Gardiner, M., 184, 185
offerings, 182, 187
Ogan, E., J. Nash, and D. Mitchell, 237

Omar, R., 17
Ong, A., 17
organizations
　agencies, 77
　civic, 159
　nongovernment. *See* NGOs (nongovernment organizations)
Orleans, L., 118
Other, 76, 110, 111
overpopulation, 124

Pacific, 5, 7, 10, 21, 28, 248, 263, 264, 266–68, 273–75, 277, 285, 286, 288, 292–94, 297, 298
　islands, 264, 266, 268, 272
　southwest, 264, 267, 275, 288, 296–98
paile (men's "communal houses," Simbo, western Solomon Islands), 240
Pai Panandiker, V. A., and P. K. Umashankar, 97–99
Pakistan, 1, 4, 58, 61, 62, 68, 69, 71–76
Pandey, G., 84, 99, 102
Pan Suiming, 132
Pan Yunkang, 124–26
Papua New Guinea, 244, 262–64, 268, 273, 277, 282, 285, 290, 291, 293–96
Parisada Hindu Dharma (quasi-government Hindu umbrella organization, Bali), 191
parish records, 157
Parker, L., 4, 14–16, 46, 180, 189
Parker, A., et al., 2, 156
Parmiti, D. P., 184
Partition, 58–61, 66, 67, 75
Pateman, C., 6, 10, 13–15, 107, 156, 159
paterfamilias, 11, 60, 68
Patiala (India), 70
patriarchy, 118, 213
　patriarchal, 10, 11, 14, 15, 19, 25, 79, 107, 111, 167, 204
patrilineal, 48, 180, 184
　patrilineages, 15
Pauline model, 20
peasant mode of production, 179
Peng Xizhe, 120, 127
Petchesky, R. P., 17, 27

Philippines, 4, 12, 13, 154, 156, 157, 160, 164, 170, 172, 173
    gun culture, 15
Phongpaichit, P., 205
Pieris, S. J., 157, 164
PKK (Family Welfare Organization, Indonesia), 194
pleasure, 134, 140
Podhisita, C., 210
Poffenberger, M., 178, 195
polluted women, 11, 69, 180, 218, 285, 293
polygamy, 277, 285
polygyny, 182
Polynesia (Pacific), 263, 268, 273
Population Council, 38, 41, 43, 219, 220
population, 4, 5, 10, 18, 23, 26, 36–39, 47, 48, 53–55, 90, 92, 97, 98, 101, 103, 104, 108, 111, 127, 129–31, 141, 142, 144, 154, 178, 183, 197, 203, 204, 206, 207, 213, 235, 236, 240, 243, 251, 253, 262–64, 266–68, 272–77, 280, 286, 288, 296–98
    control, 4, 36, 37, 39, 44, 50, 296
    programs, 38, 39, 53
pornography, 134
postcolonial, 7, 78, 96, 99, 100, 101, 105, 108–10, 155, 156, 263, 264, 292
postmodern, 83
post-Partition, 75, 77–79
    state, 70
Poulsen, A., 209
poverty, 12, 18, 23, 82, 92, 111, 144, 157, 159, 204, 205, 208, 225
Prasartkul, P., and C. Sethaput, 206, 211
precolonial, 158, 172
premarital sex, 135, 137
premarriage, 128
priestesses, 158, 172
priests, 158, 160, 162, 164–67, 173
primary health care (PHC), 21
private, 6, 13, 23, 159, 172
Prizzia, R., 205
problematization of desire, 131
pronatalist, 17, 18, 26, 44, 45, 206
prostitution, 67, 211
public, 6, 7, 13, 159, 160, 187, 206, 225, 244, 248

public health, 37, 197
Pucci, I., 180
Puerto Rico, 48
Pui Lan, K., 161
Pulea, M., 248
Punjab, 58, 59, 63, 75
purdah (India), 11, 12
purity and pollution, 15
Pusey, J. R., 122

Quan Yazhi, 133
Quinn, N., 40

race, 157
Raghuram, S., and A. Rahman, 91
Rai, S., 69
Raina, B. L., 85, 106
Rallu, J.-L., 275
Ram, K., 4, 5, 11, 12, 21–23, 25, 84, 129, 155, 206
Ram, K., and M. Jolly, 8
Rao, M., 94, 107
rape, 167, 173, 219, 224
Ravindran, T. K. S., 89, 92–94
Ray, R., 65, 78
Raymond, J., 9, 49
Redemptorists, 160
Reed, A., 277
Reeler, A. V., 215
refugees, 58, 61, 64, 68
    mass widowhood, 62
    rehabilitation, 62, 64, 67
    resettling, 62
    resistance, 74
    widows, 61, 66
religion, 11, 97, 98, 101, 102, 106, 109, 111, 154, 209
    Protestant, 155
    World Council of Churches, 155
religious discourse, 164
Ren Jianying, 124
Ren Wen, 136
Ren Wen, and Yin Ming, 139
repressive hypothesis, 131
reproduction, 8, 9, 130
    choice, 25
    consciousness, 84

politics of, 8
state control over, 17
technologies, 9, 25
reproductive health, 293, 298
resistance, 4, 13, 145, 170, 222, 255
Reuther, R. R., 160
Reynolds, C. J., 205
rights, 61, 78, 172
  citizenship, 172
  civil, 77, 78
  community, 61, 77
  gender, 61
  political, 77
  poor and oppressed communities, 172
  reproductive, 27, 143
  sexual and reproductive, 26, 28
Riley, J. N., and S. Sermsri, 208
rites (*li*, China), 119
ritual(s), 210, 216, 289, 291, 294
Rivers, W. H. R., 237
Robertson, A. F., 84, 111
Robinson, K., 5, 14, 15, 17, 25, 54, 263
Rockefeller Foundation, 38, 42, 239
Romania, 9, 17
Rosaldo, M., 240
Rose, Sr. (pseud.), 162, 164
Rosenfield, A., 36, 49
Rozario, S., 11
Ruan Fangfu, 134
Rural Women's Social Education Centre (RUWSEC, India), 88, 91
Rushdie, S., 82, 83

Sa (south Pentecost, Vanuatu), 286, 288
Sadik, Nafis, 27
safe motherhood, 272
Safilios-Rothschild, C., 41, 42
Said, E., 54
Sambia (Papua New Guinea), 292
SAMIN (Sisters Association in Mindanao, Philippines) 156, 159, 163, 164, 170
Samoa, 240
Sangari, K., 84
Sanger, Margaret, 105
Santo Niño (little Jesus), 165

sarkar (ruler, "government," India), 62, 75
satria (caste classification, Bali) 181
satyagraha (truth force, India), 12
sawah (irrigated rice fields, Indonesia), 15, 16, 183, 184
Sawicki, J., 46
SBS, 38, 50, 52, 53
Scheffler, H. W., 255
Scherer-Warren, I., 157, 163, 164, 169, 172
Scragg, R. F. R., 237
Second Vatican Council, 155, 160
secular, 77
Sen, G., 110
Sen, S., 12
seventeenth century, 158
sexuality, 1, 4, 11–13, 15, 19, 46, 48, 52–54, 60, 75–77, 88, 91, 103, 119, 121, 126, 130–32, 140, 143, 144, 154, 158, 163, 171, 173, 179, 180, 183, 189, 196–98, 209, 214, 224, 235, 238, 241, 250, 252, 272, 276–78, 281–86, 289, 290, 292, 293, 298
  commodification of, 134
  economy of pleasure, 131, 144
  equality, 144
  pleasures of sex, 24, 131, 252
  sexual, 125
  sexual desires, 1, 136, 144, 209
  sexual hygiene, 135
  sexual love (*xingai*, China), 138
  sexual pleasures (*ars erotica*), 131
  sexual politics, 235
  techniques, 131
Shah Commission of Inquiry, 94
Sheehan, B., 204
Shiva, V., 44, 45
S.I. [Solomon Islands] Census Office, 236
Sigley, G., 5, 21, 23, 24, 263
Sikhs, 10, 58, 60
Simbo (Solomons), 4, 19, 267, 282, 284, 285
Sind (Pakistan), 69
Singapore, 123
Sino-Thai, 204
sistem banjar (Bali), 16, 178, 188–90
  status of, 190

Sister Annie, 165, 168, 169, 171
Sister Daniel Mitchell, 156
Sister Josie, 165, 167–69
Sister Lydia, 169, 171
Sister Mary (Mary John), 170
Sita, abduction of, (India), 69
Sittitrai, W., 206, 207, 211
Sittitrai, W., et al., 213
Sivin, I., et al., 216
sixteenth century, 158
social change, 178
social marketing, 225
social movements, 154
social reconstruction, 64
social scientists, 83
Solomon Islands (Pacific), 4, 18–20, 264, 267, 268, 274, 275, 277, 282, 283, 296
Soni, V., 86–89, 95
Soonawala, R. P., 88, 96, 98
Soonthorndhada, A., O. Buravisit, and P. Vong-Ek, 207
Soroako (Indonesia), 46, 54
South Asia, 5
Southeast Asia, 5, 37
South Pacific Commission, 268, 273
Spanish, 172
Sparks, H., 13
Speiser, F., 275
spiritual ascetics (*jingshen jinyuzhuyi*, China), 132
Spriggs, M., 274, 275
Srikantan, K., K. Balasubramian, and S. Nikam, 89
Stannard, D. E., 275
state, 13, 76, 167. *See also* nation-states
postcolonial, 155
status, 211, 216, 219
status groups, 180
Stayapan, S., K. Kanchanasinith, and S. Varakamin, 216
sterilization, 17, 18, 22, 23, 25, 37, 43, 50, 86, 93–95, 104, 111, 144, 188, 189, 206, 211, 216, 263
Stivens, M., 8, 17
Strathern, M., 9, 17, 26, 27, 263, 288–92
Streatfield, K., 178, 180, 191, 195
structural adjustment programs, 92

Suharto government (Indonesia), 188, 197
New Order, 14, 15
Sukdis, T., P. Taendum, and R. Na Pattalung, 211
Sulawesi (Indonesia), 50
Sullivan, N., 194
Sun Yat-sen, 140
Swaminathan, P., 92
Synod of Catholic Bishops, 155

taboo, 290
Tamil Nadu (India), 88–91
Tandrup, A., 205
Taoism, 157
Taskforce Detainees (TFD), 164
Tata Institute of Social Sciences, 65
Taylorism, 43
Team Pengembangan, 184, 185
television documentaries, 5
Thai state, 205, 208, 210, 218, 225
Thailand, 4, 18, 20–22, 203, 210, 212, 219, 220, 224, 225
Baan Srisaket, 203, 204, 208, 211, 215, 216
Bangkok, 204, 205
central Thai, 19, 204, 205, 217, 218
Chinese Thai, 19, 217
Khon Kaen, 222
northeast, 204, 205, 207, 208, 210
Population and Community Development Association, 207
state, 203, 204, 214, 225
Thakur Das Bhargava, 72
Thapar, S., 12
theologies, 5, 156
feminist, 5
liberation, 5, 12
Third World, 2, 5, 12, 17, 36, 46, 47, 55, 100, 155, 157, 158, 188
Thorbek, S., 222
total fertility rate(s) (TFR), 18, 20, 178, 203, 268, 273
tourism industry, 185
transformation(s), 16, 23, 183, 196
trial marriages, 137
tribe, 82, 83, 101
Trobriands (Southwest Pacific), 285, 291

tropes of motherhood, 264
Tse, C., 159, 172
Tuzin, D., 293
TV Antony, 92

Underhill-Sem, Y., 273, 274
United Nations, 4, 100
United Nations Fund for Population Activities (UNFPA), 38
United Provinces of East Punjab (India), 70
United State of Rajasthan (India), 70
United States Operations Mission, 205
urbanization, 20, 267, 273, 294, 295
U.S. bases, 155
utopianism, 157, 163
Uttar Pradesh (India), 94
uxorilocal, 48

Vanuatu (southwest Pacific), 5, 8, 264, 267, 268, 274, 275, 277, 282, 286, 288, 289, 296
Vanuatu, National Planning and Statistics Office, 268
vasectomies, 211
Vatican II, 13, 160, 163
Veneracion, J. B., 158–60
venereal disease, 134, 275, 293
Vicziany, M., 23, 86
Vietnam, 204, 205
village medicine, 294
virginity, 158

wage-labor, 179, 183, 194, 198. *See also* work
Wang Enfeng, 127
Wang Ling, 136, 137
Wang Lirun, 138
Wang Wei, 138
Wang Xingjuan, 136, 137
Wang Xingjuan, Xu Xiuyu, and Wang Ling, 139
wantoks (communities of people speaking the same language, Tok Pisin, Papua New Guinea), 294
Ward, K., 40

Warren, C., 189, 190, 195
war zones, 168, 169
Weiner, A., 281, 291
West, 158, 159
West Bengal (India), 65
Western political theory, 107
western Solomons, 282
West Punjab (India), 62, 73
White, G., 285
white Australia, 14
Whitehead, H., 291
Whittaker, A., 4, 9, 18, 19, 25, 43, 49, 54, 204, 206, 208
whore, 162
widows, 184
witches (*brujas*), 158
Women in Development (WID), 39
women, 1
    autonomy, 18
    body commoditization, 28
    childless, 9, 12, 13
    economic autonomy, 16
    emancipation, 24, 28
    and knowledge, 219
    medicalization of, 19
    purity, 12
    repatriation of, 1, 5
    rights, 7
    status, 141
    status as citizen, 15
    targets of state control, 21
    as victims, 11
    widow burning, 11
    women's business, 18
Women's Federation (DCAPRC) (China), 128, 135
women's health, 84
women's movement, 154
Women's Resource and Training Centre (Delhi, India), 4
Women's Section (India), 61, 62, 64
work, 11, 164. *See also* wage-labor
Working Group on Women's Rights (India), 84
World Bank, 100, 206
World Fertility Survey, 46
Wu Yishi, and Wu Ling, 138

Xu Xiuyu, 136, 137

yaa dong lau (pickled medicine, Thailand), 221
Yan Fu, 122
Yang, C. K., 118
Yang Lingling, 126, 133, 134, 142
Yan Shi, 128
Yeager, D. M., 157, 162
yin and *yang* (China), 133
Yin Ming, 136
Young India, 105
Yue Ping, 137

Yu Jing, 138
Yuval-Davis, N., and F. Anthias, 8, 11, 159

Zaire, 276
Zhang Xiyu, 137
Zhang Xiyu, et al., 137
Zhao Pinghe, 136
Zheng Xiaoyang, and Chen Yuhan, 139
Zhong Jiaoshou, 138
Zhou Xizhang, 126
Zhu Junlun, 138
Zhu Xi, 120